ESSENTIALS OF
VETERINARY BACTERIOLOGY
AND MYCOLOGY

ESSENTIALS OF VETERINARY BACTERIOLOGY AND MYCOLOGY

G. R. Carter, D.V.M., M.S., D.V.Sc.

Division of Pathobiology and Public Practice
Virginia-Maryland Regional College of Veterinary Medicine
Virginia Tech
Blacksburg, Virginia

With Chapters By

G. William Claus, B.S., Ph.D.

Microbiology Section
Department of Biology
College of Arts and Sciences
Virginia Tech
Blacksburg, Virginia

Yasuko Rikihisa, M.S., Ph.D.

Division of Veterinary Biology and Clinical Studies
Virginia-Maryland Regional College of Veterinary Medicine
Virginia Tech
Blacksburg, Virginia

THIRD EDITION

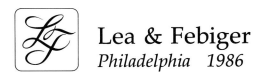

Lea & Febiger
Philadelphia 1986

Lea & Febiger
600 Washington Square
Philadelphia, PA 19106-4198
U.S.A.
(215) 922-1330

Library of Congressa Cataloging in Publication Data

Carter, G. R. (Gordon R.)
 Essentials of veterinary bacteriology and mycology.

 Bibliography: p.
 Includes index.
 1. Veterinary bacteriology. 2. Veterinary mycology.
I. Claus, G. William. II. Rikihisa, Yasuko. III. Title.
SF780.3.C37 1985   636.089'6014   85-10420
ISBN 0-8121-1004-8

PRINTED IN THE UNITED STATES OF AMERICA

Print No.   4   3   2   1

To

Jane, Marion and Nick

PREFACE

Veterinary bacteriology and mycology are traditionally taught by means of lectures and laboratory exercises. This text was prepared to provide veterinary students with the more important facts of introductory and pathogenic bacteriology and mycology for the lecture portion. In the interest of economy the number of illustrations has been kept to a minimum. If laboratory exercises are adequate, students will have an opportunity to observe and study the microscopic and cultural characteristics of the various microorganisms.

I have found that the teaching of the pathogenic portion of the course can be made more interesting and relevant to veterinary practice by the use of "Clinical Examples" of the kind shown in the Appendix. These can be used as the principal means of conveying the lecture material or can be employed on occasion to stimulate interest. The "Clinical Examples" may involve a brief case report or description of a disease outbreak.

A number of references are listed at the end of each chapter for students interested in additional information and greater depth in a particular topic. A number of standard works can be used for supplementary reading on various microbial agents and the diseases they cause. Rather than list them after each chapter, they are all listed in the Appendix under, "Suggested Sources for Reference and Supplementary Reading."

I would like to express my appreciation to the Information Processing staff of our College for their fine effort in typing the manuscript and to the College Media Center for preparation of illustrations. Thanks is also due to Mrs. Cheryl Owens for reading portions of the manuscript and assisting in the preparation of some of the tables.

The help of my publisher Lea & Febiger and their editorial staff in the editing of the manuscript is gratefully acknowledged.

I am also much indebted to Professors C. William Claus and Yasuko Rikihisa for contributing chapters that have considerably strengthened the Introductory Microbiology portion of the book.

Blacksburg, Virginia   G. R. Carter

CONTENTS

PART I INTRODUCTORY MICROBIOLOGY

PART II BACTERIA

PART III FUNGI

Part I

INTRODUCTORY MICROBIOLOGY

1

Classification and Morphology of Bacteria and Fungi

Yasuko Rikihisa

PROCARYOTES AND EUCARYOTES

In terms of intracellular organization, the cells of all living things are either *eucaryotes* or *procaryotes* (Fig. 1–1). The eucaryotic cells have a membrane-bound nucleus (i.e., a true nucleus), whereas in the procaryotic cells nuclear material is not enveloped by a membrane. Bacterial cells are procaryotes and cells of all other living organisms are eucaryotes. *Protists* are undifferentiated unicellular organisms that do not form specialized tissues and organ systems as do higher plants and animals. The protists are divided into eucaryotic (higher) and procaryotic (lower) protists. Eucaryotic protists are divided into algae, fungi, and protozoa. *Algae* have chlorophyll and cell walls. *Fungi* have cell walls but lack chlorophyll. *Protozoa* have neither chlorophyll nor cell walls.

BACTERIA

The bacteria, or procaryotes, are single-celled organisms that are distinguished from the eucaryotic organisms by the characteristics listed in Table 1–1.

In volume 1 of *Bergey's Manual of Systematic Bacteriology*, published in 1984, the kingdom *Procaryotae* is proposed to contain four divisions:

I. Gracilicutes (*gracilis.* [L.] thin) have a gram-negative type cell wall.

II. Firmicutes (*firmus.* [L.] strong) have a gram-positive type cell wall.

III. Tenericutes (*tener.* [L.] soft) lack a cell wall and are commonly called the mycoplasmas.

IV. Mendosicutes (*mendosus.* [L.] having faults) are members of *Archaeobacteria* such as methanogens, halophiles, and thermoacidophiles, which live in somewhat extreme environments. Archaeobacteria are so called because of their apparent primitiveness and dissimilarities in comparison to other bacteria.

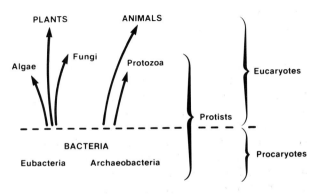

Figure 1–1. Relationships of living organisms.

3

Table 1–1. Differences Between Procaryotic and Eucaryotic Cells

Characteristics	Procaryotic Cells	Eucaryotic Cells
Nucleoplasm bounded by a membrane	–	+
Nucleolus	–	+
Chromosome number	1	>1
Reproduction	asexual	sexual or asexual
Mitotic nuclear division	–	+
D-amino acids, diaminopimelic acid, and muramic acid	+*	–
Cytoplasmic ribosomes	70S	80S
Endoplasmic reticulum	–	+
Mitochondria	–	+
Chloroplasts	–	+†
Golgi apparatus	–	+
Cytoplasmic streaming	–	+
Cytoplasmic membrane	sterols generally absent	sterols present
Organelles with nonunit membrane	+	–

*Except for mycoplasmas and chlamydiae.
†Plants and algae.

All other bacteria are referred to as *Eubacteria*. The bacteria that are associated with or cause disease in animals are included among Eubacteria: Divisions I, II, and III. Eubacteria are more conveniently grouped as consisting of *blue-green algae* and other *bacteria*.

Blue-Green Algae (Cyanobacteria)

This group has been treated as one of the algae; however, their typically procaryotic cell structure identifies them as bacteria. The cyanobacteria perform oxygen-elaborating photosynthesis and possess plant-type chlorophylls in thylacoid membranes. They are different from photosynthetic bacteria, which perform nonoxygenic photosynthesis and possess bacteriochlorophyll but not thylacoid membranes. On occasion livestock, pets, and wild animals may ingest toxic cyanobacteria and be fatally poisoned.

Other Bacteria

Conventional Bacteria. These include the rest of the free-living bacteria, e.g., the phototrophic, gliding, sheathed, and appendaged bacteria; rod, coccal, and spiral-shaped bacteria; and gram-positive and -negative. The phototrophic bacteria (purple bacteria and green bacteria) perform anoxygenic photosynthesis and possess a unique pigment system containing bacteriochlorophyll.

Rickettsiae and Chlamydiae. These organisms differ from conventional bacteria in that they are smaller (0.2 to 0.5 μm in diameter) and they are obligate intracellular parasites. They resemble bacteria because they contain both DNA and RNA, multiply by binary fission, have muramic acid (except for chlamydiae), and are sensitive to some antibacterial drugs.

Mycoplasmas. Most of these organisms are parasitic on plants or animals, lack cell walls, are highly pleomorphic, are resistant to penicillin, and are the smallest of the free-living organisms.

METHODS EMPLOYED FOR OBSERVING BACTERIA

The microscope is an essential investigative tool of microbiology. The units of measurement employed in microbiology are the micron (μ) or micrometer (μm = 10^{-6}m), the nanometer (nm = 10^{-9}m) and the angstrom (Å = 10^{-10}m). The two types of microscopes available are light and electron. These types differ by the ray they use to effect magnification, i.e., light and electron beams, respectively.

MICROSCOPE

Light Microscope

Bright-Field Microscope. The conventional microscope has three objectives: low power, high power (high dry) and oil-immersion. The latter, with the usual ocular lens × 10 providing a total magnification of approximately × 1000, is used for the routine examination of stained bacterial smears and wet preparations under coverslips. The resolution of the light microscope is limited by the wavelength of visible light, which is about 0.5 μm; images less than 0.2 μm cannot be clearly resolved.

Dark-Field Microscope. This type of illumination can be used in the conventional microscope by substituting a dark-field condenser for the conventional condenser. The special condenser obliquely reflects a powerful source of light onto a wet preparation. Very small objects, including microorganisms, scatter the light and can be seen as brilliant images against a dark background. By this method very small and very slender organisms, such as the spirochetes, which cannot be seen with the conventional microscope, can be readily visualized. Living organisms and their movement can be seen.

Fluorescence Microscope. Although various fluorescent dyes are used to stain microorganisms, the technique known as immunofluorescence (fluorescent antibody or FA procedure) is much more widely used in clinical microbiology, mainly for the identification of organisms. Fluorescent antibody reagents are prepared by coupling a fluorescent dye to a specific antibody. This conjugate will unite with its corresponding bacterial or viral antigen. The union is visually detectable by the presence of characteristic fluorescence when it is excited by the ultraviolet light of a fluorescence microscope. An indirect procedure is also used in which the conjugated antibody (2°) is prepared against the globulin, which includes specific antibody (1°) to identify the organism. This conjugate can thus recognize whether or not the specific antibody (1°) has united with the microorganism.

Phase-Contrast Microscope. When the light waves pass through transparent objects, such as cells, they emerge in different phases, depending on the properties of the materials through which they pass. In phase contrast microscopy, a phase condenser and phase objective lens convert differences in phase into differences in intensity of light. Thus some structures appear darker than others. This method is useful in studying the fine detail of unstained living microorganisms.

Electron Microscope

The principle of this instrument is analogous to that of the light microscope. Instead of visible light, the electron microscope employs a beam of electrons that is focused by an electromagnetic field instead of by glass lenses. Because of the short wavelength, it can resolve objects as small as 0.0004 μm.

Because biologic materials are mainly composed of the elements carbon, hydrogen, nitrogen, and oxygen, which have low electron scatter-deflecting ability, special techniques are necessary to make specimens stand out against background.

Thin Sectioning. Most microorganisms are too thick for direct examination of the internal structure by the electron microscope. To make them transparent to the electron beam, thin sectioning is employed. Before sectioning, the specimen must be fixed, dehydrated, and embedded to preserve specific structures. Positive staining of the thin section with heavy metal elements is used to increase the contrast of specimens.

Negative Staining. Negative staining sets specimens against an electron-dense heavy metal element. The procedure provides a high resolution of viral and other small particles. The technique is very simple, quick, and economical, and it is often used as a quantitative device to enumerate viral particles and as a diagnostic procedure to identify the virus in stools, urine, cerebrospinal fluid, tears, blood, lavages, and blister fluids.

Freeze Fracture. In the freeze-fracture procedure, specimens are quick-frozen in freon, split or cleaved, and the carbon replica of the fractured surface is prepared at liquid nitrogen temperature. The replica surface is shadow-cast with a heavy metal to provide contrast. Chemical fixation, embedding and sectioning procedures, and accompanying artifacts are thereby avoided. This technique is especially valuable for viewing the internal structure of the biologic membrane, since fracture often occurs between the outer and inner leaflets of a unit membrane.

Localization Techniques. To determine the cellular site of enzymes and their activities, or to be able to follow the formation or incorporation of specific structures within a cell, *enzyme cytochemistry* and *autoradiography* are used. In enzyme studies, the reaction product of an enzyme is precipitated and made electron-dense, so that the position of the enzyme can be identified. Autoradiography may be defined as a method for locating radioactive substances by use of modified photographic techniques. The microorganism is incubated with a radioactive precursor and allowed to use this precursor in its normal metabolic pathways. The tissue to be examined is then fixed and routinely sectioned for electron microscopy. The section of tissue is coated with a thin film of photographic emulsion. Rays released by radioactive decay expose silver grains in the emulsion that are subsequently developed, fixed, and viewed in the microscope.

To identify the position of specific antigens, either within or on the surface of a cell, *immunolabeling* by antibody coupled with ferritin, gold particles, or peroxidase is used. Ferritin and gold particles are electron-dense and readily recognizable under the electron microscope. Peroxidase enzyme forms a complex with the substrate hydrogen peroxide. This complex reacts with an electron donor, such as diaminobenzidine tetrahydrochloride, to form an electron-dense precipitate.

High Voltage Electron Microscopy. The thicker specimens can be examined to obtain a stereo image. Because of the higher accelerating voltage, the resolution and penetration power are better at a voltage of 1000 kV (1 mV) or higher, whereas the conventional electron microscope is operated at 60 to 80 kV.

Scanning Electron Microscopy (SEM). The object is scanned with a flying spot of electrons, and the emergent secondary electrons are collected and shown on a screen of the cathode-ray tube. Three-dimensional images are obtained, but internal detail is not provided by SEM.

X-Ray Microanalysis. When an electron hits a specimen, characteristic x-rays are released from each element. In x-ray spectroscopy, an x-ray detector is used to monitor the distinct x-ray pattern produced by the interaction between the electron beam of the microscope and the chemical elements in specific areas of the specimen. This method is especially suitable for localizing specific elements in the microorganism.

STAINING PROCEDURES

Staining methods are used to determine the morphologic form of bacteria and their affinity for certain dyes. Bacteria are divided into two major groups on the basis of the Gram stain. Briefly, the procedure for the Gram stain is as follows: The cells are first fixed to a glass slide by heat, then stained with a basic dye (e.g., crystal or methyl violet) that is washed off with an iodine-potassium iodide solution (mordant), and then washed with water and cautiously decolorized with acetone or ethyl alcohol. The smear is then counterstained with safranin.

Gram-positive organisms retain the basic dye following "decolorization" with acetone or alcohol and appear deep violet. The gram-nega-

tive organisms, on the other hand, do not retain the violet stain but take up the counterstain (safranin) and stain red to pink. As a general rule, organisms that give a doubtful reaction are gram-positive. The gram-positive cell wall is not stained but presents a permeability barrier to elution of the dye-iodine complex by the decolorizer. Aging gram-positive cells become gram-negative because autolytic enzymes attack the cell wall.

There are differences between gram-positive and gram-negative organisms in the structure of the cell wall.

1. Gram-negative organisms have more lipid in their cell wall.
2. Gram-positive bacteria have a thicker peptidoglycan layer, which renders them more resistant to mechanical damage. Because of these structural differences, the two groups vary in their reaction to Gram stain and their susceptibility to enzymes, disinfectants, and antimicrobial drugs.

Not all bacteria can be satisfactorily stained by the Gram method. The cell walls of mycobacteria contain lipids and waxy substances (mycolic acid) that make them difficult to stain. However, when they are stained by a special procedure called an *acid-fast stain*, they retain the carbolfuchsin even after exposure to a strong acid alcohol (HCl and ethanol) solution.

The leptospira and treponemes are very slender and cannot be satisfactorily resolved following Gram staining, but they can be demonstrated by *negative staining* employing nigrosin or India ink. The organisms appear clear and unstained, surrounded by the dark inert particles. Negative staining is also used for demonstrating capsules. For demonstrating flagella (around 0.02 to 0.03 μm in diameter), a *mordant* is used before staining; this precipitates on flagella and thus thickens them.

BACTERIAL STRUCTURE

SHAPE AND SIZE OF BACTERIA

The three basic morphologic forms of bacteria are the straight rod (bacillus), the sphere (coccus), and the spiral or curved rod (spirochete, spirillum, vibrio). There is considerable variation in these basic forms; coccobacillary, ovoid, and filamentous forms are frequently seen.

The cocci are found in different arrangements, depending upon their dividing planes. The staphylococci occur in bunches or clusters, the streptococci form chains, and the pneumococci are predominantly paired. Some of the micrococci occur in groups of four or tetrads *(Aerococcus viridans)*; others are grouped in packets of eight *(Sarcina)*.

The various species of the Enterobacteriaceae occur as rather regular rods, but some of the smaller organisms such as *Pasteurella, Brucella,* and *Haemophilus* are both bacillary and coccobacillary. Some members of the genera *Bacillus* and *Clostridium* have rods in chain formation. The corynebacteria are remarkably pleomorphic and produce club-shaped forms. The actinomycetes *(Actinomyces* and *Norcardia)* have both bacillary and filamentous branching forms. The anaerobic *Fusobacterium* has a characteristic elongated, spindle shape. Among the spiral forms are those that are curved, comma, or S-shaped *(Vibrio* and *Campylobacter)* and those that are tightly or loosely coiled *(Treponema* and *Leptospira)*. There is considerable variation in the size of bacteria. Most rod forms range from 2 to 5 μm in length to 0.5 to 1 μm in width; spirochetes may be longer (up to 20 μm) and narrower (0.1 to 0.2 μm). Cocci are approximately 1 μm in diameter. The size of bacteria varies somewhat, depending upon the medium and the growth phase. They are usually smallest in the logarithmic phase of growth. An *Escherichia coli* bacterium has a volume of $\sim$ μm^3 and a weight of $\sim$ 10^{-12}g, whereas a liver cell has a volume of $\sim$ 1,000 μm^3 and a weight of $\sim$ 10^{-9}g. For convenience, bacteria can be roughly grouped according to size as follows:

Large: Spirochetes, *Bacillus, Clostridium*
Medium: Enterobacteriaceae *(Escherichia coli, Proteus)*, pseudomonads
Small: *Brucella, Pasteurella, Haemophilus*
Very small: *Rickettsia, Chlamydia, Mycoplasma*

BACTERIAL ULTRASTRUCTURE

Bacteria are enclosed by the cell envelope, which is made up of two or three layers, depending upon the organism. All, except mycoplasmas, have a *cell wall* internal to which is the cell or *cytoplasmic membrane,* and some have *capsules* external to the cell wall. Many bacteria have *flagella* and some gram-negative varieties have *pili or fimbriae.*

The cytoplasmic membrane surrounds the body of the organism, which consists principally of cytoplasm. Ribosomes, granular inclusions, and in some bacteria, mesosomes (infoldings of

plasma membrane), are found distributed within the cytoplasm. Bacteria do not have a membrane enveloped nucleus as do the eucaryotes, although with appropriate staining nuclear structures can be seen. The principal structural features of bacteria are shown in Figures 1–2 and 1–3.

Cell Envelope

Capsules and Slimes. These are amorphous, polymeric, often gelatinous materials lying outside the cell wall. Most are polysaccharides but several are polypeptides; some bacteria, such as *Bacillus megaterium,* have both compounds in their capsule. Special staining procedures, including negative stains, are used to demonstrate capsules. The capsules of mucoid strains of *Pasteurella multocida* and *Streptococcus equi* consist almost wholly of hyaluronic acid. Virulence may depend to some extent on the antiphagocytic properties of the capusle, e.g., *Bacillus anthracis, Brucella abortus,* and *Streptococcus pneumoniae.*

Cell Wall. There are basic differences between the cell walls of gram-positive and gram-negative bacteria. The cell wall makes up approximately 20% of the total dry weight of the bacterium. It gives the organism shape and a rigid structure that protects the cell proper from severe chemical and physical actions.

The cell wall is permeable and the cytoplasmic membrane is selectively semipermeable, determining which molecules will be excreted from the cell and what concentration of the different solutes will be maintained. Movement of substances across the membrane takes place by simple diffusion and by more complex transport systems.

The supporting role of the cell wall can be demonstrated if its formation is prevented by penicillin or destroyed by *lysozyme.* The struc-

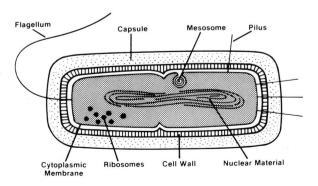

Figure 1–2. Principal structures of bacteria.

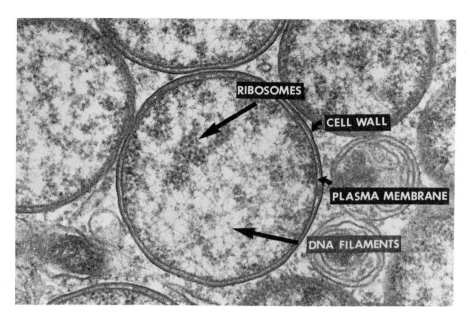

Figure 1–3. Transmission electron micrograph of *Rickettsia*.

tures that remain are bound by the cytoplasmic membrane only and are called *protoplasts* (gram-positive) or *spheroplasts* (gram-negative). Unless placed in a hypertonic milieu, protoplasts and spheroplasts swell and burst.

STRUCTURE AND CHEMICAL COMPOSITION OF CELL WALLS. *Peptidoglycans* provide the cell wall's rigid structure. These very large polymers are composed of two kinds of building blocks: (1) *N*-acetylglucosamine and *N*-acetylmuramic acid disaccharide polymers, and (2) peptides consisting of four or five amino acids, namely, L-alanine, D-alanine, D-glutamic acid, and either lysine or diaminopimelic acid (Fig. 1–4). These are unique to bacteria.

GRAM-POSITIVE BACTERIA. The cell walls range from 150 to 800 Å in thickness. In addition to the peptidoglycan, some gram-positive organisms possess polysaccharides and *teichoic acids*.

Table 1–2 compares some major envelope structures of gram-positive and gram-negative bacterial cells. A diagram of the cell walls of both types of organisms is shown in Figure 1–5.

GRAM-NEGATIVE BACTERIA. The cell wall is approximately 100 Å in thickness, high in lipid content (11 to 22%), and appears as a unit membrane; thus, it is called the outer membrane. A major protein of the outer membrane is called "porin," which forms transmembrane pores or diffusion channels that allow passage of small hydrophilic molecules through the outer membrane. A relatively small amount of peptidoglycan is present in the inner rigid layer, but a large amount of a lipopolysaccharide (LPS), often referred to as *endotoxin*, occurs external to the outer membrane. Endotoxin is important in the pathogenesis of some diseases. The serologic specificity of the O-antigens of gram-negative bacteria

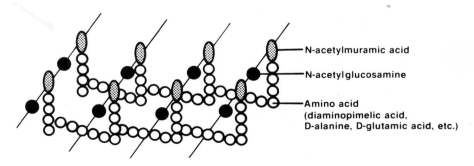

Figure 1–4. Schematic peptidoglycan structure.

Table 1–2. Principal Components of the Cell Walls of Gram-Positive and Gram-Negative Bacteria*

Component	Gram-Positive	Gram-Negative
Peptidoglycan	+ (thick)	+ (thin)
Teichoic acid and/or teichuronic acid	+	–
Lipopolysaccharide	–	+
Polysaccharide	+	+
Protein	Present or absent	+
Lipid	–	+
Lipoprotein	–	+

*Modified from Mandelstam, J., and McQuillen, K. (eds.): *Biochemistry of Bacterial Growth* 3rd Ed. New York, John Wiley & Sons, 1982.

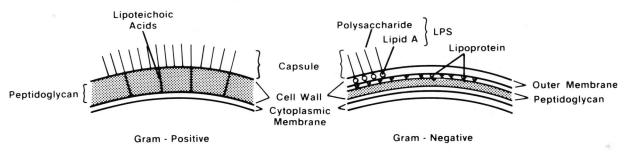

Figure 1–5. Diagram of gram-positive and gram-negative envelope structures.

resides in the determinants of polysaccharide. The lipid moiety of the LPS, called lipid A, is the toxic component. The basic structure of *Salmonella* LPS is shown in Figure 1–6.

Periplasm. The periplasm is the space between the plasma membrane and cell wall and is visible in gram-negative but difficult to see in gram-positive bacteria. The periplasm contains various hydrolytic enzymes and binding proteins that specifically bind sugars, amino acids, and inorganic ions. These enzymes and proteins aid transport of various compounds into and out of the bacterial cytoplasm, and they are released by osmotic shock.

Appendages

Flagella. These are long whip-like structures of locomotion. They are composed of three parts: filament, hook, and basal body. The basal body is embedded in the plasma membrane and gives the flagella rotary motion, which propels the organism. The distribution of flagella on the cell is of significance in taxonomy. *Monotrichous* bacteria have a single polar flagellum; *lophotrichous* bacteria have tufts of several flagella at one pole; *amphitrichous* bacteria have flagella at both poles; and *peritrichous* organisms have a number of flagella distributed all around the cell surface. The diameter of a flagellum is 10 to 20 nm, and special staining procedures are used to demonstrate flagella. They are composed mostly of a protein monomer called *flagellin*. Flagella contain H-antigens and are thus useful in serologic identification of some bacterial species.

Most of the organisms that produce capsules, e.g., species of *Klebsiella, Haemophilus, Pasteurella,* and *Bacillus,* are nonmotile. None of the cocci of medical importance is motile. Motility

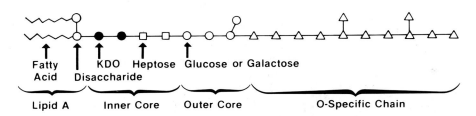

KDO: 2-keto-3-deoxyoctonic acid

Figure 1–6. Schematic diagram of lipopolysaccharide structure.

is determined in the laboratory by the examination of wet preparations from cultures under the microscope (hanging-drop method) and by observing the kind of growth obtained when a semisolid agar medium is stabbed with an inoculum of the organism being examined. Diffuse growth into the agar indicates motility.

Axial Filament. This is a flagellum-like filament located in the periplasmic space between the inner and outer membranes of spirochetes. The spiral organisms move by a traveling helical wave along axial filaments.

Pili (Fimbriae). These are shorter, thinner, and straighter than flagella and are attached to the plasma membrane of gram-negative bacteria, with the exception of *Corynebacterium renale.* They are composed of a protein monomer called *pilin,* which is 4 to 20 nm in diameter and can only be seen by electron microscopy. The pili enable some bacteria to adhere to epithelial cells, thus leading to colonization of mucous membranes.

The sex pili (see Chapter 3) occur in fertility (F) factor (+) cells found among the Enterobacteriaceae and a few other bacteria. They adhere to F (−) cell surfaces and make possible the transfer of genetic material from F (+) to F (−) cells in conjugation.

Endospores

Members of the genera *Clostridium* and *Bacillus* have the capacity to produce highly resistant, thick-walled spores. They occur when vegetative cells are deprived of some factor or nutrient necessary for growth, e.g., they may appear in the later stages of artificial cultivation. In anthrax, spores are produced when the organisms are exposed to oxygen.

Spore formation begins with realignment of DNA material into filaments and invagination of plasma membrane, forming a structure called the *forespore.* The forespore is further surrounded by the plasma membrane. The facing side of these two plasma membranes is the peptidoglycan synthesizing side, and *spore cortex,* a poorly polymerized peptidoglycan, is synthesized in the space between the two layers of plasma membranes. *Spore coat,* a keratin-like protein rich in cysteine, is formed outside the spore cortex. In some microorganisms, an *exosporium* is formed outside the spore coat. When spore formation is completed, the mature spore is released by the disintegration of the envelope of the mother cell, or *sporangium.* Each spore germinates into a single vegetative cell when conditions for growth are favorable. In gram-stained preparations, spores appear as ovoid, refractile, nonstaining objects either within the cell or free of it. Figure 1–7 contains a diagram of an endospore.

The location of the mature spore in the cell may be central, terminal, or subterminal, depending upon the organism, and is useful for identification of the microorganism.

The remarkable heat resistance of spores is thought to be due to the dehydration of the spore protoplast. The irradiation resistance may be related to a high level of cystine disulfide bonds in the spore coat protein, and dehydration resistance is due to keratin-like spore coat protein.

Relatively large amounts of calcium and a compound unique to spores, *dipicolinic acid,* derivatives of diaminopimelic acid (a component of peptidoglycan), occur in the spore.

BACTERIAL TAXONOMY AND CLASSIFICATION

Taxonomy is defined as the science of classification (orderly arrangement of organisms). *Nomenclature* is the assignment of names to the taxonomic groups according to international rules.

PRACTICAL (PHENOTYPIC) CLASSIFICATION

The bacteria are placed in groups in *Bergey's Manual of Systematic Bacteriology,* volume 1, 1984, based on a few readily identifiable characteristics such as morphologic characteristics, reaction to Gram stain, and oxygen requirements. *Bergey's Manual,* the standard reference work for microbiologists, contains detailed descriptions of most known bacteria. Many different characteristics, including morphologic, cultural, biochemical, and nucleic acid (DNA base compositions, DNA homologies), are used, often in a rather inconsistent manner.

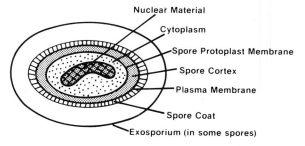

Figure 1–7. Schematic diagram of endospore structure.

Nomenclature. The classic binomial (Linnaean) system whereby organisms are given a genus and species name is used. The taxonomic levels or ranks used in the current *Bergey's Manual* are hierarchical ones. A specific suffix is used for each category:

Class (-al): A class consists of related orders.

Order (-ales): An order contains a group of related families.

Family (-aceae): In this category are placed closely related genera or tribes.

Tribe (-ieae): A tribe contains closely related genera.

Genus: This most important category contains closely related species.

Species: Included in the same species are strains of organisms that have many characteristics in common, e.g., different strains of *Escherichia coli* will give substantially the same reactions to many biochemical tests.

Subspecies: Some species may be further subdivided into subspecies on the basis of small but consistent differences, e.g., *Campylobacter fetus* subsp. *fetus*, subsp. *intestinalis*, subsp. *jejuni*.

Strain: A strain consists of the descendants (clone) of a single isolate in pure culture. For each species there is a *type strain,* which usually is the particular culture from which the species description was originally made. Type strains are available in various culture collections.

In addition to generic and species names, well-known trivial names, such as tubercle bacillus *(Mycobacterium tuberculosis),* often appear in medical literature. When a generic (genus) name is vernacularized in English, such as bacillus and salmonella, it is neither capitalized nor italicized.

Bergey's Manual has evolved since the publication of the first edition in 1923. The manual provides a key that may be used for the identification of bacteria. It is not widely used in diagnostic laboratories except for very uncommon organisms. Microbiologists in diagnostic laboratories usually use simplified schemes to place an unknown organism into a particular genus from relatively small choices, and then reference is made to tables or flow diagrams for the identification of a species within the genus. A modified presentation of the classification of medically important bacteria according to the 1984 *Bergey's Manual of Systematic Bacteriology,* volume 1, is given in Table 1–3.

Since 1980, valid names of all bacterial species have been published in the *International Journal of Systematic Bacteriology.*

GENETIC BASIS FOR CLASSIFICATION

Genetic information is coded in DNA base sequence. As organisms drift apart by mutation, recombination, transduction, and selection in different environments (i.e., evolution), their genomes change in size, nucleotide base composition, and nucleotide base sequence.

DNA Base Compositions. The proportions of the four DNA bases in the total DNA of an organism can be assayed. By convention the base composition of a DNA preparation is expressed as the mole percentage of guanine-cytosine (GC) to the total. Since GC + AT (adenine-thymine) = 100%, if the GC content is 40%, the AT = 60%. Determination of GC% is relatively simple and is of some value in taxonomy, e.g., all the Enterobacteriaceae from *E. coli* to *Salmonella* have GC%'s ranging from 50 to 54. Similarity of base composition, however, does not necessarily signify DNA homology. The genomes of all vertebrates have a GC% of 44, which is the same as some microorganisms.

DNA Hybridization. DNA sequence homology between two organisms can be quantified by procedures that determine the extent of formation of molecular hybrids from two DNA strands of different origin. This approach has been useful in demonstrating relative order and degree of DNA similarity of closely related groups of bacteria. However, this technique is too specific for studying the relationships of dissimilar bacterial groups. Hybridization between DNA molecules of two *E. coli* strains would be close to 100%, but hybridization of *E. coli* with a *Salmonella* would be about 70%.

Ribosomal RNA Hybridization. r-RNA exhibits more homology among widely dissimilar organisms than does DNA. Thus it is useful in comparing distantly related organisms. r-RNA similarity values have contributed to the establishment of Division IV, Mendosicutes, in the kingdom Procaryotae.

NUMERICAL TAXONOMY

In numerical taxonomy each physiologic and biochemical characteristic is given equal weight. Bacterial strains being studied are subjected to about 50 different tests, and each strain is listed as giving a positive or negative result on each test. With a large number of strains and tests

Table 1–3.   Classification Outline of Medically Important Bacteria

Kingdom Procaryotae*
   Division I.   Gracilicutes: Procaryotes that have a rigid or semirigid cell wall containing peptidoglycan and a negative rection to Gram stain.
     Class I.   Scotobacteria
      Section I.   Spirochetes
       Order I.   Spirochaetales
        Family I.   Spirochaetaceae
         Genus I.   *Spirochaeta*
         Genus III.   *Treponema*
         Genus IV.   *Borrelia*
        Family II.   Leptospiraceae
         Genus I.   *Leptospira*
      Section 2.   Aerobic-Microaerophilic, Motile, Helical-Vibroid Gram-Negative Bacteria
        Genus   *Spirillum*
        Genus   *Campylobacter*
      Section 3.   Nonmotile (or Rarely Motile) Gram-Negative Curved Bacteria
      Section 4.   Gram-Negative Aerobic Rods and Cocci
       Family I.   Pseudomonadaceae
        Genus I.   *Pseudomonas*
       Family VI.   Legionellaceae
        Genus I.   *Legionella*
       Family VIII.   Neisseriaceae
        Genus I.   *Neisseria*
        Genus II.   *Moraxella*
       Other Genera
        Genus   *Flavobacterium*
        Genus   *Alcaligenes*
        Genus   *Brucella*
        Genus   *Bordetella*
        Genus   *Francisella*
      Section 5.   Facultatively Anaerobic Gram-Negative Rods
       Family I.   Enterobacteriaceae
        Genus I.   *Escherichia*
        Genus II.   *Shigella*
        Genus III.   *Salmonella*
        Genus IV.   *Citrobacter*
        Genus V.   *Klebsiella*
        Genus VI.   *Enterobacter*
        Genus VII.   *Erwinia*
        Genus VIII.   *Serratia*
        Genus IX.   *Hafnia*
        Genus X.   *Edwardsiella*
        Genus XI.   *Proteus*
        Genus XII.   *Providencia*
        Genus XIII.   *Morganella*
        Genus XIV.   *Yersinia*
       Family II.   Vibrionaceae
        Genus I.   *Vibrio*
        Genus III.   *Aeromonas*
       Family III.   Pasteurellaceae
        Genus I.   *Pasteurella*
        Genus II.   *Haemophilus*
        Genus III.   *Actinobacillus*
       Other genera
        Genus   *Chromobacterium*
        Genus   *Streptobacillus*
        Genus   *Eikenella*
        Genus   *Gardnerella*
        Genus   *Calymmatobacterium*
      Section 6.   Anaerobic Gram-Negative Straight, Curved, and Helical Rods
       Family I.   Bacteroidaceae
        Genus I.   *Bacteroides*
        Genus II.   *Fusobacterium*
        Genus III.   *Leptotrichia*
      Section 7.   Dissimilatory Sulfate- or Sulfur-Reducing Bacteria
      Section 8.   Anaerobic Gram-Negative Cocci
       Family I.   Veillonellaceae
        Genus I.   *Veillonella*
        Genus II.   *Acidaminococcus*
        Genus III.   *Megasphaera*

Table 1–3.   *Classification Outline of Medically Important Bacteria* **Continued**

       Section 9.   The Rickettsiae and Chlamydiae
        Order I.   Rickettsiales
           Family I.   Rickettsiaceae
              Tribe I.   Rickettsieae
                 Genus I.   *Rickettsia*
                 Genus II.   *Rochalimaea*
                 Genus III.   *Coxiella*
              Tribe II.   Ehrlichieae
                 Genus IV.   *Ehrlichia*
                 Genus V.   *Cowdria*
                 Genus VI.   *Neorickettsia*
              Tribe III.   Wolbachiae
                 Genus VII.   *Wolbachia*
                 Genus VIII.   *Rickettsiella*
           Family II.   Bartonellaceae
              Genus I.   *Bartonella*
              Genus II.   *Grahamella*
           Family III.   Anaplasmataceae
              Genus I.   *Anaplasma*
              Genus II.   *Aegyptianella*
              Genus III.   *Haemobartonella*
              Genus IV.   *Eperythrozoon*
         Order II.   Chlamydiales
           Family I.   Chlamydiaceae
              Genus I.   *Chlamydia*
       Other Sections: Gliding Bacteria, Sheathed Bacteria, Budding and/or Appendaged Bacteria
     Class III.   Oxyphotobacteria
        Order I.   Cyanobacteriales
        Order II.   Prochlorales
     Class II.   Anoxyphotobacteria
        Order I.   Rhodospirillales
        Order II.   Chlorobiales
Division II.   Firmicutes: procaryotes that have a rigid or semirigid cell wall containing peptidoglycan and a positive reaction
        to Gram stain.
     Class I.   Firmibacteria
     Section I.   Gram-Positive Cocci
        a. Aerobic and/or facultatively anaerobic
           Family I.   Micrococcaceae
              Genus I.   *Micrococcus*
              Genus II.   *Staphylococcus*
              Genus III.   *Planococcus*
           Family II.   Streptococcaceae
              Genus I.   *Streptococcus*
              Genus III.   *Pediococcus*
              Genus IV.   *Aerococcus*
              Genus V.   *Gemella*
         b. Anaerobic
           Family III.   Peptococcaceae
              Genus I.   *Peptococcus*
              Genus II.   *Peptostreptococcus*
              Genus III.   *Ruminococcus*
              Genus IV.   *Sarcina*
     Section II.   Endospore-Forming Rods and Cocci
          Family I.   Bacillaceae
              Genus I.   *Bacillus*
              Genus II.   *Clostridium*
     Section III.   Gram-Positive, Asporogenous Rod Bacteria
          Family I.   Lactobacillaceae
              Genus I.   *Lactobacillus*
              Genera of Uncertain Affiliation
              Genus   *Listeria*
              Genus   *Erysipelothrix*
              Genus   *Caryophanon*

Table 1–3.   Classification Outline of Medically Important Bacteria Continued

```
        Class II.   Thallobacteria and Related Organisms
                    Coryneform Group of Bacteria
                        Genus I.   Corynebacterium
        Order I.    Actinomycetales  - Actinomycete any organism in this order.
            Family I.   Actinomycetaceae
                Genus I.   Actinomyces
                Genus V.   Rothia
            Family II.   Mycobacteriaceae
                Genus I.   Mycobacterium
            Family V.   Dermatophilaceae
                Genus I.   Dermatophilus
            Family VI.   Nocardiaceae
                Genus I.   Nocardia
            Family VII.   Streptomycetaceae
                Genus I.   Streptomyces   Genus II - micromonospora
Division III.   Tenericutes: Procaryotes that do not have a rigid or semirigid cell wall.
    Class I.   Mollicutes
        Order I.   Mycoplasmatales
            Family I.   Mycoplasmataceae
                Genus I.   Mycoplasma
            Family II.   Acholeplasmataceae
                Genus I.   Acholeplasma
                Genera of Uncertain Affiliation
                Genus   Thermoplasma
                Genus   Spiroplasma
Division IV.   Mendosicutes: Procaryotes with unusual walls, membrane lipids, ribosomes, and RNA sequences.
    Class I.   Archaeobacteria
```

*Adapted from Krieg, N.R., and Holt, J.G. (eds.): Bergey's Manual of Systematic Bacteriology. Volume 1. Baltimore, Williams & Wilkins, 1984, and Buchanan, R.E., and Gibbons, N.E. (eds.): Bergey's Manual of Determinative Bacteriology. 8th Ed. Baltimore, Williams & Wilkins, 1974.

the data are analyzed by computer, making possible a comparison of each strain with all other strains to detect similarities and differences. Similarity coefficients are calculated that indicate the relatedness of each strain to another. Numerical taxonomy has little practical significance, but it is a convenient way of detecting and quantifying the finer differences among fairly closely related bacteria.

CLASSIFICATION OF FUNGI

Kingdom Mycetae

Division Mastigomycota: motile spore (zoospore)
Division Amastigomycota: nonmotile spore
   Subdivision Zygomycotina: Nonseptate mycelium, asexual and sexual reproduction
      Order Mucorales: Asexual reproduction by sporangia, bread mold (*Rhizopus, Absidia, Mucor*)
      Order Entomophthorales: Asexual reproduction by conidia
   Subdivision Ascomycotina: Septate mycelium, sexual reproduction by a sac-like structure (ascus). *Neurospora*, morels, truffles, and yeasts (*Saccharomyces cerevisiae*). *Emmonsiella capsulata.*

   Subdivision Basidiomycotina: Septate mycelium, sexual reproduction by a basidium. Poisonous mushrooms, rusts, smuts, *Filobasidiella neoformans.*
   Subdivision Deuteromycotina (Fungi imperfecti): Septate mycelium, sexual reproduction has not been discovered. *Penicillium, Aspergillus.* Most pathogens did belong or belong here, e.g., *Coccidioides immitis.*

SUBCELLULAR STRUCTURE OF FUNGI

Fungal growth and structure are described in the section on fungi. Fungi include unicellular yeasts and multicellular molds.

In general fungal cells are larger than most bacteria and are eucaryotic. Thus, they possess all the cytoplasmic organelles indicated in Table 1–1, with the exception of chloroplasts (Fig. 1–8). They are not photosynthetic. The medically important structures of a fungus are the capsule, cell wall, and cytoplasmic membrane.

Capsule. Some fungi produce an external coating of slime or a more compact capsule. The capsule, or slime layer, is composed of amorphous polysaccharides that may cause the cells to adhere and clump together. The fungal cap-

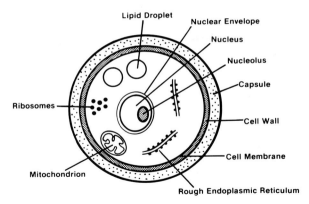

Figure 1–8. Schematic drawing of a yeast cell.

sule may be antigenic and antiphagocytic, as in *Filobasidiella* (formerly *Cryptococcus) neoformans.*

Cell Wall. The cell wall is the major structure of a fungus and it determines its shape and the process of fungal morphogenesis (e.g., sporulation or yeast-mold dimorphism). It lies immediately external to the cytoplasmic membrane. Unlike that found in bacteria, most of the fungal cell wall is a thatchwork of polysaccharide (chitin, glucan, mannan, cellulose) chains called *microfibrils.* The rest is protein and glycoprotein, which cross-link the polysaccharide chains. Since a wide variety of species of fungi share the same polysaccharides, many have common surface antigens. However, many unique antigenic determinants resulting from the different branching patterns of the polysaccharides are also found within a certain group. These anti-

gens are useful for classification. Detection of species-specific surface antigens in solution provides a sensitive identification of slow-growing or poorly sporulating pathogenic fungi or both.

Cytoplasmic Membrane. Fungi possess a bilayered membrane similar in structure and composition to the cell membranes of higher eucaryotes. Unlike the bacterial membrane (except for the mycoplasmas), but similar to that of other eucaryotes, the fungal membrane contains sterols. The principal fungal sterols are *ergosterol* and *zymosterol* (mammalian cell membrane possesses *cholesterol).* This difference has been exploited in the successful use of the polyene antibiotics (e.g., amphotericin B), which have greater affinity to fungal sterol than to cholesterol.

SOURCES FOR FURTHER READING

Joklik, W.K., Willett, H.P., and Amos, D.B. (eds.): Zinsser Microbiology. 18th Ed. Norwalk, Conn., Appleton-Century-Crofts, 1984.

Skerman, V.D.B., McGowan, V., and Sneath, P.H.A. (eds.): Approved lists of bacterial names. Int. J. Syst. Bacteriol., 30:225, 1980.

Davis, B.D., Dulbecco, R., Eisen, H.N., and Ginsbery, H.S. (eds.): Microbiology. 3rd Ed. New York, Harper & Row, 1980.

Webster, J.: Introduction to Fungi. 2nd Ed. Cambridge, Cambridge University Press, 1980.

Deacon, J.W.: Introduction to Modern Mycology. New York, John Wiley & Sons, 1980.

Moore-Landecker, E.: Fundamentals of the Fungi. Englewood Cliffs, New Jersey, Prentice-Hall, 1982.

Krieg, N.R., and Holt, J.G. (eds.): Bergey's Manual of Systematic Bacteriology, Volume 1. Baltimore, Williams & Wilkins, 1984.

2

Microbial Nutrition, Metabolism, and Growth

G. William Claus

CHEMICAL AND PHYSICAL REQUIREMENTS FOR GROWTH

An infection occurs whenever a particular microorganism carries out an active metabolism, grows, and exerts a harmful effect within the tissue of an animal's body. Whether or not this happens depends upon the environment provided by that tissue. Many microorganisms will never cause an infection simply because the host tissue does not provide the physical or chemical conditions necessary to support that microbe's metabolism and subsequent growth. On the other hand, some tissues provide an excellent environment for the growth of a few harmful microorganisms. Therefore, a knowledge of the chemical and physical requirements for the growth of various microorganisms is important to the overall understanding of the infection process. In addition, one must understand these requirements in order to grow a suspected pathogen in vitro in the laboratory.

Nutritional Categories

From a nutritional standpoint, microorganisms may be divided into three major categories according to their ability to use various forms of energy and carbon for biosynthesis (Fig. 2–1).

Photosynthesis and Autotrophs. Photosynthetic microorganisms are those capable of using light as a sole energy source and either carbon dioxide or more reduced organic molecules as a carbon source for growth. Autotrophic (chemolithotrophic) microorganisms are those that cannot use light as an energy source but can use inorganic molecules as the sole source of energy, and they may use either carbon dioxide or more reduced organic molecules as a carbon source for synthesis and growth. There are no known strict photosynthetic or autotrophic microorganisms that are animal pathogens.

Heterotrophs. Heterotrophic microorganisms are those that are incapable of using either light or inorganic compounds as an energy source and also cannot use carbon dioxide as the sole source of carbon for synthesis and growth. Instead, the heterotrophs use reduced organic molecules (like sugars, amino acids, fatty acids, and nucleic acids) both as a source of energy and of carbon for synthesis and growth. There are only a few heterotrophs that cannot be cultivated in artificial (synthetic) media in the laboratory, that is, outside the animal's body. Most heterotrophs are considered saprophytes because they can be cultivated on media in the laboratory. All pathogenic microorganisms, both

16

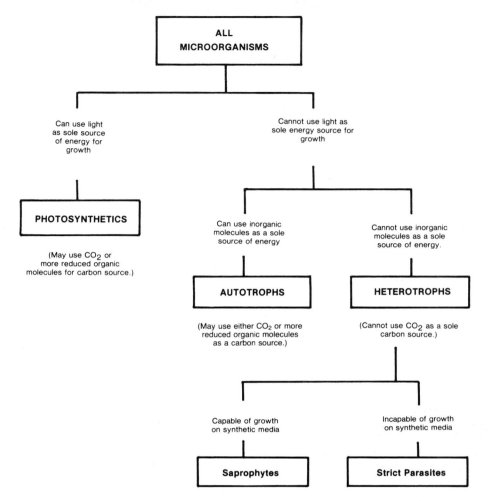

Figure 2–1. Major nutritional categories of all microorganisms. Note that the majority of microorganisms having veterinary significance are saprophytic heterotrophs.

opportunistic and strict pathogens, are heterotrophs, and the large majority of these are saprophytes.

Nutrient Requirements

Nutrients for microbial growth may be divided into two classes: (1) essential nutrients, without which a cell cannot grow; and (2) nonessential nutrients, which are used if present. All essential nutrients must be provided in an artificial medium for in vitro cultivation of a microorganism.

All cells must have a source of carbon and a source of energy to grow. In addition, all cells must have a nutritional source of nitrogen, phosphorus, sulfur, sodium, potassium, iron, magnesium, manganese, and trace quantities of many other minerals. These nutrients are essential for the growth of all microorganisms.

Some microorganisms are able to grow on media that contain only those nutrients just listed. For example, some enterobacteria will grow in a medium containing only glucose (as a carbon and energy source), ammonium ion (as the sole nitrogen source), phosphate ion (as a phosphorus source), and trace amounts of other minerals. This means that these cells can make all the polysaccharides, fats, proteins, and nucleic acids necessary for growth solely from the carbon and energy available in glucose. Thus, these cells have a very complex metabolism with powerful biosynthetic capabilities.

Other microorganisms require the presence of many other complex organic compounds to grow. For example, they may require the presence of certain amino acids, fatty acids, nucleotides, or vitamins before growth is possible. This means that these microbes are not able to make these compounds from a simple carbon and energy source (like glucose); therefore, these compounds must be supplied in the growth medium. These organic compounds are called preformed nutrients because they must be offered to the cells in a "preformed" state. Some microbes require many preformed nutrients for growth, and these microorganisms are called fastidious. Since many nutrients need to be preformed for the growth of these cells, this indicates that they lack powerful synthetic capabilities.

Even though a microorganism is capable of making everything it needs from a simple sugar like glucose, it will usually grow more rapidly in the presence of many preformed nutrients. For example, *Salmonella* species are capable of growth on glucose, mineral salts medium, but they will grow many times faster if provided with the preformed nutrients found in yeast and beef extracts. These extra nutrients are called nonessential because their presence is helpful but not necessary. In general, microorganisms will preferentially take in preformed nutrients rather than making them on their own because this saves them large amounts of energy.

Microorganisms that coexist with or are pathogenic for animals seem to range all the way from those able to grow in only a glucose, mineral salts medium to those that are extremely fastidious.

Hydrogen Ion Concentration

Some bacteria of veterinary significance are acidoduric, that is, they have the ability to survive (endure) for short periods of time in very acidic environments. For example, gastric fluids may have a pH value of 1.0, and gastrointestinal (GI) pathogens must first survive these stomach fluids before growing and exerting their adverse effects in the intestines. Although some microbes are acidoduric, very few are able to grow at these extremes in pH.

Each microorganism has a pH range within which growth is possible, and each usually has a well-defined optimum pH at which the cells grow at their maximum rate. Most bacteria of medical or veterinary significance grow best at a neutral or slightly alkaline pH (pH 7.0 to 7.5), the pH of most mammalian fluids and tissue.

For cultivating bacteria in the laboratory, it is sometimes necessary to first adjust the pH (hydrogen ion concentration) of the medium with an inorganic acid or base so that the pH will be

appropriate to allow growth. In addition, it is desirable to maintain a relatively constant pH during microbial growth. In many synthetic laboratory media, this is not possible without the addition of artificial buffers. Buffers are salts of weak acids or bases that are added to a medium to help keep the pH constant. During growth, many bacteria excrete organic materials that alter the pH of the medium. Buffers placed in the medium respond to the excretion of acid or alkaline materials by taking up or giving off hydrogen ions, thereby keeping the pH constant. Amino acids are good buffers, and they are naturally present in many complex laboratory media that contain extracts of living tissue or fluids. Therefore, artificial buffers need not be added to maintain an appropriate pH for the cultivation of bacteria in most complex laboratory media.

Carbon Dioxide Concentration

All microorganisms require carbon dioxide (CO_2) for both survival and growth. This is supplied either exogenously (from the environment outside the cell; the earth's atmosphere normally contains about 0.03% CO_2) or endogenously (from within the cell; produced by decarboxylation reactions during catabolism).

Some microorganisms initiate growth in the laboratory and reproduce at a more rapid rate when the CO_2 concentration is increased in the atmosphere above the medium. This phenomenon is characteristic of many pathogens of veterinary significance. These microbes may be grown in a "CO_2 incubator" by using compressed CO_2 to replace about 10% of the inside air. Alternatively, one may seal the inoculated cultures inside a jar with a lighted candle (candle jar) and allow the candle to burn to extinction; this method decreases the amount of O_2 available and raises the CO_2 levels from 0.03% to about 3%. Often it is not clear whether it is the decreased O_2 concentration or the elevated CO_2 levels that stimulate growth (see Microaerophils further on).

Oxygen Concentration

When oxygen is dissolved in fluids, it forms a variety of ions, such as the toxic superoxide radical. As a consequence of metabolism in the presence of O_2, hydrogen peroxide is also formed, and this, too, is toxic. Therefore, cells capable of growth in the presence of O_2 must have a way to detoxify these harmful forms of oxygen. Microorganisms accomplish this by producing enzymes that break down the toxic molecules or change them into a form that is less toxic. Superoxide dismutase, catalase, and peroxidase (Fig. 2–2) are examples of such enzymes. Cells that grow in the presence of air usually use O_2 to support a respiratory type of metabolism. Other types of microbes normally live where there is only a small amount of O_2; consequently, they have only a limited ability to detoxify oxygen radicals, and their cultivation in the laboratory must be under conditions in which the O_2 concentration is artificially lowered. Still other microbes live only in environments that lack O_2; these microbes usually lack this detoxification ability, and their laboratory cultivation must be in the complete absence of O_2. The terms that follow reflect an organism's ability to grow in the presence of O_2, and, in some cases, to even use O_2 to their metabolic advantage.

Strict (Obligate) Aerobes. These are microorganisms that can only grow in the presence of air (O_2), and the more O_2 available, the better they grow. All filamentous fungi but only a very few bacteria are in this category. Strictly aerobic pathogens are not very common but occur on the mucosa of the upper respiratory tract. They have an unusually high capacity to detoxify the toxic forms of O_2, that is, they produce large amounts of extremely active catalase and superoxide dismutase. Strict aerobes are usually cultivated on the surface of solid media or in well-aerated liquid media. These microbes are incapable of supporting growth from the energy supplied by fermentation. They accomplish a respiratory type of metabolism and use only O_2 as a terminal electron acceptor.

Facultative Anaerobes. These microbes are able to grow in either the presence or the absence of air (O_2), but they grow better in its presence. All yeasts and a large number of bacteria fit this description. Facultatively anaerobic pathogens are very common. They may begin to grow in well-oxygenated tissue (or laboratory media), rapidly use the dissolved oxygen, and then continue to grow in the absence of O_2 but at a slower rate. Since facultative anaerobes are

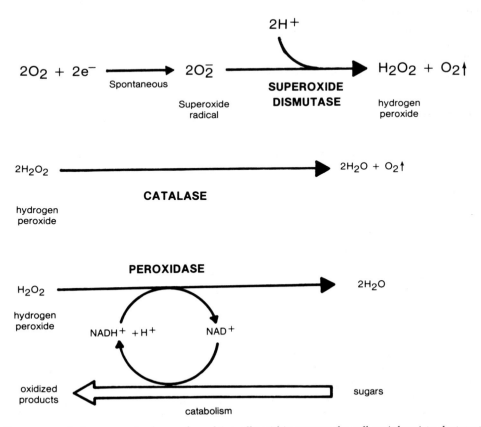

Figure 2–2. Enzymes made by some microbes and used (usually within or near the cell periphery) to destroy toxic forms of oxygen, such as the superoxide radical and hydrogen peroxide.

able to grow in the presence of air, they must have the ability to detoxify the toxic forms of O_2. In the laboratory, facultative anaerobes are usually cultivated under aerobic conditions, but they may grow in the complete absence of O_2 and at all oxygen concentrations in between. These microbes are able to support growth from the energy supplied by either fermentation or a respiratory type of metabolism. While respiring, some may use inorganic ions other than O_2 for a terminal electron acceptor to support respiration. In other words, some may continue to respire, even under anaerobic conditions, if an alternate terminal electron acceptor is available.

Microaerophiles. These microbes are strict aerobes, but they will not grow in an atmosphere containing the level of oxygen present in air (20%). Only a few bacteria are microaerophiles, but some of these are important animal pathogens, such as *Actinomyces* and *Campylobacter* species. They grow in body cavities and tissues having reduced O_2 concentrations. It is believed that microaerophiles will not tolerate normal atmospheric oxygen concentrations because they have a limited ability to detoxify the toxic forms of O_2. Cultivation in the laboratory is often achieved on liquid or solid media in an atmosphere containing about 6% oxygen, but this is not necessary if one uses semisolid media containing 0.1 to 0.4% agar. The gelling agent prevents oxygen from freely mixing through the tube. Oxygen can only diffuse from the surface; thus the medium is stratified with an oxygen gradient having the most oxygen-rich layer at the surface. After inoculation of the medium by stabbing deeply with a loop or needle, microaerophiles begin to grow in a discrete band located a few millimeters or centimeters below the surface, where the oxygen concentration is the most favorable. Microaerophiles have a strictly respiratory type of metabolism, with O_2 being the only terminal electron acceptor used.

Strict Anaerobes. These microbes lack the ability to grow in the presence of air, and often even the smallest amounts of O_2 are toxic. In healthy animals, anaerobic environments are found in the oral cavity (especially between the teeth and gums) and in the intestines (where the facultatively anaerobic microbes scavenge all available O_2). Strict anaerobes are among the normal microflora of these environments. Most infections of other tissues initially contain a mixed culture, and the facultative bacteria quickly use up the available O_2. This leaves an anaerobic environment that favors the growth of strict anaerobes. So far as is now known, only a few microbial types are strictly anaerobic. The best known types having veterinary significance are in three genera: *Bacteroides*, *Clostridium*, and *Fusobacterium*. The reasons why strict anaerobes are intolerant to O_2 are not completely clear, but it currently appears that they lack the ability to remove toxic forms of oxygen (most lack superoxide dismutase). For this reason, anaerobes are cultivated in an artificially reduced medium and under an atmosphere that contains little or no oxygen. Reducing agents such as sodium thioglycolate or dithiotreitol are added to the medium to depress and poise the oxidation-reduction (redox) potential of the medium at a correct state of reduction. A satisfactory anaerobic atmosphere is often achieved with a GasPack (BBL Microbiology Systems, Cockeysville, MD) that uses an H_2 and CO_2 generator; the H_2 reacts with O_2 inside the sealed container to form H_2O, thereby reducing the gaseous O_2. Although some strict anaerobes are capable of anaerobic respiration (using inorganic terminal electron acceptors other than oxygen), those of veterinary significance appear to support growth only from energy supplied by fermentation.

Temperature

Temperature is one of the most important environmental factors affecting the growth and survival of microorganisms. At very low temperatures, metabolic rates are very slow, and cells will survive for long periods of time (Fig. 2–3). As the temperature rises, enzymatic reactions inside the cell proceed at faster rates and

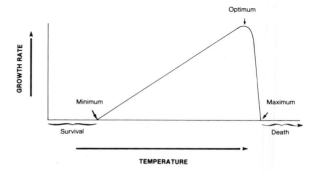

Figure 2–3. Effect of temperature on microbial survival and growth. Cell viability is preserved by temperatures below that supporting minimal growth. As temperature is increased, growth rate is also increased. As temperatures increase above that which is optimum for growth, the rate of growth decreases and then stops. Death occurs at temperatures above the maximum that will support growth.

growth also becomes more rapid until the optimum growth rate is achieved. Just above that temperature, however, proteins, DNA, RNA, and other critical cell components become irreversibly inactivated, and the growth rate falls rapidly to zero. Subsequent increases in temperature may kill the microbe.

All microorganisms have an optimum growth temperature. That of most microbes associated with mammals is from 35 to 37°C, but some (such as *Yersinia* species) still grow well at room temperature (25°C). Microbiologists classify these cells as mesophiles (optima from 28 to 38°C), and this category contains almost all known microorganisms.

Those pathogens that have an optimum growth rate at the body temperature of one animal may not grow or may be killed when transferred to another animal that has a normal body temperature just a few degrees higher. This may help to explain the species specificity of some microbial pathogens. Also, in the inflammatory response, the localized temperature increase provides an environment that is less favorable for microbial growth, and this allows enough time for the body's natural defense mechanisms (e.g., phagocytosis) to overcome the invading microorganisms.

If the temperature is elevated above the maximum at which growth is possible, then vegetative cells (but not endospores) die. Our knowledge of these lethally elevated temperatures is used in the pasteurization of liquids to make them safe for human consumption and in the boiling or autoclaving of instruments to kill most or all of the contaminating microorganisms.

The effect of cold temperatures on microorganisms is also of considerable significance. As the incubation temperature is lowered, enzymatic reactions inside the cell proceed at slower rates, and growth rates are decreased until cells reach the minimum temperature at which growth is possible. Unlike elevated temperatures, however, temperatures below the minimum growth temperature cause no damage. On the contrary, cold temperatures preserve microorganisms. Storing cultures in a refrigerator, or, with special handling, in a freezer (about −10°C), or in a container with liquid nitrogen (about −196°C) is a commonly used method for the long-term preservation of microbial cultures.

MOVEMENT OF NUTRIENTS INTO CELLS

Translocation Across the Capsule and Cell Wall

The capsule surrounding many microorganisms and the cell wall of gram-positive bacteria appear to be a loose matrix that permits the diffusion of all soluble molecules but does not allow transfer of colloid-sized particles. Thus, the capsule around all bacteria and the cell wall of gram-positive bacteria do not prevent the entry of most available nutrients into the cell.

The outer membrane of gram-negative cell walls, however, is thought to be a barrier. Interspersed throughout this outer membrane are a large number of only a few types of proteins (Fig. 2–4). The concentration of each protein type in the outer membrane can vary considerably, depending upon the types of nutrients in the environment. One type, almost always present in large numbers, is called matrix protein or porin. The porin molecules appear to form water-filled channels that span across the outer membrane, and these channels are of sufficient diameter to allow passage of molecules having a molecular weight up to 800 to 900 daltons. Therefore, small hydrophilic nutrients (like inorganic ions, mono- and disaccharide sugars, amino acids, and di- and tripeptides), as well as small non-nutrient molecules (like penicillin), can easily diffuse through these channels (pores). Thus, it is believed that the outer membrane of the gram-negative cell wall acts as a molecular sieve.

Other proteins present in the outer membrane of the gram-negative cell wall occur in smaller numbers than the porins. A number of these minor proteins seem to be receptor proteins that facilitate entry of molecules too large to pass through the pores (such as iron chelates, vitamin B_{12}, and degradation products of nucleic acids). These receptor proteins occur in larger amounts when their substrate is present in the medium. Still other minor outer membrane proteins appear to have a structural function.

The outer membrane of the gram-negative cell wall or the cytoplasmic (plasma) membrane (Fig. 2–4) should not be thought of as a static structure. There is evidence that optimal cell growth occurs only when these two membranes are in a semifluid state.

In the region between the outer membrane

Introductory Microbiology

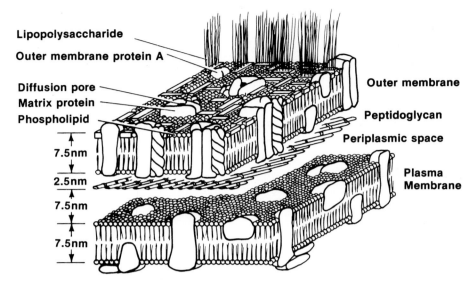

Lipopolysaccharide
Outer membrane protein A
Diffusion pore
Matrix protein
Phospholipid
7.5nm
2.5nm
7.5nm
7.5nm
Outer membrane
Peptidoglycan
Periplasmic space
Plasma Membrane

Figure 2–4. Suggested molecular architecture of the *Escherichia coli* cell envelope (cell wall and plasma membrane). For simplicity, only one sheet of the peptidoglycan is shown, and only a few of the polysaccharide side chains on the lipopolysaccharides are shown as hair-like projections. (From Ingraham, J.L., and Maaløe, O.: Growth of the Bacterial Cell. Sunderland, MA, Sinauer Associates, Inc., 1983 as modified from DiRienzo, J.M., Nakamura, K., and Inouye, M.: Annu. Rev. Biochem., 47:481, 1978.)

and the plasma membrane of the gram-negative cell, there is a rigid, girder-like polymer called peptidoglycan (Fig. 2–4). This region (or that between the peptidoglycan and the plasma membrane) is referred to as the periplasmic space. Residing within the periplasmic space are three types of proteins. First, there are hydrolytic enzymes, such as proteases, RNA and DNA nucleases, phosphatases, phosphodiesterases, and lactamases that destroy the β-lactam antibiotics like penicillin. The function of these enzymes is to cleave intermediate-sized nutrients so that they are small enough to pass through the plasma membrane. Second, there are binding proteins that specifically bind sulfate, some sugars, and amino acids and act in concert with the plasma membrane to help translocate these nutrients into the cell. Finally, there are the chemoreceptor proteins that allow motile gram-negative cells to detect certain nutrients in the environment, so that they may direct their movement toward the nutrient source. Thus, periplasmic proteins play a predominant role in both detecting nutrients and transferring them into the cell.

Translocation Across the Plasma Membrane

Most microorganisms function best when surrounded by water that contains dissolved inorganic ions and many also require organic molecules. In order for the cell to use these nutrients, they must first be translocated across the plasma membrane. The term translocation is used here to indicate the general movement of nutrients across the plasma membrane regardless of whether energy is required to accomplish that movement. Translocations that are accomplished without the expenditure of energy are called diffusion, whereas those that require energy are called transport.

Passive and Facilitated Diffusion. Passive diffusion is probably the simplest method of translocating nutrients into or out of the cell. It allows the free flow of nutrients across the plasma membrane, it requires no carrier protein within the membrane, and it requires no energy. But passive diffusion is slow, and the nutrient concentration eventually becomes equal on both sides of the membrane. Therefore, both the intercellular concentration and the rate of nutrient uptake depend upon the extracellular concentration. There are probably few, if any, nutrients that are translocated across the plasma membrane by passive diffusion.

Facilitated diffusion is similar to passive diffusion in that it requires no energy and the nutrient concentration inside the cell is never greater than on the outside. However, facilitated diffusion differs from passive diffusion in two important ways: (1) facilitated diffusion uses carrier proteins in the plasma membrane, often called permeases which specifically bind the nutrient and facilitate its translocation, and probably because of this, (2) facilitated diffusion is more rapid than passive diffusion. At present, it appears that facilitated diffusion of nutrients is rare in bacteria. Glycerol is the only nutrient known to enter *Escherichia coli* by facilitated diffusion, and it appears that the same mechanism is also used for glycerol translocation in *Salmonella typhimurium* and species of *Klebsiella, Shigella, Pseudomonas, Bacillus, Nocardia,* and every other bacterium studied to date.

Both passive and facilitated diffusion probably play minor roles in nutrient translocations. This is suspected because the concentration of most nutrients is much greater inside the cell than it is in the environment outside the cell. The higher intercellular concentration of nutrients allows the cell to keep its enzymes saturated with substrates, so that biochemical reactions are accomplished at the maximum possible rate. But a higher intracellular concentration of nutrients also means that they are translocated against a concentration gradient, and this requires energy. Energy-requiring translocations are only accomplished by actively metabolizing cells, and these types of translocations are usually referred to as transport mechanisms.

Mechanisms of Transport. To date, there are two types of energy-requiring transport mechanisms known: one type is called active transport and the other is known as group translocation.

ACTIVE TRANSPORT. There are three main features of active transport: (1) like facilitated diffusion, active transport requires membrane-bound carrier proteins (also called permeases) that specifically bind one type of nutrient and assist in its translocation across the membrane; (2) also like facilitated diffusion, the nutrient translocated by active transport enters the cell in an unaltered state; and (3) unlike facilitated diffusion, active transport requires energy, and this energy is provided by the protonmotive force. Before we consider how the protonmotive force drives active transport, we must first briefly consider a few key features of the metabolic process called electron transport. Note, however, that electron transport is covered in more detail later in this chapter.

The internal breakdown (oxidation) of a nutrient serving as the respiring cell's energy source (such as glucose) provides the cell with high-energy electrons that are given to a series of membrane-bound proteins collectively known as the electron transport system (Fig. 2–5). As these energy-rich electrons are passed from one electron transport protein to the next, the energy in those electrons is used to translocate protons (H^+) from the inside to the outside of the plasma membrane. Since the plasma membrane is relatively impermeable to both H^+ and OH^-, electron transport creates a strong positive charge (H^+) on the outside of the membrane and a more negative charge (OH^-) on the inside. This difference in charge (pH) across the membrane is called the proton gradient, and the amount of energy available in a membrane having a proton gradient is called the protonmotive force. The energy in the protonmotive force can apparently be used for doing useful work, such as translocating ions and uncharged molecules into the cell against a concentration gradient. This process may be likened to an energy-driven pump that pushes the nutrients "upstream," that is, against a concentration gradient.

There are at least two ways that this proton-driven pump may work. The first is called symport (Fig. 2–5). With this mechanism, the carrier protein transports both the nutrient and one or more protons into the cell. In so doing, the electrochemical (proton) gradient is somewhat diminished, but the cell has accomplished some useful work. It has pumped a nutrient inside the cell against a concentration gradient. At present, it appears that symport may be a primary mechanism for transporting nutrients into the cell.

The second active transport mechanism is called antiport (Fig. 2–5). With this mechanism, the carrier protein simultaneously transports two things in opposite directions. Once again, one or more protons enters the cell, along with the transport of another substance from the inside to the outside. It is conceivable that antiport may be used by cells in the excretion of toxic waste products against a concentration gradient.

GROUP TRANSLOCATION. There are three main features of group translocation: (1) like facilitated diffusion and active transport, group translocation requires a membrane-bound carrier protein to specifically bind one type of nutrient and assist in its translocation across the membrane; (2) like active transport, group translocation requires energy, but this energy comes from a high-energy metabolic intermediate rather than the protonmotive force; and (3) unlike active transport, the nutrient enters the cell in a chemically altered (usually phosphorylated)

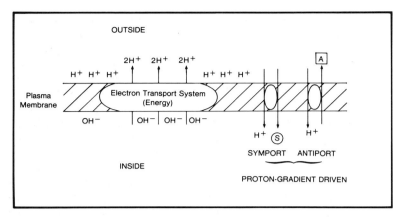

PROTONMOTIVE FORCE

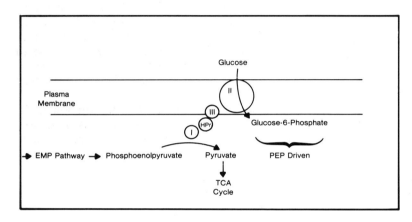

GROUP TRANSLOCATION

Figure 2–5. Two types of energy-requiring mechanisms of transport. In active transport, the cell uses the electron-transport system to translocate protons (H^+) outside the cell, thus creating a proton gradient. The energy established by the proton gradient (the protonmotive force) can be used to drive substrates (S) into the cell. With group translocation of glucose by *Escherichia coli*, the high-energy phosphate bond of phosphoenolpyruvate (PEP) serves as the initial energy source for transport, and four different proteins (I, HPr, II, and III) are also involved.

state (Fig. 2–5). Since the transported material is chemically different from that found outside the cell, technically speaking there is no concentration gradient produced. However, the cell does accumulate a useful nutrient in much greater concentration than its precursor on the outside, so the overall effect appears similar to that accomplished by active transport.

The best studied examples of group translocations involve certain sugars, such as β-glucosides, fructose, glucose, N-acetylglucosamine, and mannose. Each of these appears to be phosphorylated during transport by the phosphotransferase system (PTS). The mechanism (Fig. 2–5) involves at least four separate proteins that carry the high-energy phosphate group from phosphoenolpyruvate (a common catabolic intermediate) to the incoming sugar. The first two (proteins I and HPr) contain histidine, have a low molecular weight, and reside as soluble mol-

ecules inside the cell. These two proteins are subject to genetic regulation and are formed in greater amounts when the PTS-transported nutrient occurs in the environment. The next one (III) appears to be a peripheral protein located on the inner surface of the plasma membrane. The last protein to carry the high-energy phosphate (II) exists tightly bound within the membrane and also serves as a carrier protein to bring the phosphorylated nutrient across the membrane.

Since group translocation does not require intermediates that are produced in great quantities only during respiration (ATP and high-energy electrons), this transport mechanism is thought to occur predominantly in fermenting organisms. Most strict aerobes, such as *Azotobacter*, *Micrococcus*, *Mycobacterium*, and *Nocardia*, appear to lack a phosphotransferase system. Facultative anaerobes of veterinary significance known to contain a PTS include *Escherichia, Salmonella, Staphylococcus,* and *Vibrio;* the strict anaerobes include *Clostridium* and *Fusobacterium.*

CELLULAR METABOLISM

Metabolism is a term that refers to the integration of all chemical reactions occurring within the living cell. Metabolism starts with nutrients brought in from the environment, and the ultimate product is a new cell. For the sake of discussion, metabolism is often divided artificially into two parts: catabolism and anabolism (Fig. 2–6). Catabolism refers to those metabolic reactions that break down the nutrient serving as the cell's chemical energy source. Anabolism defines those metabolic reactions that make new cellular materials and use the energy provided by catabolism.

Catabolic pathways are exergonic, that is, they yield energy, and this is often trapped in the formation of new high-energy phosphate bonds, like adding energy to ADP and inorganic phosphate (Pi) to form ATP. Catabolic pathways are oxidative, i.e., some reactions remove electrons ($2H^+ + 2e^-$) but save these high-energy electrons for later use by giving them to the reduction of NAD^+ or $NADP^+$. Catabolic pathways produce intermediates (building blocks) for biosynthesis at many steps during the oxidation process. Finally, when the cell can oxidize the carbon and/or energy source no further, the product of the last reaction is excreted as waste, such as CO_2 (the most oxidized form of carbon), various organic acid or neutral compounds, or oxidized inorganic molecules.

Anabolic pathways are endergonic, that is, they require energy, and this is frequently supplied by the hydrolysis of the high-energy phosphate bond in ATP. Anabolic pathways are also reductive; some reactions use electrons ($2H^+ + 2e^-$) supplied by reduced NAD^+ and $NADP^+$ ($NADH_2$, $NADPH_2$). Anabolic pathways begin with intermediates produced by catabolism and then use these to form building blocks such as amino acids, fatty acids, sugars, purines, and pyrimidines. These building blocks are then polymerized into new cellular materials, such as proteins, lipids, polysaccharides, and nucleic acids.

Catabolism is integrated with anabolism in three major ways: (1) the energy (ATP's) produced by catabolism is used to drive anabolic

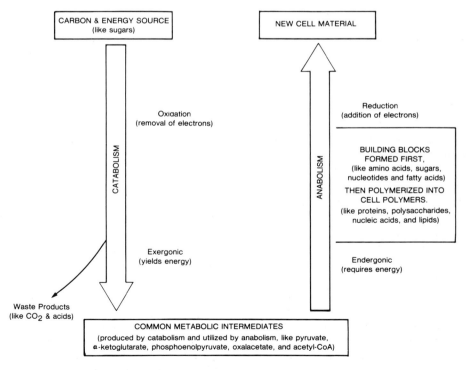

Figure 2–6. An overview of cellular metabolism. Catabolism provides the energy and electrons needed to drive anabolism. Catabolism also provides many if not all of the organic intermediates (building blocks) needed for biosynthesis of polymers during anabolism.

pathways; (2) the electrons (hydrogens) removed during oxidative catabolism and carried by $NADH_2$ or $NADPH_2$ are used to support the reductive (hydrogen-requiring) anabolic pathways; and, as previously mentioned, (3) some of the intermediates produced during catabolism are used to start anabolic pathways.

The following three sections present a brief overview of the metabolism of microorganisms having veterinary importance. They begin with a consideration of the two major types of catabolism (fermentation and respiration) and end with a succinct examination of how anabolism is integrated with microbial catabolism.

Fermentative Catabolism

Pasteur described fermentation as "life without air." Indeed, we now know that fermentative catabolism is carried out by most (but not all) bacteria and fungi growing in anaerobic environments, such as the rumen or the gut, or deep within infected tissue. Anyone who has smelled rumen fluid or the exudate from many infections has sampled a few of the many rich odors that often result from fermentations. Although not limited to fermentations, the excretion of gases and volatile organic compounds is very common to this form of catabolism.

Common Characteristics. Fermentative catabolism shows two common characteristics. First, small amounts of ATP are formed by a process known as substrate-level phosphorylation. Oxidative phosphorylation does not occur during fermentation. Second, organic intermediates of fermentative catabolism serve as the cell's terminal electron acceptor, and the reduced organic product is excreted into the surrounding medium.

To illustrate these characteristics of fermentation, let us use what is perhaps the simplest example: the homolactic fermentation of glucose accomplished by *Streptococcus faecalis*. Like many fermenting microbes, these bacteria are quite fastidious; that is, they will only grow in a nutritionally rich medium. Therefore, most of their biosynthetic intermediates are supplied by the growth medium, most of the glucose is oxidized only for energy, and most of the carbons from glucose end up in products excreted by the cell. Most of the excreted material is lactic acid, but there are also small quantities of acetic acid, formic acid, and ethanol formed. These bacteria use the Embden-Myerhoff-Parnas (EMP) pathway (sometimes called glycolysis) to oxidize glucose to pyruvate. This pathway is not limited to fermentation or to *S. faecalis*; it is found in both eucaryotic and procaryotic cells and is common to many fermentative and respiratory forms of catabolism.

The general scheme for the EMP pathway and for lactic acid formation by *S. faecalis* is shown in Figure 2–7. This serves to illustrate the two major characteristics of fermentative catabolism. The first is that ATP is formed only by substrate-level phosphorylation. This usually occurs as a two-step process: (1) the incorporation of inorganic phosphate into a catabolic intermediate to form a high-energy phosphate bond, followed by (2) the subsequent transfer of that phosphate to ADP to form ATP. In the EMP pathway, inorganic phosphate is incorporated into glyceraldehyde-3-phosphate to form a new high-energy phosphate bond attached to the first carbon. In the next step, this high-energy phosphate is transferred from the first carbon of 1,3-DPG to phosphorylate ADP. Thus, one more ATP is added to the cell's ATP pool in the ab-

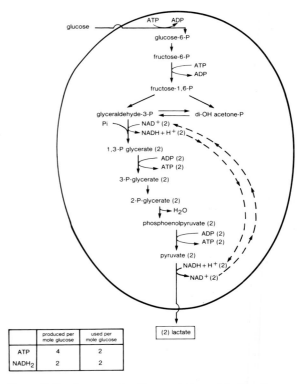

	produced per mole glucose	used per mole glucose
ATP	4	2
$NADH_2$	2	2

Figure 2–7. An example of fermentative catabolism (homolactic fermentation) illustrating two common characteristics: (1) ATP is formed only by substrate-level phosphorylation; and (2) catabolic intermediates (e.g., pyruvate) serve as the terminal electron acceptor, and the reduced organic product (e.g., lactate) is excreted into the surrounding medium.

sence of electron transport and coupled oxidative phosphorylation. When one molecule of glucose is oxidized to two molecules of pyruvate, the cell uses two ATP's (to form fructose-1,6-diphosphate), but it gains four ATP's (as two glyceraldehydes are oxidized to two pyruvates); therefore, the net gain is two ATP's for each glucose oxidized to two pyruvates. To emphasize the inefficiency of fermenting glucose, compare this yield with the 36 to 38 ATP's produced in oxidizing one molecule of glucose with a respiring catabolism!

From the preceding paragraph, it is evident that fermenting microbes are not very efficient in converting their nutrients into usable forms of energy (ATP). To compensate for this inefficiency, they oxidize great quantities of their energy source. This brings us to the second characteristic of fermentative catabolism: catabolic intermediates serve as the cell's terminal electron acceptor and the reduced organic product is excreted into the surrounding medium. The explanation focuses on the idea that all cells seem to produce only a limited quantity of electron carriers (NAD$^+$ and NADP$^+$). During oxidative catabolism, these electron carriers accept hydrogens as they are being removed from the energy source. Some but not all of these reduced carriers give up their hydrogens to support reductive anabolic reactions. This reoxidizes a few of them, so that they can once again accept hydrogens given off during oxidative catabolism; however, most of the electron carriers would remain in the reduced state in a fermenting cell if it were not for the catabolic intermediate's acceptance of electrons from the reduced carriers. In *S faecalis* (Fig. 2–7), pyruvate is reduced to lactic acid when it accepts hydrogens from NADH$_2$, and the lactic acid is excreted. For every glucose molecule fermented, two glyceraldehyde-3-phosphates are oxidized to two pyruvates, and this generates two molecules of NADH$_2$. To reoxidize both electron carriers, both molecules of pyruvate could be reduced to lactic acid. This accomplishes two things for the cell: (1) it reforms the NAD$^+$ needed for continued glucose oxidation, and (2) it gets rid of unneeded hydrogens (protons and electrons) in the form of reduced pyruvate (lactic acid).

The fermentative production of lactic acid from sugars by the EMP pathway and the excretion of large quantities of lactic acid are characteristic of the lactic acid bacteria. These bacteria are part of the natural microflora of the mouth and intestinal tract of mammals and occur on the surfaces of plants, and they are taxonomically placed in the following genera: *Streptococcus, Leuconostoc, Pediococcus,* and *Lactobacillus.* Depending upon the species, these bacteria may also produce varying quantities of acetic and formic acids as well as carbon dioxide, ethanol, glycerol, diacetyl, acetoin, and butanediol in addition to lactic acid. Some species are predominantly responsible for the controlled fermentation of harvested plant materials (e.g., silage production). In this process, the lactic acid (produced by the lactic acid bacteria) lowers the pH of the plant material, and this inhibits growth of plant-decaying microorganisms. Thus, the lactic-acid fermentation of plant materials preserves valuable vegetation so that it may be stored for later use as an animal food source. Other species grow between the teeth and gums, and produce acid from sugars in the animal's diet; the acid erodes the tooth enamel and causes dental caries. Still other species are opportunistically pathogenic and may cause soft tissue infections (see Chapter 9, Streptococci).

Other Fermentations. Similar catabolic characteristics for fermenting sugars are found in most other fermentations, although the exact metabolic pathways used and the catabolic intermediate that is reduced and excreted vary widely (Table 2–1).

Although the preceding discussion centers on the microbial fermentation of sugars, it should be emphasized that amino acids, fatty acids, purines, and pyrimidines are also fermented by microorganisms living in anaerobic environments. Other metabolic pathways are involved, but the same common characteristics appear in these other fermentations. For example, the proteolytic clostridia produce and excrete enzymes that break down proteins to a size where short chains of amino acids can enter the cell. Once transported inside, the amino acids are fermented, and malodorous fermentation end-products are usually excreted (e.g., mercaptans, and skatole). The fermentation of dead animal and plant tissue is a necessary part of the decay process, and decay is essential for the recycling of nutrients in our environment!

Respiratory Catabolism

Common Characteristics. Respiratory catabolism has four common characteristics. First, large quantities of ATP are formed (much more per molecule of energy source is oxidized than

Table 2–1.   End-Products Excreted by Microorganisms Fermenting Sugars

Fermentation Type	Microorganisms*	Products Formed
Lactic acid	*Lactobacillus* *Streptococcus* *Leuconostoc* *Pediococcus* *Sporolactobacillus* *Bifidobacterium*	Lactic, acetic, and formic acids, ethanol, glycerol, diacetyl, acetoin, butanediol, and CO_2
Ethyl alcohol	*Saccharomyces cerevisiae* *Zymomonas* *Sarcinia ventriculi* *Erwinia amylovora*	Mostly ethyl alcohol
Butyric acid and acetone-butanol	*Clostridium butyricum* *C. kluyveri* *C. butylicum* *C. acetobutylicum* *C. pasteurianum* *C. perfringens* *Neisseria* species *Bacteroides* species *Fusobacterium* species *Eubacterium* species *Butyrivibrio* species	Varying amounts of butyric and acetic acids, butanol, acetone, ethanol, isopropanol, H_2, and CO_2
Mixed acid	*Escherichia, Salmonella, Shigella, Proteus,* and *Klebsiella*	Primarily lactic, acetic, succinic, and formic acids with little H_2, CO_2, and ethanol
Butanediol	*Enterobacter, Serratia, Erwinia, Aeromonas, Bacillus polymyxa,* and *Klebsiella*	Lots of butanediol, with some CO_2, H_2, and ethanol and only slight amounts of mixed acids
Propionic acid	*Propionibacterium* *Clostridium propionicum* *Corynebacterium diphtheriae* *Veillonella* *Neisseria* species	Primarily propionic, acetic, and succinic acids and CO_2

*If the fermentation type appears to be characteristic of the entire genus, the genus name only is given. When characteristic of several species the word "species" is used. If characteristic of only one species, the entire species name is used.

in fermentation), and most of that ATP is formed by oxidative phosphorylation (coupled with electron transport). A small proportion of ATP is also formed by substrate-level phosphorylation, just as it is with fermentation, because some of the same catabolic pathways are used. Second, inorganic compounds (such as O_2 or NO_3^-) are transported into the cell and used as the terminal electron acceptor, and the reduced inorganic products (such as H_2O or NO_2^-) are excreted into the surrounding medium. Third, many more reduced electron carriers (such as $NADH_2$ and $NADPH_2$) are formed than with fermentative catabolism. Fourth, the organic energy sources used by the cell for catabolism are usually completely oxidized to CO_2 by a cyclic oxidative pathway (such as the TCA cycle).

The following sections will consider (1) the pathways common to respiratory catabolism, (2) how the hydrogens removed during this oxidation are used to make ATP, and (3) the involvement of the electron transport system and the types of terminal electron acceptors it uses.

Glucose catabolism will be used because it occurs in most microbes, and the oxidation of other compounds usually leads into the pathways used for glucose oxidation.

Pathways of Respiratory Catabolism. Respiring microorganisms usually use one or more of the following pathways for the catabolism of glucose to acetyl-coenzyme A: the Embden-Meyerhoff-Parnas (EMP) pathway, the Entner-Doudoroff (ED) pathway, and the hexose-monophosphate (HMP) pathway. In many cases, microbes seem to use either the HMP or the ED pathway along with the HMP pathway to meet the cell's needs. Only rarely is one of these pathways used exclusively. Each of these three pathways oxidizes glucose only to acetyl-CoA, then acetyl-CoA is further oxidized by the tricarboxylic acid (TCA) cycle. Therefore, complete oxidation of glucose to CO_2 requires the participation of *either* of the three pathways (EMP, ED, or HMP) *and* the TCA cycle. We will consider how each mechanism serves the cell and meets the four characteristics for respiratory catabolism. For comparative purposes, one molecule of glucose will be completely oxidized to CO_2 for each catabolic sequence.

EMP PATHWAY COUPLED WITH THE TCA CYCLE. The EMP pathway is widely distributed among many different types of microorganisms. Perhaps the most important group of bacteria of veterinary significance is the family *Enterobacteriaceae*, which contains genera such as *Escherichia, Enterobacter, Salmonella, Shigella, Klebsiella, Proteus, Yersinia,* and *Serratia*. Note that the EMP pathway shown in Figure 2–8 is essentially identical to that shown for fermentation by the lactic acid bacteria, with one exception: pyruvate is not reduced and excreted as lactic acid. Instead, pyruvate is oxidized further to acetyl-CoA, which in turn enters the TCA cycle. When one glucose molecule is oxidized by the EMP pathway to acetyl-CoA, the following compounds are formed: (1) four molecules of ATP (but two are used in the formation of glucose-1,6-diphosphate, so the net gain is only two molecules of ATP by substrate-level phosphorylation); (2) four molecules of $NADH_2$; (3) two molecules of CO_2 (which are excreted); and (4) two molecules of acetyl-CoA (which individually enter the TCA cycle). So at this point in the catabolism, the cell has started with one six-carbon molecule (glucose), broken off and excreted two one-carbon molecules (CO_2), and two two-carbon molecules (acetyl-CoA) remain for further oxidation through the TCA cycle.

To begin the TCA cycle, the cell must have one molecule of oxalacetate, but notice that a new molecule of oxalacetate is regenerated after each turn, so this initial molecule can be considered "catalytic." Note also that one molecule of acetyl-CoA supports one "turn" of the TCA cycle. One turn of the cycle releases two molecules of CO_2, so two turns of the cycle will complete the oxidation of the glucose molecule and the release of all carbons as CO_2. Two turns of the cycle also produce two molecules of ATP by substrate-level phosphorylation, so the cell now has a total of four ATP's produced by this method from each glucose molecule. This is twice the number formed by substrate-level phosphorylation when one glucose is oxidized during the lactate fermentation and most other fermentations. In addition, two turns of the cycle also form six molecules of $NADH_2$ and two molecules of $FADH_2$, so the cell has now produced a total of 12 molecules of reduced electron carriers per glucose molecule. This large pro-

duction of reduced electron carriers by cells carrying out a respiratory catabolism is one of the major ways in which they differ from fermenting cells. But, before we consider how these electron carriers are used, let's examine the two other major mechanisms of glucose oxidation found in respiring cells.

ED PATHWAY COUPLED WITH THE TCA CYCLE. The ED pathway shown in Figure 2–9 is quite different from the EMP pathway. The enzymes supporting this pathway are widely distributed among the bacteria; those having veterinary importance are all *Pseudomonas* species and *Alcaligenes* species.

When one glucose molecule is oxidized by the ED pathway to acetyl-CoA, glucose is first phosphorylated to glucose-6-phosphate (using one ATP), then oxidized to gluconolactone-6-phosphate, and then it undergoes several rearrangements to form ketodeoxyphosphoglucose (KDPG). Next, KDPG is split into pyruvate and glyceraldehyde-3-phosphate (G-3-P). The G-3-P molecule is then oxidized to pyruvate by the same reactions used in the lower half of the EMP pathway. Note that this produces two molecules of pyruvate, both of which may be oxidized to acetyl-CoA.

When one glucose molecule is oxidized by the ED pathway to two molecules of acetyl-CoA, the following compounds are formed: (1) two molecules of ATP (one glyceraldehyde-3-phosphate is oxidized to pyruvate), but one ATP is used in the formation of glucose-6-phosphate, so the net gain is only one ATP (by substrate-level phosphorylation); (2) four molecules of $NADH_2$, (3) two molecules of CO_2 that are excreted; and (4) two molecules of acetyl-CoA that individually enter the TCA cycle. Therefore, the net gain up to this point is very similar to that achieved by the EMP pathway, except that the ED pathway produces two less ATP's per molecule of glucose. However, there are still two molecules of acetyl-CoA that may be oxidized by the TCA cycle.

Just as with oxidation of glucose by the EMP pathway and the TCA cycle, oxidation of one molecule of glucose by the ED pathway will produce two molecules of acetyl-CoA, and these will support two turns of the TCA cycle. Two turns of the cycle will produce the following: four molecules of CO_2, two molecules of ATP, and eight molecules of reduced electron carrier. Thus, cells using the ED pathway and TCA cycle have a net gain of three ATP's produced by sub-

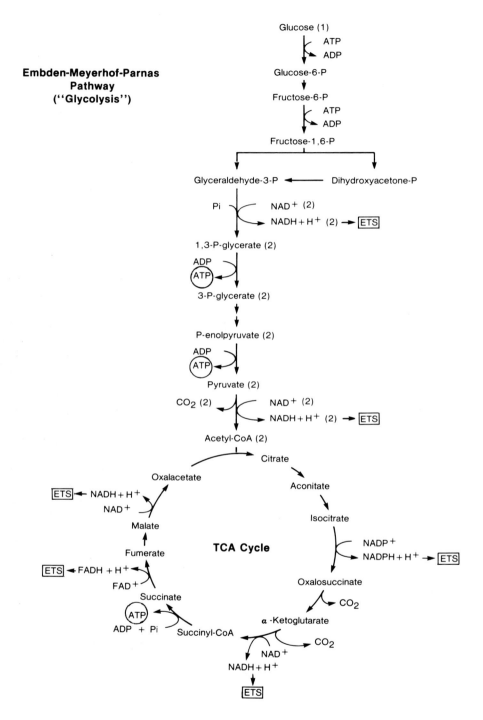

Figure 2–8. Respiratory catabolism of glucose to acetyl-CoA by the Embden-Meyerhof-Parnas (EMP) pathway and further catabolism of acetyl-CoA to CO_2 by the tricarboxylic acid (TCA) cycle. Note how oxidation of glucose through the EMP pathway and TCA cycle illustrates the four characteristics common to all respiratory catabolism (see text).

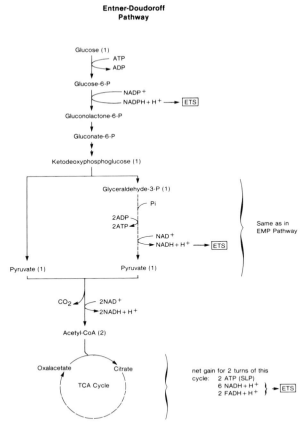

Entner-Doudoroff Pathway

Figure 2–9. Respiratory catabolism of glucose to acetyl-CoA by the Entner-Doudoroff (ED) pathway and further catabolism of the acetyl-CoA to CO_2 by the tricarboxylic acid (TCA) cycle. Note how oxidation of glucose through the ED pathway and TCA cycle illustrates the four characteristics common to all respiratory catabolism (see text).

strate-level phosphorylation and 12 reduced electron carriers coming from the complete oxidation of one molecule of glucose to CO_2. In comparison with the EMP + TCA system, the ED pathway coupled with the TCA cycle produces one fewer ATP and the same number of reduced electron carriers. Remember that respiring cells may use these reduced electron carriers to proudce many more ATP molecules by using a process known as oxidative phosphorylation. But, before we examine that process, let's comparatively examine the third major type of oxidative pathway used by cells carrying out a respiratory catabolism of glucose.

HMP PATHWAY COUPLED WITH THE TCA CYCLE. It is well known that the HMP pathway, shown in Figure 2–10, is used to form the five-carbon sugar called ribose, which is a precursor in the formation of all nucleic acids and one amino acid. The HMP pathway also produces the four-carbon sugar erythrose, which is a precursor for the synthesis of the aromatic family of amino acids in bacteria. Thus, the HMP pathway serves a synthetic (anabolic) function in most bacteria. In addition, the HMP pathway appears to serve a catabolic function for many bacteria, particularly when growing in an aerobic environment. According to some research, facultatively anaerobic microorganisms growing on sugars shift from the EMP pathway (without the TCA cycle) to the HMP + TCA pathway when their extracellular environment goes from the absence to the presence of oxygen.

The oxidative HMP pathway may, for the sake of discussion, be divided into three parts: formation of pentose phosphate, the pentose-phosphate cycle, and oxidation of glyceraldehyde-3-phosphate to acetyl-CoA (Fig. 2–10).

In the first part of the HMP pathway, glucose (a six-carbon sugar or hexose) is first phosphorylated and then oxidatively decarboxylated to xylulose-5-phosphate (a five-carbon sugar or pentose). This accomplishes three things: (1) it produces two reduced electron carriers ($NADPH_2$), (2) it breaks off and excretes one molecule of CO_2, and (3) it forms the pentose called xylulose-5-phosphate (X-5-P), which continues on into the pentose-phosphate cycle.

The pentose-phosphate cycle is the second part of the HMP. To start this cycle, assume that the cell has one catalytic molecule of ribose-5-phosphate (R-5-P), just as we did with the catalytic molecule of oxalacetate in beginning the TCA cycle. An enzyme called transketolase (TK) reacts with the two pentoses (X-5-P and R-5-P), transfers part of one to the other, and forms a seven-carbon and a three-carbon molecule. The products of this reaction are acted upon by an enzyme called transaldolase (TA) to produce a four-carbon sugar (erythrose-4-phosphate) and a six-carbon sugar (fructose-6-phosphate). Note here that the fructose-6-phosphate (F-6-P) is then oxidized to X-5-P in the same way described for the first part of the HMP, and this process accomplishes the same three things: release of one more CO_2, production of two more-$NADPH_2$'s, and formation of X-5-P. The X-5-P and erythrose-4-phosphate are converted to F-6-P and glyceraldehyde-3-phosphate (G-3-P). Once again, the F-6-P is converted to glucose-6-phosphate, which is then oxidized to X-5-P in the same way described for the first part of the HMP, and, once again, the cell produces two more $NADPH_2$'s, releases one more CO_2, and forms R-5-P. Formation of this R-5-P completes the cycle and regenerates the R-5-P required to

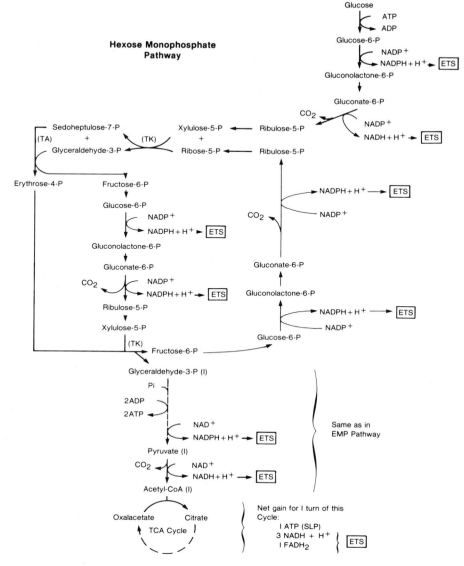

Figure 2–10. Respiratory catabolism of glucose to acetyl-CoA by the hexose monophosphate pathway (HMP) and further catabolism of the acetyl-CoA to CO_2 by the tricarboxylic acid (TCA) cycle. Note how oxidation of glucose through the HMP pathway and TCA cycle illustrates the four characteristics common to all respiratory catabolism (see text).

react with the X-5-P that starts the cycle over again. Thus, one turn of the pentose-phosphate cycle accomplishes three major things: (1) it releases two molecules of CO_2; (2) it yields four molecules of $NADPH_2$; and (3) it produces one molecule of glyceraldehyde-3-phosphate that can be oxidized further.

Oxidation of glyceraldehyde-3-phosphate (G-3-P) to acetyl-CoA can be considered the third and final part of the HMP pathway. One G-3-P molecule is formed, and this is oxidized to one molecule of acetyl-CoA in the same way as accomplished by the EMP and ED pathways.

When one glucose molecule is oxidized by the HMP pathway to one molecule of acetyl-CoA, the following compounds are formed: (1) two molecules of ATP (one glyceraldehyde-3-phosphate is oxidized to pyruvate), but one ATP is used in forming glucose-6-phosphate (in the first part of the HMP pathway), so the net gain is only one ATP (by substrate-level phosphorylation); (2) eight molecules of reduced electron carrier (two from part one, four from part two, and two from part three of the HMP); (3) four molecules of CO_2 that are excreted; and (4) one molecule of acetyl-CoA (which enters the TCA cycle). Therefore, the net gain in ATP production by the HMP pathway is similar to that of the EMP and identical to that produced with the ED pathway. On the other hand, there are twice as many reduced electron carriers produced by the HMP and twice as many CO_2's released by the HMP compared with the EMP and ED pathways. Note, however, that there is only one acetyl-CoA formed by the HMP pathway, so that only one turn of the TCA cycle is supported per glucose oxidized by the HMP pathway.

This one turn of the TCA cycle will produce only two molecules of CO_2, one molecule of ATP, and four molecules of reduced electron carrier. Thus, cells using the HMP pathway and TCA cycle to completely oxidize glucose to CO_2 have a net gain of two ATP's, produced by substrate-level phosphorylation, and 12 reduced electron carriers.

Thus, all three pathways for respiratory catabolism of glucose (EMP + TCA, ED + TCA, and HMP + TCA) have very similar gains both in ATP (from substrate-level phosphorylation) and in reduced electron carriers. One of the important features of respiratory catabolism, when compared with fermentative catabolism, is the large number of reduced electron carriers produced. It is the ability to produce and efficiently use these reduced electron carriers that allows respiratory catabolism to be so much more energy-efficient in catabolism. Let us now examine how respiring cells use these reduced electron carriers.

Electron Transport Coupled with Oxidative Phosphorylation. Electron carriers (actually hydrogen carriers like NAD^+, $NADP^+$, and FAD^+) accept hydrogens ($2H^+ + 2e^-$) that have high-energy electrons, and this happens during the oxidation of the cell's energy source such as glucose. Perhaps the most important way in which the energy in these electrons is used is the process called electron transport (Fig. 2–11). The NAD^+ and $NADP^+$ molecules are soluble and found inside the cell. Once reduced, these carriers interact with catalytic proteins that make up the electron transport chain or system (ETS) and are part of the cell's plasma membrane. The hydrogens (containing high-energy electrons) are passed from the $NAD(P)H_2$ to the first membrane protein of the ETS, and then either the hydrogens or electrons are sequentially passed from one protein to the next in sort of a bucket-brigade process.

The type of proteins found in the electron-transport chains of respiring microorganisms vary greatly, depending upon the type of microorganism and the conditions of growth. Perhaps the most common types (listed in the approximate order of their accepting hydrogens or electrons in the ETS) are flavins (flavoproteins); quinones (quinoproteins); and b-type, c-type, a-type, o-type, and d-type cytochromes. As the electrons are passed along the chain, it appears that much of their energy is used to create a proton gradient across the plasma membrane (see Mechanisms of Transport: Protonmotive Force earlier). The electron used to reduce the final electron acceptor of the ETS contains no more usable energy, so it is used to reduce an inorganic molecule such as oxygen. This inorganic molecule is called the terminal electron acceptor, because its function is to accept the energy-weak electron at the terminus of the ETS. The product of that final reduction (e.g., H_2O for aerobic respiration) is discarded by the cell as a waste product.

It is now believed that part of the energy in the proton gradient, which is established by cells carrying out respiratory catabolism, is used to form new molecules of ATP by a mechanism known as oxidative phosphorylation. Current evidence suggests that oxidative phosphorylation requires the formation of a proton gradient. The way in which a proton gradient is used to accomplish oxidative phosphorylation is schematically illustrated in Figure 2–12 and described in the following way. Reduced electron carriers, such as $NAD(P)H_2$, give hydrogen molecules (containing high-energy electrons) to the first electron-transport protein, such as a flavoprotein (FP). The FP accepts the entire hydrogen molecule ($2H^+ + 2e^-$), but it passes along only the electrons to the next electron-transport protein, which is an iron/sulfur-containing protein (Fe/S). The two protons ($2H^+$) that remain are placed on the outside surface of the cell's plasma membrane. The electrons now on the reduced Fe/S protein have slightly less energy, and these weaker electrons are next given to a quinoprotein (Q). Since the quinoprotein is able to carry both electrons and protons, it also picks up protons from the inner surface of the plasma membrane, and two complete hydrogen molecules are carried to cytochrome-$_b$. However, cytochrome-$_b$ is able to carry only one electron, so it takes two of these cytochromes to carry these two electrons, and the two protons ($2H^+$) that remain are placed on the outside surface of the

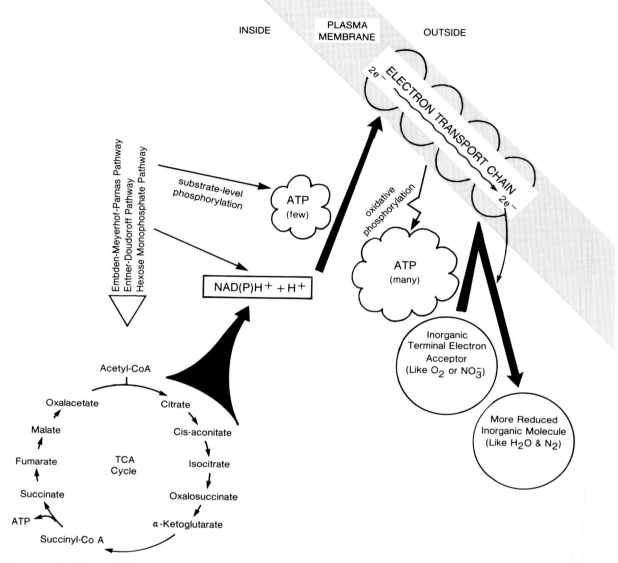

Figure 2–11. Flow of hydrogens (electrons plus protons) from catabolic pathways of respiring organisms to NAD(P)$^+$ and through the electron transport system (ETS), also called the electron transport chain. After passing through the ETS, the energy-weak electrons (e$^-$) combine with protons (H$^+$) to reduce the inorganic terminal electron acceptor. An important consequence of this electron flow during respiratory catabolism is the large amount of ATP produced by oxidative phosphorylation. The type of electron flow and ATP production is characteristic to all types of respiratory catabolism (see Fig. 2–12).

cell's plasma membrane. The electrons now carried by the two cytochrome-$_b$ molecules have slightly less energy. These weaker electrons are next given to the terminal cytochrome (the cytochrome oxidase). This reduced cytochrome gives these energy-weak electrons to two protons and an atom of oxygen to form water. Thus, oxygen serves as the terminal electron acceptor and functions in trapping these weak electrons in a molecule (water) that can easily diffuse from

the cell. In addition, electron transport has established a proton gradient, and this proton-motive force functions in part in ATP formation.

An enzyme called ATPase also exists within the cell's plasma membrane. One function of this reversible enzyme is to catalyze the phosphorylation of ADP to form ATP (Fig. 2–12). Strong evidence now suggests that this energy-requiring reaction obtains the needed energy from the proton gradient. Since it took energy

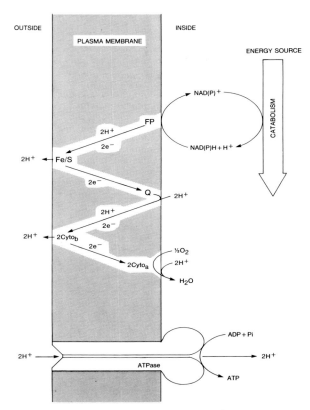

Figure 2–12. Production of a proton gradient as a consequence of electron transport resulting from respiratory catabolism, and the use of protons from that gradient to drive ATP synthesis. This mechanism of ATP formation is called oxidative phosphorylation.

to establish the proton gradient (energy coming from high-energy electrons), a collapse of this gradient would yield energy. It now appears that two protons pass into the cell through the ATPase protein and that this releases enough energy to phosphorylate ADP. Note in Figure 2–12 that the flow of one pair of electrons down this theoretical electron transport chain causes the translocation of two pairs of protons, so the flow of one pair of electrons through this ETS could conceivably support the generation of two molecules of ATP.

This type of ATP generation is referred to as "oxidative phosphorylation," and this is a very important part of respiratory catabolism. This is the way in which the energy in the electrons (hydrogens) is removed from the nutrient serving as the cell's carbon and energy source and converted to a form that can be used in synthesizing new cell materials (ATP). Note, however, that oxygen is not required by all microorganisms that carry out oxidative

phosphorylation as part of respiratory catabolism.

Terminal Electron Acceptors for Anaerobic Respiration. Although O_2 appears to be the most common terminal electron acceptor for the oxidation of $NAD(P)H_2$ by electron transport systems, a few microorganisms can use other electron acceptors. This is still part of the process known as respiratory catabolism, but the use of acceptors other than O_2 is called anaerobic respiration. Some terminal electron acceptors are known to be part of a system that generated ATP by oxidative phosphorylation; among these are nitrate (NO_3^-), nitrite (NO_2^-), sulfate (SO_4^{2-}), and fumarate (an intermediate of the TCA cycle).

Many different types of bacteria reduce nitrate if oxygen is not available, but they prefer to use O_2 as a terminal electron acceptor. These microbes are only capable of respiratory catabolism. Some reduce nitrate to nitrite and release the latter into the surrounding medium; other bacteria will continue to reduce nitrite to nitrous oxide and then reduce nitrous oxide to dinitrogen (N_2), which escapes into the atmosphere. If reduction goes all the way to N_2, this microbial process is called denitrification because it accounts for the loss of agriculturally important nitrates from the soil.

A few bacteria use sulfate as a terminal electron acceptor and reduce it to hydrogen sulfide (H_2S). Most if not all sulfate-reducing bacteria are strict anaerobes, because they are unable to alter the toxic forms of oxygen. These bacteria are often found in anaerobic muds and account for the black color and rotten-egg smell when these muds are disturbed. They play a significant part in the microbial degradation of plant tissue.

A wide variety of bacteria, under anaerobic conditions, are able to use fumarate (a TCA cycle intermediate) as a terminal electron acceptor at the end of an ETS, and they form succinate as the reduced product. This ability has been reported in *Escherichia coli* as well as in some clostridia and in *Vibrio succinogenes*, *Desulfovibrio gigas*, and *Proteus rettgeri*.

Although at present it is debated, there is evidence that CO_2 may also serve as a terminal electron acceptor for microbial electron transport chains that accomplish oxidative phosphorylation. The product of CO_2 reduction is methane (CH_4), and the microbes that accomplish this are called methanogens or methanogenic bacteria. Even though quinones and cytochromes are not found in the methanogen's plasma membrane, the membrane does contain a newly discovered type of electron carrier called F_{420}, and this may participate in an ETS-resulting oxidative phosphorylation. The methanogens are widely distributed in extremely anaerobic environments such as mud, the intestinal tract, the rumen, and anaerobic digestors of sewage treatment plants. Ruminant animals are of particular interest, because they establish a mutualistic relationship with microorganisms. Although these animals are herbivores, they cannot produce the enzyme cellulase but rather depend upon the microbes within the rumen to break down the cellulose. Various anaerobic microorganisms within the rumen convert cellulose, starch, and other polysaccharides to low-molecular-weight organic acids, CO_2, and H_2. The organic acids formed (such as acetate, propionate, and butyrate) are quickly absorbed through the wall of the rumen and enter the bloodstream, where they are oxidized aerobically to produce ATP that supports the animal's energy requirements. The methanogens appear to autotrophically use hydrogen (produced in large and otherwise toxic quantities by other microorganisms) as their primary energy (high-energy electron) source, and they use CO_2 (produced by other microbes) as their terminal electron acceptor, resulting in CH_4 as the reduced product. The ruminant then rids itself of methane by belching.

Although not a predominant form of catabolism, anaerobic respiration does play an important role in the cycling of nutrients within our ecosystem.

Anabolism

Anabolism (biosynthesis) is the second major part of metabolism. Unlike catabolism, anabolism is the building up of reduced organic molecules, ultimately resulting in the formation of a new cell. Anabolism requires energy, and this is provided by the ATP and hydrogens (on reduced electron carriers) that result from catabolic pathways. In addition, anabolism requires building blocks that are provided either by translocating them as nutrients or by making them as intermediates in their catabolic pathways. The term building block refers to the starting materials from which cellular polymers are made, such as amino acids, fatty acids, purines, pyrimidines, and sugars. If their presence is not required in the medium as an essential nutrient, this means that the microbe is able to make that

building block from intermediates resulting from catabolism of the carbon source.

Let us assume that we are working with a bacterium capable of growing in a medium containing only glucose and inorganic sources of nitrogen, phosphorus, and sulfur plus smaller quantities of other mineral salts. Since glucose is the only carbon source available to the cell, this means that all cellular polymers must be made from intermediates formed during the catabolism of glucose. It now appears that most microorganisms, whether or not they are pathogens, use similar if not identical catabolic intermediates to form these building blocks.

Many gram-negative enteric bacteria are capable of using both the EMP and the HMP pathways coupled with the TCA cycle to carry out respiratory catabolism. In the absence of a terminal electron acceptor, the TCA-cycle enzymes no longer function as a cyclic pathway, but most still function to produce the catabolic intermediates that are essential for biosynthetic pathways. Figure 2–13 schematically shows the EMP

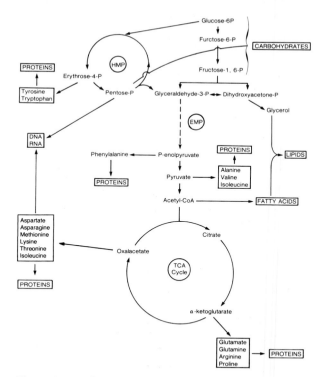

Figure 2–13. Common metabolic intermediates produced by respiratory catabolism and used as the starting point for anabolic (biosynthetic) pathways. Note that anabolism is often considered in two stages: (1) pathways for the production of building blocks (e.g., amino acids) from catabolic intermediates, and (2) mechanisms for the proper covalent bonding of these building blocks into polymers (e.g., proteins).

and HMP pathways with the TCA cycle and indicates the catabolic intermediates that appear to be the most common ones for producing building blocks necessary for forming each cellular polymer.

Note that in an actively growing microorganism, a pathway like the EMP + TCA cycle does not function solely for catabolism or energy production. One molecule of glucose may indeed be entirely oxidized to CO_2, but the next molecule of glucose may be oxidized only so far as pyruvate and from there it may support synthesis of the amino acid alanine and ultimately the synthesis of proteins. Therefore, the "catabolism" of glucose appears to be a dynamic process that supports both the cell's need for energy and its need to produce building blocks for biosynthesis.

The ultimate function or consequence of biosynthesis is growth, or, as microbiologists define growth, the production of new cells. All cells are composed of four types of polymers: protein, lipid, RNA, and DNA. Synthesis of the building blocks to support construction of these polymers and the polymerization process itself requires the expenditure of large quantities of energy. About 70% of the dry weight of the *Escherichia coli* cell is protein, and it is estimated that about 88% of all energy obtained from glucose catabolism goes into making that polymer. In comparison, these same bacteria contain only about 10% RNA, 10% lipid, 5% polysaccharide, and 5% DNA, and the remaining 12% of the energy gained from glucose oxidation is used to support the synthesis of these polymers.

ESTABLISHMENT AND GROWTH OF PURE CULTURES

Pure Culture Isolation

The establishment and maintenance of pure cultures are absolute requirements of a microbiologist who wishes to study the characteristics or the effects on the environment of one type of microorganism. Indeed, Koch's postulates require the use of pure cultures in establishing the cause and effect relationship between a microorganism and an infection. In nature, however, pure cultures are rare. Therefore, a microbiologist spends considerable amounts of time and energy purifying single types of microorganisms from the environment. Sometimes this may be accomplished simply by physically separating (streaking or spreading) the culture on the surface of a general-purpose medium. Many times, however, other microbes will grow faster and outcompete the suspected pathogen on such a medium; or the suspected pathogen may be present in such small numbers that it would never appear as an isolated colony on a streak or spread plate. This common situation requires the use of either selective media or enrichment culture to isolate the suspected pathogen.

Selective Media. An ideal selective medium is one that will preferentially grow only one (or a very few) type(s) of microorganism(s). One must first determine the type of microbe that is suspected, then choose a medium that will both encourage the growth of the suspected pathogen and inhibit the growth of all other organisms common to that environment. In order to choose a satisfactory selective medium for that microbe's growth, one must make sure that all the cell's nutritional requirements are supplied by that medium. Then one can select the type of inhibitory agent that will prevent the growth of the other microbial competitors.

There are many kinds of selective media, but most employ some chemical agent that is added to the growth medium. To be selective, the organism you wish to isolate (i.e., the suspected pathogen) must be resistant to that chemical, and the organisms whose growth you wish to inhibit (i.e., the normal flora) must be susceptible. Antibiotics, dyes, detergents, and sodium chloride are commonly used agents for the selective growth inhibition of unwanted microbes. If a medium contains a substance like blood or an acid-base indicator that only certain types of microbes will respond to in a characteristic way, that is called a differential medium. Sometimes a medium may be both differential and selective, for example, a medium that contains both blood (to differentially detect α- and β-hemolysis produced by streptococcal colonies) and an antibiotic (that will selectively inhibit growth of other gram-positive cocci). Occasionally a physical agent (like high temperature) is used in combination with chemical agents to selectively allow the growth of one type and inhibit most others. For example, selective growth of enteropathogenic *Escherichia coli* is accomplished by using a temperature of 44.5°C and a medium that contains a detergent and a dye along with the required nutrients (Difco m-FC medium).

When microbiologists use the term selective medium they usually are referring to a solid medium contained in a Petri dish or test tube. These are usually inoculated with a loop or a small volume of liquid. Therefore, the microbe one is searching for must be present within that small volume. This is not always the case. Larger volumes may need to be examined for the suspected microorganism, and this is the purpose of enrichment.

Enrichment Culture. This culturing technique is used for the growth of microbes that are present in very small numbers and may represent only a very small proportion of the types of microorganisms present in a mixed culture. Usually, a relatively large volume (from 1 to 10 ml) is inoculated into a type of broth that provides a selective environment favoring the growth of one kind of microorganism. For example, one often enriches for *Shigella* species with GN-Hajna broth, *Salmonella* species with selenite broth, and fluorescent *Pseudomonas* species with asparagine broth. The types of chemical added to these broths to make them selective, however, are often identical to those used in "selective agars." The purpose of both selective agars and enrichment broths is to enable the microbiologists to isolate a particular type of microbe so that it may be purified and studied.

Determination of Culture Purity. A pure culture is defined as one that contains cells of only one type. One can attain this by microscopic separation and subsequent cultivation of a single cell, but this method is extremely time-consuming and usually impractical. Perhaps the most practical method for obtaining a pure culture is called the streak plate. Using this method, one can theoretically start with a mixed culture and physically spread this over the surface of a solid medium until each cell is physically separated from all the others. Upon incubation, the cells grow and colonies of macroscopic size are formed. If a colony results from the growth of a single cell on the surface of a solid medium, then that is a pure culture by definition.

From a practical standpoint, however, many microorganisms adhere tightly to one another and sometimes to others of another type. Cells frequently do not become detached from one another after division, and this results in the chains, packets, or irregular clusters of cells that are characteristic and help to identify certain microbial types. Often, cellular adherence appears to be caused by extracellular (capsular) material surrounding the cell. Capsular material is adhesive, and this property allows the producing cell to stick to other things such as its own progeny, solid surfaces in its environment, or cells of another type. Therefore, the appearance of a well-isolated colony is no absolute guarantee that it arose from a single cell or even from cells of a single kind of microorganism.

On the other hand, a pure culture obtained by the streak-plate method is considered adequate in the clinical or diagnostic microbiology laboratory if it meets two criteria: (1) all cells from that culture should have the same size, shape, and Gram reaction; and (2) all subsequent streak plates should exhibit colonies of the same type. It is important, therefore, to Gram stain and streak clinical-laboratory cultures occasionally to make sure they remain pure.

Bacterial Growth Characteristics

Biologic growth is generally defined as an increase in size or mass. Because of the small size of the bacterial cell and the time-consuming properties of determining the dry weight of a bacterial population, however, this general definition for growth is not practical for the bacteriologist. When referring to growth, the bacteriologist usually means an increase in cell numbers.

For bacterial numbers to increase, the medium must have the minimum number of essential nutrients, and the environment surrounding the medium must provide the minimum physical conditions for that cell type. Both the rate of growth and the final numbers achieved at the end of growth will increase when any one of the following conditions is raised above minimum levels: the concentration of any one essential nutrient; the temperature; the hydrogen-ion concentration; and the concentration of oxygen (unless the bacterium is microaerophilic or strictly anaerobic). Also, growth rate and final numbers will often increase after the addition of a nonessential nutrient, because cells prefer to use environmentally supplied nutrients instead of making their own. On the other hand, the rate of growth will either decrease or stop when essential or nonessential nutrients are depleted, when waste products accumulate to toxic levels, or when the concentration of heat, hydrogen-ions, or oxygen (for some) is lowered below optimal levels. The same conditions that slow or stop growth may also cause cell death. The factors mentioned previously that affect growth rates and final population density or cell viability also appear to exert similar effects regardless of whether bacteria are growing on solid or liquid media.

Growth in Liquid Media. When a small number of cells from a pure culture are inoculated into a liquid medium (broth), the cells exhibit a characteristic growth curve that can be thought of in four phases (Fig. 2–14). Note that Figure 2–14 shows the change in viable cell numbers versus time.

During the lag phase, cells are shifting their metabolism so that they will be able to grow on the new medium. There are two important characteristics of the lag phase: (1) cells are rapidly making new DNA and RNA and inducing the synthesis of new enzymes needed for cell division, and thus there is a great deal of metabolic activity (including synthesis) taking place; and (2) as shown in Figure 2–14, there is no increase in cell numbers. The initiation of cell division marks the transition between the lag phase and the exponential growth phases.

During the exponential growth phase, cell division occurs at a maximum rate for the growth conditions provided by that medium. This is called the exponential phase, because cell numbers are increasing (doubling) at an exponential rate. In other words, the logarithm of the cell numbers increases linearly with time. The rate of cell division during exponential growth is often called the doubling time. This is the time that it takes for one doubling in cell numbers. The doubling time of any culture is affected greatly by the environmental (nutritional and physical) conditions provided. The doubling time is also affected by the cell's genetic ability to carry out efficiently catabolic and anabolic

pathways; therefore, growth rates are often characteristic of microbial cultures. For example, *Escherichia coli* has a doubling time of 20 minutes in nonsynthetic media under optimal conditions, whereas the doubling time of *Mycobacterium tuberculosis* may be as long as 24 hours in nonsynthetic media under optimal conditions.

This rate of cell division does not continue indefinitely, however. A test tube, flask, or plate is a closed system, that is, each contains a limited amount of medium. Eventually, the cells may run out of nutrients, or cellular waste products may build up to toxic levels, or the population density may become so great that the rate of diffusion of nutrients between cells becomes limiting. When the rate of cell division slows below exponential levels, the cells make a transition from exponential growth to the stationary phase.

In the stationary phase, there is no net increase or decrease in cell numbers. What happens depends upon the bacterial type. Some appear to just stop growing but fully maintain their viability. Others appear to reach a state in which the rate of new viable cell formation is exactly equal to the rate of cell death. Regardless of the cause, the effect is always a lack of change in viable numbers. The length of this phase varies greatly among the bacteria. Eventually, there is an initiation of death or an increase in the rate of death, and this marks the transition between the stationary phase and the death phase.

During the death phase, the rate of cell death in the population is also exponential. On the other hand, the rate of death is not always equal to the rate of growth of the same population. It is also important to point out that what is defined as cell death is really the loss of a cell's ability to grow (that is, to create new cells or increase in numbers). This does not mean that cells have entirely lost their ability to carry out metabolism and affect their environment.

Growth on Solid Media. Growth of microorganisms on the surface of a solid medium follows the same growth characteristics shown in Figure 2–14. However, cells usually cannot become as widely dispersed as in a liquid medium, so they remain tightly packed together after many divisions. Under these conditions, nutrients rapidly become limiting, especially at the center of the developing colony, and those cells rapidly reach the stationary phase. However, at the colony's edge, cells continue to grow ex-

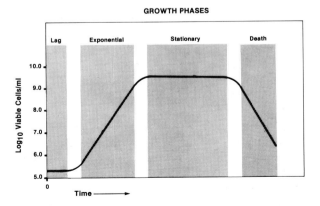

Figure 2–14. The four characteristic phases of microbial growth that occur when cells are transferred to a liquid medium in a closed container. Note that the lag phase may be eliminated if exponentially growing cells are transferred into an identical medium.

ponentially even while those at the center are in the death phase.

For reasons that are not clearly understood, bacterial colonies usually do not continue to expand indefinitely across the surface of a plate. Instead, a mature colony composed of the same type of bacteria has a well-defined edge, an elevation, a texture, and light-absorbing or light-transmitting properties that are characteristic of that bacterial type. Note, however, that these characteristics vary considerably from one type of growth medium to another; this is in part a result of differences in metabolism and changes in quantity and type of materials excreted from cells.

SOURCES FOR FURTHER READING

Atlas, R.M.: Microbiology, Fundamentals and Applications. New York, Macmillan Publishing Company, 1984.

Brock, T.D., Smith, D.W., and Madigan, M.T.: Biology of Microorganisms. 4th Ed. Englewood Cliffs, N.J., Prentice-Hall, 1984.

Gerhardt, P., *et al.* (eds.): Manual of Methods for General Bacteriology. Washington, D.C., American Society for Microbiology, 1981.

Gottschalk, G.: Bacterial Metabolism. New York, Springer-Verlag, 1979.

Ingraham, J.L., Maaloe, O., and Neidardt, F.C.: Growth of the Bacterial Cell. Sunderland, Massachusetts, Sinauer Associates, 1983.

3

Molecular Genetics and Genetic Variation in Bacteria and Bacterial Viruses

G. William Claus

STRUCTURE AND FUNCTION OF THE BACTERIAL GENOME

Structure and Chemistry of the Bacterial Nucleus

The term nucleus is defined as a membrane-bound organelle within a cell that contains chromosomes and nucleoli. Eucaryotic cells contain such a structure but bacteria do not. However, bacteria do contain genetic material, and its function is the same as the nucleus of eucaryotic cells. The genetic material inside a bacterium is often called a nucleoid, nuclear body, nuclear region, or bacterial nucleus.

The bacterial nucleus may be seen with the brightfield microscope after cells are stained with the DNA-specific Feulgen reagent. The bacterial nucleus may also be seen with the phase-contrast microscope when cells are suspended in a concentrated protein solution that matches the refractive index of the protoplasm, because this enhances the differences in contrast between the nuclear region and its surroundings. When observed in these ways, the appearance of the nuclear region(s) varies from condensed to diffuse, often depending upon the rate of

growth. The bacterial nucleus is amorphous and lacks the limiting nuclear membrane that is characteristic of eucaryotic cells.

Investigators have succeeded in isolating the nuclear region of *Escherichia coli* and other bacteria over the last 20 years, and the chemical analyses of all isolated nucleoids have been similar. Each is composed of about 80% DNA, 10% RNA (mostly nascent), and 10% protein (mostly RNA polymerase).

In 1963, John Cairns developed a special technique that allowed him to isolate and spread out the chromosomes from the nucleoids of *Escherichia coli* so their structure could be examined under an electron microscope. He found that the *E. coli* chromosome was a circular strand that had the same width as one double-stranded DNA molecule and a circular length of about 1 mm. Since the chromosome's length was about 1000 times longer than the entire cell, it was immediately recognized that the molecular organization of the chromosome within the nuclear region must be very complex. More recent evidence shows that this DNA molecule (the chromosome) is supercoiled, and this accounts for its efficient packing inside the cell. In order for the double-stranded helical DNA molecule to be supercoiled, one strand must first be broken (nicked) so that the helical molecule can be twisted upon itself (supercoiled). Studies suggest that there are 18 to 20 loops of DNA in the *E. coli* chromosome and that each loop is supercoiled, so that the entire molecule is reasonably compact inside the cell.

Genetic Elements of Bacteria—Chromosomes and Plasmids

Microbiologists use the term genome to mean the complete set of genetic elements occurring within a cell or virus particle. Although the chromosome is the primary genetic element in bacteria, many also contain small pieces of genetic material called plasmids that are physically separate from the chromosome. Therefore, when considering the genomic material of bacteria one must include both the chromosomes and the extrachromosomal plasmids. For the time being, however, let us concentrate on the bacterial chromosome, while remembering that much of what we say about that structure also applies to plasmids.

Most nongrowing eucaryotic cells are diploid, that is, they contain two copies of each chromosome per cell (pairs of matching genes). Eucaryotic chromosomes are structurally complex, and they have a number of different types of chromosomes per cell.

In contrast with eucaryotes, procaryotic cells (bacteria) have simple genetic systems. Bacterial chromosomes are single DNA molecules. Nongrowing cells are haploid, they contain only one chromosome (DNA molecule) per cell (one set of genes). During growth, however, the bacterial cell contains at least one partial copy of its chromosome at any one time, because DNA synthesis must provide two complete copies just prior to cell division.

Overview of Molecular Genetics

Genetic processes require at least three types of polymers: deoxyribonucleic acid (DNA), ribonucleic acid (RNA), and proteins. During cell growth, all three types of macromolecules are made. Since the steps leading from DNA to RNA to protein require the transfer of information, these are often called informational macromolecules to distinguish them from other large molecules such as lipids and polysaccharides.

The characteristics of each protein molecule synthesized by the cell during growth are determined by its amino acid sequence. There are 20 different amino acids commonly found in proteins, and there are often at least 100 amino acids in each protein molecule. The cell's genes determine the order of placement for each amino acid during the synthesis of a protein molecule.

One gene consists of a sequence of triplet purine and pyrimidine bases on the DNA molecule that eventually codes for a sequence of amino acids as the protein molecule is being made. The base sequence in each base triplet of the DNA is very critical, because a change in even one base may alter the eventual amino acid sequence or even cause cessation of protein synthesis.

DNA does not function directly in protein synthesis, however, but through an intermediate molecule called messenger RNA (mRNA). During mRNA synthesis, the DNA serves as a template, so that the purine and pyrimidine bases on the mRNA are arranged in the proper order. Each mRNA molecule is composed of a series of triplet bases that are complementary to those found on the DNA molecule. The triplets on the mRNA are called codons. The process of transferring information from DNA to an mRNA molecule as it is being made is called transcription. Once mRNA synthesis is complete and the new molecule binds to a ribosome, the mRNA serves as a template for protein synthesis.

Another RNA molecule made by the cell is called transfer RNA (tRNA). The tRNA molecule has two critical sites: one that will specifically bind only one type of amino acid, and another (on the opposite end of the molecule) that consists of three purine or pyrimidine bases that are complementary to only one codon on the mRNA (the triplets on the tRNA are called anticodons). The tRNA functions to specifically bind an amino acid and to specifically bind itself to the mRNA found on the ribosome complex, so that the amino acid will be inserted in the proper order during protein biosynthesis. This process of translating the code found on the mRNA into the sequence of amino acids in a protein is called translation. Bacterial cells use complex systems to determine if protein synthesis will take place and to regulate the rates of protein synthesis once it does take place. This is probably because not all proteins are always needed by the growing cell and some proteins are needed in greater quantities than others.

DNA Structure and Synthesis

A DNA molecule consists of two strands, each of which contains alternating units of phosphate

(PO$_4^{2-}$) and a sugar called deoxyribose (Fig. 3–1). Each phosphate attaches to either the 3' or the 5' position of adjacent deoxyribose molecules (ester linkages), forming what is commonly called the "sugar-phosphate backbone" of one DNA strand. At the end of each strand, the sugar phosphate has a free 3' hydroxyl, and it has a free 5' hydroxyl at the other end. Thus, it is common to refer to either the 3' or the 5' end of a single DNA strand. Attached to each deoxyribose on each strand is one of four possible purine or pyrimidine bases: adenine, thymidine, guanine, or cytosine. Replication (synthesis) always begins at the 5' end and progresses toward the 3' end of each DNA strand.

The single bacterial chromosome contains two complementary (not identical) DNA strands that are wound around one another in a helical fashion, with the ends covalently bonded together to form a circular macromolecule. The purine and pyrimidine bases of each strand are arranged such that the guanine on one strand is always across from a cytosine of the adjacent strand and a thymine is always across from an adenine (see upper half of Fig. 3–2). These adjacent bases are held close to one another by hydrogen bonding. Replication occurs by unwinding the existing helix and then adding individual sugar-phosphate-base units (called nucleotides) so that a new complementary DNA strand is built adjacent to the old existing strand (see bottom half of Fig. 3–2).

The point at which the two strands unwind is called the replication fork, the growing point, or the replicon, and it is believed that the bacterial chromosome is attached to the cell's

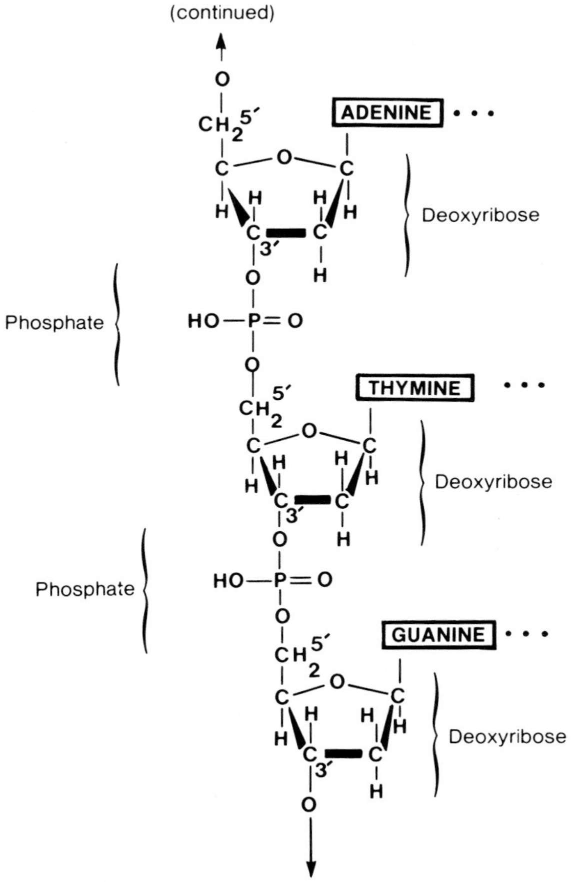

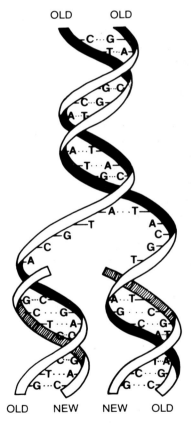

Figure 3–1. A small segment of DNA showing alternating molecules of deoxyribose and phosphate covalently bonded together to form one strand of the double-stranded DNA molecule. Each purine or pyrimidine base is covalently bonded at the 1' position of the ribose and loosely associated by hydrogen bonding (· · ·) to a complementary base on the adjacent strand (not shown).

Figure 3–2. The double-helix structure of DNA during the replication process. At the top of this drawing, each sugar-phosphte strand is shown as a continuous band with the bases adenine (A), cytosine (C), guanine (G), or thymine (T) covalently bound (—) to each sugar. The two strands are held together by hydrogen bonding (· · ·) between each complementary base pair. During replication, the old strands separate, and one new strand is formed that is complementary to each of the old strands.

plasma membrane at this DNA replication site. Here, during bacterial chromosome (DNA) replication, each nucleotide unit is added at the 3' hydroxyl end of the new DNA strand. Therefore, replication of each strand must run in opposite directions (Fig. 3–3).

When the double helix opens up to begin replication, an enzyme called primase initiates the synthesis of a short DNA (primer) strand. Once the first nucleotide is in place, then another enzyme (one type of DNA polymerase) continues to covalently bond each additional nucleotide to the 3' hydroxyl end of the newly developing strand. This new DNA forms in short chains (called Okazaki fragments), and then the adjacent fragments are covalently bonded together by an enzyme called DNA ligase. With the addition of each new nucleotide, the old DNA strand acts as a template (preformed pattern) for the formation of the new strand, so that complementary base pairing occurs during this synthesis. The end result of this synthesis is two double-stranded DNA molecules (one bacterial chromosome). Each one contains one strand

from the old molecule and a new, complementary strand.

Once replicated, each chromosome is then supercoiled. Supercoiling is believed to be an important factor in both the replication of DNA and its transcription. Enzymes called topoisomerases appear to regulate the degree of DNA supercoiling and thus its ease of replication and transcription. Each time that DNA is supercoiled, it is put under strain. Because it is under strain, it unwinds more easily than if it were not supercoiled. The topoisomerase that promotes DNA supercoiling (and thus controls unwinding) at the replication fork is called DNA gyrase.

A highly schematic and oversimplified illustration of chromosome replication and the subsequent division of these two DNA macromolecules prior to cell division is shown in Figure 3–4. The exact manner in which the two chromosomes are physically moved into each new cell is not known, but it is believed that the site of attachment of the chromosome to the plasma membrane plays an important part in this partitioning process. There is also evidence to suggest that rapidly dividing cells have more than one growing point (site of replication), because the time between cell divisions is shorter than the time it takes to replicate an entire chromosome. If this is true, then at any one time during rapid growth there would be at least one complete chromosome and many partial copies at various stages of completion.

RNA Structure and Synthesis

Like DNA, the bacterial cell's ribonucleic acids (RNAs) also play an important part in gene expression. Therefore, RNA must be understood in order to completely comprehend genetic variation in bacteria.

There are three major differences between the chemistry of RNA and that of DNA. First, macromolecules of RNA contain the sugar ribose instead of deoxyribose. Second, RNA has a base called uracil instead of the base thymine. And finally, *cellular* RNA is not a double-stranded molecule (but there are some double-stranded viral RNAs). Like all other cells, bacteria contain three major types of RNA: messenger RNA, transfer RNA, and ribosomal RNA.

Messenger RNA Synthesis. The function of messenger RNA (mRNA) is to copy (transcribe) the genetic code from the gene (chromosomal DNA) and to move that message to the site of protein synthesis (the ribosome). Transcription

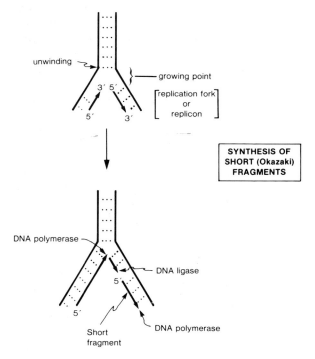

Figure 3–3. Mechanism of DNA replication. Unwinding occurs at the growing point (replication fork or replicon). The enzyme DNA polymerase connects each nucleotide only to the 3' end of each short fragment. These short (Okazaki) fragments are subsequently joined together by the enzyme DNA ligase.

of the genetic code occurs during mRNA synthesis.

The site on the chromosome where mRNA synthesis begins is called the promoter region, and each gene (or set of genes) on the chromosome has its own promoter. An enzyme called RNA polymerase binds to the promoter region, and this causes the two DNA strands to uncoil, so that the code may be read (transcribed) from one strand (the sense strand). The RNA polymerase then moves along the DNA sense strand while it simultaneously bonds together the ribonucleoside building blocks (adenosine triphosphate or ATP, cytosine triphosphate or CTP, guanosine triphosphate or GTP, and uridine triphosphate or UTP) to form the new mRNA molecule. The order in which the ribonucleosides are inserted into the developing mRNA is determined by the sequence of bases on the single-stranded DNA molecule. In other words, the bases on the single DNA strand act as a template for the assembly of complementary ribonucleosides, and RNA polymerase covalently bonds these ribonucleosides together and releases one pyrophosphate for each nucleoside that is bound. Therefore, the transcription process translates the genetic code from the DNA (gene) to the mRNA. As the RNA polymerase moves progressively down the DNA molecule, the double-stranded helix continues to open up; it recloses after the message has been transcribed.

Termination of mRNA synthesis also occurs at a specific (termination) site on the DNA molecule. This termination site determines how long the mRNA will be, and, as we will see, this in turn determines how large the protein molecule will be. Several types of termination sites on the DNA molecule have been identified, and both effectively stop the action of RNA polymerase (thus mRNA synthesis). The resulting complete, functional mRNA molecule is linear and single-stranded.

Not all mRNA molecules code for synthesis of a single protein molecule. In bacteria, some mRNAs code for synthesis of several or many related enzymatic proteins whose synthesis is coded for on adjacent genes. For example, the genes that code for all of the enzymes needed in the synthetic pathway for formation of one amino acid may be sequentially arranged on the DNA. Instead of having one termination site at the end of the code for each enzyme, the DNA may have one termination site for the entire se-

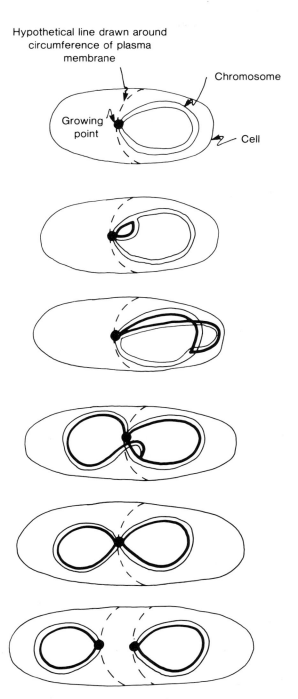

Hypothetical line drawn around
circumference of plasma
membrane

Chromosome

Growing
point

Cell

Figure 3–4. Replication of the bacterial chromosome. Each of the old strands of chromosome is represented by thin lines, and the new strands are shown with heavy lines. Sites of attachment to the plasma membrane are also sites for DNA replication (growing point). Separation of growing points may allow for partitioning of each new chromosome prior to cell division.

quence of genes. Thus, one long mRNA molecule could be transcribed so that it would code for the simultaneous synthesis of all enzymes required for that synthetic pathway.

Several important antibiotics appear to interfere with mRNA synthesis. Actinomycin inhibits mRNA synthesis by binding to the DNA molecule such that the binding blocks further mRNA synthesis. Two groups of antibiotics, the rifamycins and the streptovaricins, are effective against bacteria because they appear to bind to the RNA polymerase molecule and inhibit its activity. The rifamycins seem to be highly specific for the procaryotic RNA polymerase.

Transfer RNA Structure and Function. The molecular structure of a transfer RNA (tRNA) molecule (Fig. 3–5) closely reflects its function. It is a single-stranded molecule that contains double-stranded regions as a result of the molecule folding back upon itself. These folded regions have complementary bases across from each other, and hydrogen bonding holds these adjacent strands together. The structure of tRNA is generally drawn like a cloverleaf, with three distinct loops (of unpaired bases) and a stem having two open ends.

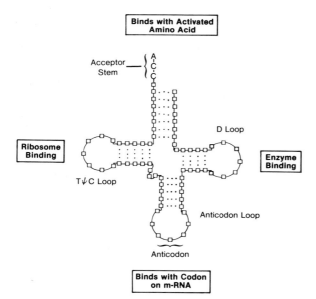

Figure 3–5. Molecular structure of a transfer RNA (tRNA) molecule showing a cloverleaf arrangement. Nucleotides (boxes or letters) are covalently bound together (—) to form a long, single-stranded molecule that is folded back upon itself. The folded tRNA is held together by hydrogen bonds (· · ·) between adjacent complementary bases. Three loops are formed upon folding, and each loop has a specific function. The two ends of this single strand form the stem of the molecule that will bind one type of amino acid (see Fig. 3–6).

To function properly, a molecule of tRNA (Fig. 3–5) must do the following: (1) it binds with an enzyme that activates amino acids; (2) it specifically binds with one type of amino acid; (3) it recognizes a specific triplet code (codon) on the mRNA, and it binds with the triplet bases on that codon; and (4) it nonspecifically binds with the ribosome to which an mRNA is bound. The structure of the tRNA molecule closely reflects how it functions during protein synthesis.

The D loop on tRNA selectively binds an enzyme called an aminoacyl-tRNA synthetase. This enzyme does two things: (1) it specifically activates one type of amino acid, and (2) it binds that activated amino acid to the acceptor stem of the tRNA. To activate the amino acid, AA-tRNA synthetase cleaves pyrophosphate from an ATP molecule and covalently bonds the remaining AMP to the amino acid. Thus, an activated amino acid is an amino acid–AMP complex. The specificity of the tRNAs toward only one type of AA-tRNA synthetase should be emphasized here. It is extremely important that the correct AA-tRNA synthetase be attached to the tRNA molecule, because this enzyme determines which amino acid will be activated and bound to the tRNA, and this, in turn, determines which amino acid will be inserted in the developing protein during translation. Specific binding between a tRNA and an amino acid occurs in the soluble portion of the cell. Once the amino acid has been activated and the amino acid tRNA complex leaves the enzyme, the tRNA complex migrates through the cell to a ribosome containing an mRNA molecule.

The anticodon loop on tRNA contains three bases (the anticodon) that are complementary to three bases on mRNA (the codon). The function of the anticodon on this loop is to specifically recognize and bind it to an mRNA codon. In other words, the mRNA codon specifies which activated amino acid–tRNA complex it will bind and thereby determines which amino acid will be inserted at that point in the developing protein. Thus, the genomic message from the chromosome is transcribed by the mRNA, which then migrates to the ribosome where its message is translated by the tRNAs carrying the activated amino acids.

The TψC loop appears to bind to the 50S ribosome subunit (see next section) during the translation process to help all of these components stay in the proper configuration while the activated amino acids are being covalently bonded onto the newly developing protein molecule.

Ribosome Structure and Function. Three important types of RNA are found in all cells: messenger, transfer, and ribosomal RNA. All three types are involved in transferring information from the sequence of nucleotide bases in the DNA to the sequence of amino acids in the polypeptide chain of a protein. Almost all the proteins made by a cell are catalytically active (enzymes). One might say that the DNA carries the genetic information, the RNA translates it, and the catalytic proteins that are made express the genetic information.

In bacteria, each ribosome is constructed of two subunits. Each subunit is described by the way it sediments in a high-speed centrifuge. These sedimentation properties (abbreviated "S" for Svedberg units) are determined by the size, density, and shape of the subunit. Thus, bacteria contain a ribosome that is made up of one 50S and one 30S subunit. Each subunit is made up of a number of individual proteins as well as a special type of ribosomal RNA (rRNA). The 30S and 50S subunits exist free in the bacterial cell and come together to form a 70S particle on the mRNA. Translation of the genetic code takes place on this ribosome-mRNA complex.

The 70S ribosome provides the structural framework that supports and aligns not only the mRNA but also the tRNAs and the many proteins required for translation. Distortion of ribosomal structure, therefore, can prevent proper functioning of this entire translational complex. Certain types of antibiotics appear to be effective because of the way they alter the structure of ribosomal subunits. For example, streptomycin, neomycin, tetracycline, and spectinomycin affect the 30S subunit of bacteria in some way and therefore are specific in their action against procaryotes. Similarly, puromycin, chloramphenicol, erythromycin, and cycloheximide appear to affect the 50S procaryotic subunits. Note, however, that this is not the only mode of action of these antibiotics. Most also affect other steps in protein synthesis.

The Genetic Code

The information contained in the nucleotide sequence of the bacterial cell's chromosome (DNA) is ultimately translated into the sequence of amino acids that make up each protein. Thus, the genetic code is contained in the DNA. However, this code is transcribed from the DNA molecule to mRNA, and it is actually the mRNA that serves as a template for the assembly of amino acids during protein synthesis. Therefore, it is customary to speak of the genetic code in terms of nucleotide sequence of the mRNA molecules.

All RNAs contain four different nucleotide bases: adenine (A), guanine (G), cytosine (C), and uracil (U). Within the mRNA, three sequential nucleotide bases (triplets like CUA) are used to code for the positioning of an amino acid during translation. Each of the triplet nucleotide sequences on the mRNA strand is called a codon. Since there are four nucleotide bases and three bases in each codon, there are 64 different triplets (codons) possible. On the other hand, there are only 20 different amino acids to code for. Therefore, there are many more codons than are needed for translating genetic information from the mRNA to the developing protein. What this means is that the genetic code is redundant, with several codons capable for coding for insertion of the same amino acid into the developing protein during synthesis (such as UCU, UCC, UCG, and UCA all coding for serine insertion).

There are a few codons that do not code for any amino acids (such as UGA, UAG, and UAA); these are called nonsense codons, and they serve as a signal to stop protein synthesis when the molecule is complete. Some evidence suggests that a few codons represent only starting points for new protein synthesis. These are called initiating codons. An adequate starting point is essential so that translation begins at the proper location. Without a specific starting point, the whole reading frame might be shifted and a completely different protein (or no protein at all) would be made, depending upon the extent of the reading frame shift.

Errors in translating the messge on mRNA are probably rare under normal circumstances. However, those antibiotics that act on the 30S or 50S ribosome subunits are thought to increase translation errors to such an extent that many protein molecules are abnormal, and the cell can no longer function properly. Drastic shifts from optimum pH, temperature, and cation concentration also appear to cause translation errors during protein synthesis.

Mechanism of Protein Synthesis

Protein synthesis (translation of the genetic code from mRNA) is a continuous process that may be thought of as occurring in four steps: (1) initiation, (2) elongation, (3) termination-release, and (4) polypeptide folding.

Initiation (Fig. 3–6) requires the formation of a complex that contains mRNA, the 30S ribosome subunit, formylmethionine-tRNA, the 50S subunit, and several proteins (called initiation factors). In bacteria, tRNA binds to the 30S subunit, and the 50S subunit binds to the 30S particle, forming the 70S ribosome. The anticodon on an activated formylmethionine-tRNA recognizes and binds to the initiating codon on the mRNA strand, and this tRNA also binds to the 50S subunit of the ribosome. Streptomycin interferes with initiation, probably because of its effect upon the 30S subunit.

In bacteria, the first (initiating) codon on the mRNA strand is either AUG or GUG. When used as an initiating codon (only), these triplets code for an amino acid called *N*-formylmethionine, so this is the first amino acid in the sequence for each protein. This amino acid can later be enzymatically removed, so not all bacterial proteins have methionine at their amino terminal ends. Just preceding the initiation codon are three to nine nucleotides that bind the mRNA

to the 30S ribosome subunit (probably by base pairing with the rRNA).

Elongation, the next step in protein synthesis, is actually a repeated series of events called recognition, transfer, and translocation (Fig. 3–6). To achieve elongation, there must be a continual supply of activated amino acid–tRNA complexes, such that the mRNA (on the ribosome) will be continually bathed in amino acid–tRNAs. However, only those whose anticodons match the next codon on the mRNA will be "recognized" and bind to the mRNA. (The antibiotics streptomycin, neomycin, and tetracycline appear to adversely affect codon recognition.) Once the two amino acids are adjacent to one another (because the adjacent codons on the mRNA dictate this), then the first amino acid is transferred and covalently bonded to the second amino acid. Next, the empty tRNA on the first codon is released from the mRNA (and 50S subunit), and the tRNA molecule with its attached polypeptide chain is moved along the ribosome (translocated) to the next position. (The antibiotics cycloheximide and spectinomycin appear to interfere with ribosome translocation.) This series of events is repeated over and over again,

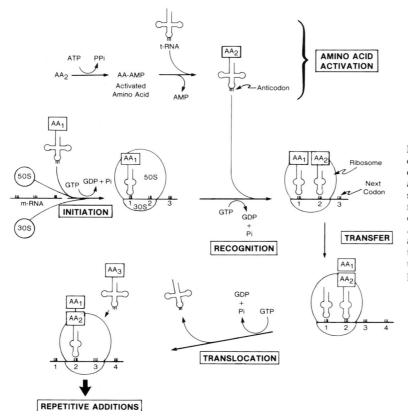

Figure 3–6. Translation of the genetic code from a messenger RNA (mRNA) molecule to the order of amino acids (AA) on a protein molecule during synthesis. Once synthesis is initiated such that the mRNA-ribosome-AA$_1$ complex is formed, the addition of each additional amino acid (e.g., AA$_2$ or AA$_3$) requires four events: amino acid activation, recognition, transfer, and translocation. These four events are continuously repeated in the elongation step of protein synthesis.

resulting in the elongation of the polypeptide chain.

Note in Figure 3–6 that each event in the elongation process, including initiation and amino acid activation, requires molecules that have high-energy phosphate bonds (adenosine triphosphate or ATP and guanosine triphosphate or GTP). For example, formation of the initiation complex (the initiation step) requires energy, and this is provided by the hydrolysis of one GTP. High energy compounds like GTP are supplied by catabolism of the cell's exogenous energy source. Catabolism (and anabolism too) is accomplished by enzymes (catalytically active proteins) that are made in the manner being described. Thus, catabolism of the energy source and synthesis of proteins are inseparably linked by the supply and demand for ATP and GTP, among other things.

Termination, part of the third step in protein synthesis, occurs when an mRNA codon is reached that does not code for any AA-tRNA. (In addition to their other activities, the tetracycline antibiotics also seem to interfere with the termination of protein synthesis.) There are three nonsense codons (UGA, UAG, and UAA) that stop polypeptide synthesis. Because no AA-tRNA binds with these nonsense codons, there is nothing to transfer the polypeptide chain to, and the chain is then released into the cytoplasm.

Once released from the ribosome-mRNA complex, the polypeptide chain is free to fold into an active, three-dimensional structure that is held in this form by weak disulfide bridges and hydrogen bonding. This is the last step in protein synthesis, known as polypeptide folding. If everything has gone correctly, the result is a functionally active enzyme that can participate in the cell's metabolism.

Regulation of Protein Synthesis

Most of the proteins in a cell are enzymes. Therefore, it is common to equate bacterial protein synthesis with enzyme synthesis. Some enzymes are always being made by the cell, so they are always present in relatively high concentration, and these are called constitutive enzymes.

Other enzymes, such as those catalyzing either the degradation or synthesis of certain compounds, are not produced under certain conditions. There are three mechanisms of genetic control that will be briefly discussed here: (1) the induction-repression mechanism, (2) catabolite repression, and (3) attenuation. Each of these control mechanisms acts at the transcription level, that is, on the gene (DNA), as its message is being transcribed to a new mRNA molecule. And each of these mechanisms functions to turn off gene expression (ultimately enzyme synthesis) when the gene product (the enzyme) is not needed for cellular metabolism. The function of repressing enzyme synthesis seems obvious, since it would be foolish for a cell to waste energy on making unneeded enzymes.

The ability to repress enzyme synthesis is now thought to be a valuable and widespread mechanism for energy conservation by all types of microorganisms. Regulating genetic expression in bacteria (procaryotes), however, appears simpler than in eucaryotic microorganisms. The following sections will deal only with genetic control mechanisms in procaryotic cells.

Induction and Repression. Control of enzyme synthesis by induction or repression usually involves not one but a set of adjacent genes on the bacterial cell's chromosome. These structural genes are responsible for the synthesis of several enzymes that usually accomplish all or part of the catabolism of a specific energy source. This set of adjacent genes forms a functional genetic unit called an operon. The operon is located right next to parts of the DNA that regulate its expression, and these DNA segments are called promoters, operators, and regulatory genes. The operon that has been most closely studied is the lactose (*lac*) operon from *Escherichia coli*. The *lac* operon is responsible for the initial stages of lactose catabolism in this bacterium, and it contains three structural genes (Fig. 3–7): (1) the "Z" gene that codes for production of an enzyme called β-galactosidase; this enzyme breaks apart disaccharide sugars that contain a galactoside molecule covalently joined by a β-glycosidic bond to another sugar; (2) the "Y" gene that codes for galactoside permease production, an enzyme within the plasma membrane that transports galactoside molecules inside so that they can be cleaved into separate monosaccharide sugars; and (3) the "A" gene that codes for production of galactoside acetylase, an enzyme whose function is not clearly understood.

Repression of the *lac* operon comes about in the following way. Transcription begins when RNA polymerase binds to the promoter. The regulator region is the first part of the DNA-sense strand transcribed. The function of the regulator gene is to code for continuous production of

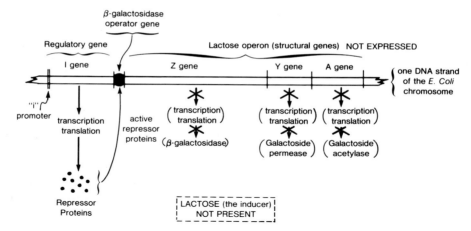

Figure 3–7. Repression of the lactose *(lac)* operon of *Escherichia coli.* In the absence of lactose, repressor proteins remain active and bind to the operator gene, thereby preventing transcription of the structural genes that make up the *lac* operon. Because these genes are not transcribed, the unnecessary proteins are not made; thus energy is conserved.

repressor proteins (see Fig. 3–7). If lactose (or another β-galactoside) is *not* present in the medium, then the repressor proteins are free to bind with the operator. In so doing, they prevent the RNA polymerase from binding to the operator region, which it must do before it can move on to transcribe the structural genes of the *lac* operon. This alteration of the operator stops further transcription and effectively inhibits synthesis of the enzymes required for lactose utilization, but note that these enzymes are not used in the absence of lactose, so this may be thought of as an energy-conservation mechanism.

For induction, a β-galactoside (like lactose) must be present in the medium, and the β-galactoside itself serves as the inducer (Fig. 3–8).

Cells probably always have a small number of galactoside transport proteins (permeases) in the membrane, even if transcription of the *lac* is repressed. Therefore, if lactose is added to the medium, a small amount is initially transported into the cell. The regulatory gene continues to code for synthesis of repressor proteins; however, lactose (the inducer) binds with these repressor proteins, so that the repressor proteins will no longer bind with the operator gene. Since the repressor proteins are now inactivated, they will no longer bind to the operator, and transcription of the operon genes by RNA polymerase can proceed. Thus, induction and repression both have the same underlying mechanism: control of the operator region, such that RNA poly-

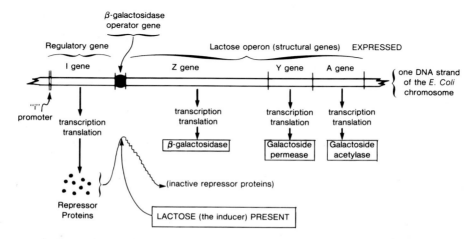

Figure 3–8. Induction of the lactose *(lac)* operon of *Escherichia coli.* When lactose is present, it binds with the repressor proteins, thereby making them unable to bind to the operator gene. This allows transcription (and subsequent translation) of the structural genes of the *lac* operon so that all the enzymatic proteins necessary for lactose utilization are made.

merase is either prevented from transcribing or is permitted to transcribe genes that are part of the operon. Since induction actually interferes with the action of the repressor proteins, some microbiologists prefer to call the induction process derepression.

Catabolite Repression. Another mechanism for control of enzyme (protein) synthesis is called catabolite repression. To understand this mechanism, it is important to know that bacteria are often capable of growing on a variety of nutrient energy sources, but some of these energy sources are used preferentially. For example, *E. coli* can catabolize either glucose or lactose to obtain energy for growth. If both are present, however, these bacteria will first use glucose until the supply is exhausted and then shift to lactose utilization. As previously described, the enzymes responsible for lactose utilization are inducible, but the synthesis of these enzymes (transcription of the *lac* operon) is also subject to catabolite repression. When glucose is preferentially used in the presence of lactose, glucose is the catabolite (substrate for catabolism) that acts as a repressor on the *lac* operon. Once the glucose supply in the medium is exhausted, there is no catabolite to serve as the repressor, and catabolite repression is abolished. Lactose can then induce the *lac* operon, and lactose catabolism can begin after a short lag.

The way that glucose acts as a catabolite repressor has only recently been determined. To understand this mechanism, it is first necessary to describe more fully how RNA polymerase binds to the sense strand of the DNA. In the previous section, it was stated that transcription (mRNA synthesis) begins when RNA polymerase binds at the promoter. However, with catabolite-repressible enzymes, binding appears to occur only if a catabolite-activator protein (CAP) has already bound to the promoter. In order for CAP to bind, it must be in the proper three-dimensional structure, and this requires a molecule called cyclic AMP (cAMP). It appears that glucose either inhibits the synthesis of cAMP or causes cAMP to be broken down. Regardless of the reason, intracellular cAMP concentrations are low in the presence of glucose. The lack of sufficient cAMP prevents CAP binding to the promoter; thus RNA polymerase does not bind, and transcription does not occur. Therefore, catabolite repression is really the result of a cAMP deficiency.

There is some evidence that glucose-controlled cAMP concentrations regulate enzyme synthesis for a number of other catabolic pathways in *E. coli*. This suggests that enzymes responsible for catabolism of energy sources other than glucose are not made in the presence of glucose (a preferred energy source for *E. coli*). Thus, once again, the cell conserves energy by stopping synthesis of unneeded enzymes. Alternatively, when the preferred energy source (glucose) is depleted, the cell starts synthesis of other enzymes used for catabolism of other substrates. Perhaps cells capable of such feats are more adaptable to changing environments and thus more likely to survive than those that lack such regulation mechanisms.

Attenuation. A third mechanism of regulation occurs in operons controlling synthesis of amino acids. The best studied seems to be the tryptophan operon. This operon contains structural genes for the five enzymes required to convert catabolic intermediates to tryptophan. The adjacent regulatory sequence includes three major regions: the promoter, the operator, and a region that seems characteristic of attenuation controlled regulatory sequences called the leader sequence. Within the leader sequence is a region called the attenuator that codes for synthesis of a peptide (small molecular weight protein) that is rich in tryptophan. This tryptophan-rich peptide is called a leader. If tryptophan is abundant in the medium and in the cell, then the leader can be assembled. On the other hand, if intracellular tryptophan concentrations are low or absent, the leader peptide cannot be made.

The critical feature of this mechanism is that synthesis of the leader peptide causes transcription of the tryptophan structural genes to stop. On the other hand, if a tryptophan deficiency stops synthesis of the leader peptide, then transcription of the structural genes will take place, and tryptophan synthesis will occur inside the cell.

Summary. Although it may appear that much is known about how protein (enzyme) synthesis is regulated, there is much more detail still to learn, and it is too early to tell if anabolic and catabolic pathways are regulated in similar or different ways. At the present time, however, it appears that *catabolic* (energy-yielding, degradative) pathways are controlled using either induction-repression or catabolite repression. Note that both of these mechanisms use the presence of the initial substrate (energy source) to turn *on* the synthesis of these catabolic enzymes. Alternatively, the attenuation mechanism appears to regulate *anabolic* (energy-requiring, biosynthetic) pathways, and this mechanism uses the presence of the end-product to turn *off* synthesis.

MUTATION AS A MECHANISM FOR GENETIC VARIATION IN BACTERIA

Introduction to Microbial Mutations

We previously examined the structure of the bacterial chromosome and how its genetic information is expressed and regulated under normal circumstances. Let us now shift attention to how the infrequent but important changes occur in the nucleotide sequence of bacterial chromosomes. But first we need to define some terms.

A microbial strain (also called a clone) is a population of cells that are genetically identical. Pure culture techniques are extremely important for isolation and maintenance of microbial strains. The genotype of a strain would be the entire set of genetic characteristics regardless of whether these genes are being expressed (transcribed and translated) at any given time. In contrast, the phenotype of a strain is that set of genetic characteristics that are readily seen or measured in any given environment; thus, phenotypic characteristics are those resulting only from those genes that are expressed under that set of environmental conditions. If the environment is changed, genetic regulation may (by induction or repression) change genetic expression, thereby also changing the apparent phenotype of that strain.

Microbiologists commonly refer to strains isolated from the environment as wild types and strains isolated from wild type strains following mutation as mutants. In the broadest sense of the term, mutation is defined as a sudden and inheritable change in the cell's chromosome that results in a phenotypic change. With microorganisms, however, it is often convenient to differentiate between two types of sudden and inheritable change in the DNA: (1) recombination, in which the change is caused by the introduction of new genes from outside the cell, and (2) mutation, in which changes occur that are not the result of introducing new genetic material from outside the cell. For the present, let us deal only with mutation and leave an explanation of recombination for later in this chapter.

Spontaneous Mutations

A spontaneous mutation is one that occurs without any direct intervention by the investigator or known cause from outside the cell. Therefore, spontaneous mutations probably most commonly result from errors made while copying the DNA during chromosome replication.

The accuracy with which DNA is copied during chromosome replication is very high (errors estimated at fewer than one in every 500,000 bases copied). Therefore, the rate of error in any one gene is very small, and the frequency of spontaneous mutation is rare. But with microbial populations, large numbers of individuals may be grown quickly and inexpensively in the laboratory, so microbes make excellent tools for studying mutation.

For any given gene, spontaneous mutation will occur at the frequency of only about one in every 10^5 to 10^9 cells. For example, streptomycin resistance may arise spontaneously in a bacterial population in one out of every 10^7 cells; therefore, one could find only 10 streptomycin-resistant cells in every 10^8 cells examined. It should be apparent that detection of spontaneous mutation in the laboratory is difficult unless selection techniques are used. For example, one could place a large number of cells ($>10^7$) in a medium containing growth-inhibiting concentrations of streptomycin (a selective medium), and only the streptomycin-resistant cells should grow.

Whether streptomycin-resistant mutants will remain at the spontaneous level of one in every 10^7 cells in the natural environment depends upon the presence or absence of streptomycin. Continual prophylactic or therapeutic use of any single antibiotic encourages the selection of spontaneous, antibiotic-resistant mutants, and the predominance of these mutants in the environment drastically decreases the effectiveness of this antibiotic in combating future infections.

Spontaneous mutation frequencies vary for different characteristics and also for the same characteristics from one species to another. For any given species or strain, however, it is important to realize that the frequency of spontaneous mutation for each gene may be different, and the occurrence of one mutation will be independent of all others. Thus, if the frequency of spontaneous mutation to streptomycin resistance in a bacterial strain is one in every 10^7, and the frequency of spontaneous mutation to penicillin resistance in that same strain is one in every 10^5 cells, then the frequency of mutation of two genes in the same cell (allowing both streptomycin and penicillin resistance) is one in every 10^{12} cells. Given these considerations, it should be obvious why dual antibiotic therapy is often preferred.

Molecular Mechanisms of Mutagenesis

All evidence indicates that mutations result from alteration in the nucleotide base sequences of the cell's genes (DNA). If we continue to define mutation as excluding recombination events, there are still many different types of mutations described in the literature. However, two mechanisms seem to help describe many (if not most) mutation events, and these are point mutations and deletion mutations.

Point Mutations. Point mutations result when there is a substitution of one deoxyribonucleotide for another during DNA synthesis. For example, a deoxyadenosine may be inserted instead of a deoxyguanosine during DNA synthesis (gene replication), and this means that adenine would replace guanine in the sequence of bases on the new DNA strand. Therefore, point mutations are alterations of only one base in the sequence of bases that make up a single structural or regulatory gene.

Whether or not a point mutation is phenotypically expressed depends upon which base is substituted and where that substitution takes place on the gene. To explain this, let us consider a point mutation occurring in the DNA triplet that codes for the amino acid serine during translation. You may recall that the genetic code is redundant, that is, there is more than one triplet that will code for serine. If the point mutation causes a substitution that alters the DNA triplet, such that the resulting mRNA codon will still code for serine, then there will be no alteration in the amino acid sequence of the protein made by this gene. Since it is the same protein, it will function the same, and there will be no phenotypic expression of this point mutation. This is called a silent mutation, because the protein produced by that gene is identical to that made before the mutation.

Alternatively, the DNA-base substitution resulting from point mutation can alter the triplet such that the mRNA (produced during transcription) will code for the insertion of another amino acid during protein synthesis (translation). If this different amino acid is in a critical location, like part of an enzyme's active site, then the function of that protein could be altered or even destroyed. If that protein were critical to the cell's survival, this point mutation could be lethal. On the other hand, if the substitution altered the amino acid sequence at a point on the protein that was not critical for its catalytic activity, then this mutation would not be phenotypically expressed. Note that this latter mutation is not silent because the amino acid sequence of the protein produced by that gene is altered.

Deletion Mutants. A deletion mutant is one in which a portion of one strand of the DNA is removed. Anywhere from one to several hundred deoxyribonucleotides (bases) may be deleted from the DNA strand. Deletion of a single base in a structural gene will probably result in a reading frame shift, because the next three bases appear to be a nonsense codon. This causes the cessation of transcription and hence a shorter mRNA. If this occurs at the terminal end of the gene, the alteration of the mRNA and the resulting protein may not drastically affect the protein's catalytic activity. If, however, the deletion occurs closer to the promoter end (5' end) of the structural gene, then the resulting (shorter) polypeptide will probably be nonfunctional and easily detected phenotypically (if this mutant strain survives). Deletion of larger segments of the DNA results in complete loss of the ability to produce the protein. Phenotypically detectable deletion mutations cannot be restored through further mutation.

Reversions. A revertant is a strain in which a wild-type phenotypic characteristic, originally lost due to mutation, is restored regardless of the mechanism. Reversions are often called back mutations because a second mutation is required to restore the original characteristic. Many mutations are revertable, and the reversion may occur in one of several ways. For example, a back mutation may occur at the same site (or close to the same site) of the original mutation, such that reading frame shift originally caused by a small deletion is corrected. Chemical or physical agents that increase the frequency of mutation (mutagens) also stimulate the frequency of reversion.

The stimulation of back mutation by mutagens

has a very practical application in the use of the Ames test for determining the carcinogenic potential of chemical mutagens. The Ames test (named for Dr. Bruce Ames, University of California, Berkeley) uses mutant strains of *Salmonella typhimurium* that are very sensitive to back mutation when subjected to chemical carcinogens. This test is much more economical and takes far less time than using laboratory animals for initial screening of suspected carcinogens.

Mutagenesis and Carcinogenesis

It is now well known that a wide variety of chemical and physical agents can induce (increase the frequency of) mutation by reacting directly with the cell's DNA. For example, some chemicals may cross-link adjacent DNA strands and cause either point mutations or deletions. Other chemicals, such as the dyes called acridine orange and ethidium bromide, may insert between two base pairs during DNA replication and cause reading frame shift mutations. Physical agents (like nonionizing or ionizing radiation) may cause pyrimidine dimer formation or actually break the DNA strands; when the cell tries to repair these DNA alterations, errors may be introduced or actual deletions in the DNA strains may occur. These chemical or physical agents may increase the frequency of mutation from 10 to 100 times compared with that which will spontaneously arise; therefore, these mutagens are frequently used in the laboratory to increase the possibility that certain mutants needed for study will be isolated.

There is good evidence that large numbers of animal cancers are caused by synthetic chemicals added to the environment. The variety of these chemicals that animals come in contact with each day is enormous. It is important to note that there is good correlation between the mutagenic capability of a chemical and its carcinogenic (cancer-causing) ability. Therefore, laboratory procedures (like the Ames test) that assess mutagenic potential are helpful tools that will inexpensively screen large numbers of suspected chemical mutagens in a short period of time. Note that it is not always true that mutagens are also carcinogens, but the correlation is quite high, and the knowledge that a chemical is mutagenic warns of a possible carcinogen. Also, if a chemical is *not* mutagenic for bacteria, this does not mean that it will not be carcinogenic for animals. Therefore, procedures like the Ames test should be used in conjunction with other tests for screening chemicals, and further confirmation of carcinogenic potential must be made with animal tests once the screening tests warn of the chemical's carcinogenic possibilities.

Effect of Mutation on Bacterial Characteristics

Even though spontaneous mutation is a rare event, it does alter phenotypic characteristics, and this may lead to difficulties in identifying pathogenic microorganisms. The clinical microbiologist is very familiar with the isolation of strains that have all of the typical characteristics of a pathogen except one or two. Indeed, it is common for clinical isolates to vary in one or more phenotypic characteristics from those described for a pathogen. It is assumed that these phenotypic variations between pathogenic strains are the result of altered environments that have allowed one or more mutants to overgrow the parental strain.

A mutation may affect a wide variety of phenotypic characteristics. The general types of changes often seen are given in Table 3–1. One type of mutation commonly seen by the clinical microbiologist is the smooth-to-rough colony alteration. The smooth appearance of the colony is usually caused by the presence of an extracellular capsule that accumulates in the developing colony to such an extent that it makes the colony appear smooth and glistening. Smooth strains are often the more virulent strains, because the presence of a capsule helps the cell resist phagocytosis; thus it will be more evasive. Repeated cultivation on artificial media will often select for mutants that lack capsules and appear dry and granular or rough. These rough strains are usually less virulent (pathogenic) than the smooth strains. However, when rough strains are placed back into the animal, this altered environment is such that nonencapsulated cells are engulfed by phagocytes, and only encapsulated mutants survive if present. Hence, animal passage selects for growth of encapsulated mutants, and this may result in the apparent restoration of a smooth strain.

GENETICS AND REPLICATION OF BACTERIAL VIRUSES

Structure of the Bacterial Virus Particle

All viruses are obligate intracellular parasites that lack a cellular structure and also lack the ability to carry out catabolic metabolism. The

Table 3–1. *Common Effects of Mutation on Bacterial Characteristics**

Category	Nature of Change	Expressed Phenotypic Characteristic
Motility	Loss of flagella or flagellar function	Compact colonies instead of flat and spreading
Capsule	Loss or modification of capsule	Rough and somewhat small colonies instead of smooth and larger
Nutritional	Loss of enzyme in anabolic pathway	Inability to grow on medium lacking that nutrient
Energy Source	Loss of enzyme in catabolic pathway	Give no evidence of metabolic activity (e.g., acid production) on media containing that energy source (e.g., sugar)
Drug-resistant	Impermeable to drug, or drug target altered, or drug detoxified	Growth on medium having a growth-inhibiting concentration of that drug
Virus-resistant	Loss of virus receptor on cell surface	Growth in presence of large numbers of virus
Heat-sensitive†	Alters an enzyme so that it becomes more heat-labile	Inability to grow at higher temperatures that normally support growth (e.g., 37°C) but does grow at lower temperatures
Cold-sensitive	Alters an enzyme so that it becomes more cold-labile	Inability to grow at a low temperature that normally supports some growth (e.g., 20°C)

*Adapted from Brock, T.D., Smith, D.W., and Madigan, M.T.: Biology of Microorganisms. 4th Ed. Englewood Cliffs, N.J., Prentice-Hall, 1984, p. 306.

†More commonly (but less descriptively) called "temperature-sensitive" in the literature.

structure of viruses is very diverse, but all virus particles share two common characteristics: (1) they contain only one type of nucleic acid—*either* DNA *or* RNA (never both)—and this nucleic acid is either single- *or* double-stranded (never both); and (2) they surround their nucleic acid with a protein coat, called the capsid (or the head) that may be composed of one or several types of protein molecules (capsomeres).

The nucleic acid (whether DNA or RNA) within all virus particles functions as the viral genome, that is, it carries the genetic information for virus replication. Where evidence is available, it seems that the nucleic acid is highly folded and tightly packed inside the capsid (head). For example, the DNA of an *E. coli* virus called T4 contains one DNA molecule with a total length of about 50 μm, whereas the entire diameter of the virus particle is about 0.095 μm by 0.065 μm.

The protein coat surrounding all viruses has at least two important functions: (1) it serves to protect the genome from destructive cellular enzymes (like DNAse and RNAse); and (2) the individual protein molecules of the virus coat (capsomeres) have enzyme-like specificity that recognizes and specifically binds with surface components on the susceptible host cell. This binding occurs during the attachment step of the replicative cycle, and it is so specific that a given virus will usually only recognize and bind to one species (or one type of tissue within one species in the case of a multicelled animal or plant).

Bradley has categorized bacterial viruses (called phage or bacteriophage) into six cate-

gories, depending upon their structure and genomic content:

1. Icosahedral head (looks round at low magnification but has 20 triangular faces) containing double-stranded DNA (dsDNA) with a contractile tail having fibrils on the distal end.
2. Icosahedral head containing dsDNA with long (often thin and flexible) noncontractile tail lacking fibirls.
3. Icosahedral head containing dsDNA with short (often apparently rigid) noncontractile tail lacking fibrils.
4. Much smaller icosahedral head (composed of large capsomeres) containing single-stranded DNA (ssDNA) with no tail.
5. Equally smaller icosahedral head (composed of small capsomeres) containing single-stranded RNA (ssRNA) with no tail.
6. Filamentous (long, hollow, flexible rod-shaped) structure (no head) containing ssDNA (forms a central spiral surrounded by the protein capsomeres).

Thus, it can be seen that the structure and genomic content of bacteriophage vary widely. It appears that most (if not all) structural types occur within any one genus of bacteria, but the significance of these structural and genomic variations is not yet clear.

Replication of Lytic Bacterial Viruses

Since viruses are strict intracellular parasites, they all must be capable of directing the living and infected host cell to make virus particles instead of more cells. The replication cycle of all lytic (cell-destroying) viruses appears similar, and this cycle is usually thought of as occurring in six separate steps (Fig. 3–9): (1) attachment (specific adsorption) of the virus particle to the susceptible host's cell surface; (2) penetration of either the nucleic acid (all bacteriophage) or the entire virus particle (many animal and plant viruses); (3) eclipse, in which the viral nucleic acid shuts down cellular synthesis and host-cell DNA is degraded; (4) replication, in which the altered host cell's metabolism is now directed to make each viral component; (5) assembly of the nucleic acid and protein capsomeres into fully infective virus particles; and (6) release of the new virus particles from the cell.

With bacterial cells, this process of viral (phage) replication is called the replicative cycle or the lytic cycle, because the infecting virus genome produces many new viruses and because the infecting units are released upon lysis (breaking apart) of the host cell. In contrast, many virus-infected plant or animal cells do not lyse at the end of their replicative cycle. Instead, virus particles are slowly released from these eucaryotic cells by a mechanism resembling pinocytic or phagocytic engulfment, except that the viruses move out of rather than into the cell. This "blebing" process usually results in a virus particle coated with a piece of the eucaryotic cell's membrane.

A feature of the bacterial-virus replicative cycle that appears unique occurs at the penetration step. Note that it is only the nucleic acid that penetrates the bacterial cell, and the protein coat (capsid) remains attached to the outside surface of the bacterial cell wall. With the animal or plant viruses, however, the entire virus particle enters the cell by a pinocytosis-like process.

Lytic phage are detected and enumerated by spreading an infected culture of a susceptible host on the surfce of an appropriate growth medium, such that confluent growth will occur. Wherever lytic phage attacks host cells, lysis will occur and the released phage will continue to infect and lyse adjacent cells until culture growth stops. This results in a clear area on a surface of otherwise confluent growth, and this clear area of lysis (containing many virus particles) is called a plaque. Lytic viruses may be serially diluted and spread-plated with a susceptible host to enumerate the number of lytic phage in the undiluted culture.

Temperate Bacterial Viruses and Lysogeny

Many bacterial viruses do not carry out a lytic replicative cycle as just described. Instead, the viral genome is inserted into the host cell's chromosome, and that insertion (called a prophage) is replicated along with host DNA between cell divisions (Fig. 3–10). Note that only the viral genome is transferred to new progeny cells at each generation. Viruses capable of this phenomenon are called temperate, and the bacterial cell that is able to carry and replicate the prophage is called a lysogenic bacterium. The entire process of infection of a lysogenic bacterium with a temperature-phage particle and the subsequent reproduction of the prophage is called lysogeny.

In the case of lytic phage, the virus genome carries and expresses genes for the synthesis of certain enzymes and other types of proteins that are essential to virus reproduction. In contrast, temperate phage carry similar information, but the expression of these genes is temporarily blocked by a specific repressor coded for by the virus. When this repressor is inactivated, synthesis of the entire virus particle occurs, but note that only temperate phage are produced. Once

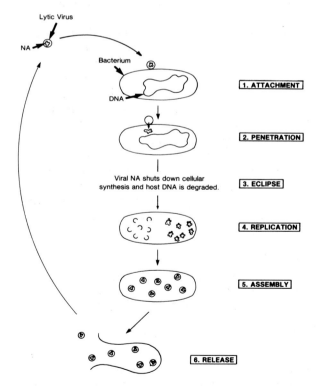

Figure 3–9. Replicative cycle of lytic bacterial viruses. Although the illustrations represent characteristics of bacterial viruses, these six steps are common for all types of lytic viruses. The virus particle is illustrated as the capsid proteins or coat surrounding the viral nucleic acid (NA).

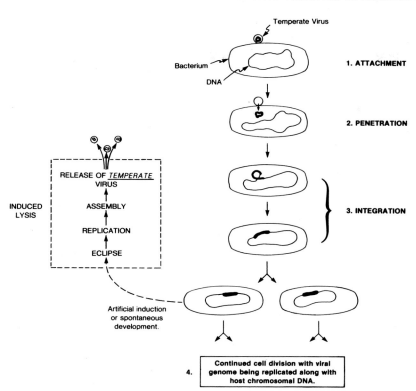

Figure 3–10. Consequences of infecting a lysogenic bacterium with a temperate virus. Attachment and penetration occur just as in the replicative cycle, but once inside the cell, the viral DNA (heavy line) becomes integrated into the host's chromosome. Expression of the integrated viral nucleic acid is normally repressed, but it is replicated along with the host's DNA. If repression is lifted (dotted arrow), the remaining steps in the replicative cycle will occur (box); however, only temperate viruses are produced.

mature virus particles are assembled inside the host, the host cell will lyse and release temperate phage that can infect new cells but only establish lysogeny.

Usually, lysogenic bacteria appear uninfected, but note that they carry the hereditary ability to produce complete, infective phage particles. If a culture of lysogenic bacteria is treated with mutagens known to damage DNA and activate the repair process, such as ultraviolet light or nitrosoguanidine, then most if not all of the cells carrying prophage will produce mature temperate phage and lyse. This treatment is called phage induction. It is presumed that the DNA damage somehow disturbs the repression mechanism, and this allows the replicative cycle to continue and the cell to produce mature temperate phage particles. Note that this process produces only temperate phage, even though the host cell lyses. This is because the prophage that is induced to complete the replicative cycle codes only for production of temperate phage.

However, induction is not always necessary to produce mature, fully infective, temperate phage particles. In any lysogenic bacterial culture, some small fraction of the prophage-infected cells (e.g., only one in every 1000 or less) will produce mature, infective, temperate phage and lyse. This is why infected lysogenic cultures exhibit a few cloudy (not clear) plaques on spread plates containing confluent growth.

Many strains of bacteria isolated from nature are found to carry temperate phage, and the large majority of bacterial viruses isolated from the natural environment are temperate rather than lytic. Therefore, it currently appears that lysogeny is a common microbiologic phenomenon. Yet, one could reasonably ask why bacteria tolerate temperate phage infections. In the following section, one may see that lysogeny is an advantage not only to the geneticist but also to the bacteria themselves, because a special type of lysogeny (called transduction) may give the host a survival advantage in a constantly changing environment.

RECOMBINATION AS A MECHANISM FOR GENETIC VARIATION IN BACTERIA

Introduction to Recombination Events

We have previously defined bacterial recombination as a ". . . sudden and inheritable change caused by the introduction of new genetic material (of cellular origin) from outside the cell." Recombination in bacteria involves the insertion of a genetically different piece of DNA (coming from a donor cell) into a recipient cell. Often, but not always, this foreign piece of DNA is then inserted into the chromosome of the recipient cell and replicated along with the recipient's own chromosome. Insertion of the foreign DNA by recombination may occur in one of three different ways among the bacteria: (1) transformation occurs when free chromosomal DNA (presumably released upon lysis of another bacterial cell) is inserted directly into another (competent) recipient cell; (2) transduction occurs when chromosomal DNA is also packaged inside a temperate bacterial virus, and transfer of this DNA occurs along with the viral DNA after the virus adsorbs to an appropriate lysogenic host cell; and (3) conjugation (mating) occurs after actual cell-to-cell contact between donor and recipient cells.

Some knowledge of recombination mechanisms in bacteria is necessary to understand certain types of drug resistances and toxin formation in bacteria and for an understanding of how bacteria are genetically "engineered" with genes from animal and plant cells. The next few paragraphs will deal with the three different types of bacterial recombination events, and then the following section will show how these principles are used in genetic engineering.

Transformation

Of the three known recombination mechanisms, transformation is the only one that appears to have evolved solely for the purpose of exchanging chromosomal DNA among bacterial cells. The others accomplish an exchange of chromosomal DNA only as a consequence of errors in phage growth (transduction) or plasmid transfer (conjugation).

To obtain transformation, one must have two important things: an appropriate source of free DNA (from a donor strain), and competent recipient cells that are capable of binding, translocating, and integrating this DNA into its own chromosomal DNA.

Nature of Transformable DNA. The long, continuously closed, supercoiled, helix of double-stranded DNA that serves as the single chromosome within the bacterial cell does not stay in that form when the cell is lysed. Even with gentle lysis under laboratory conditions, the chromosome will break into 100 or more pieces, each piece containing about 50 genes (one average gene has a molecular weight of about 10^6 with about 1000 base pairs). A competent cell will usually incorporate only a few of these DNA fragments, so that only a small portion of genes from a donor cell can be transferred to another cell by transformation.

Natural Competence. Unaltered cells (recipients) that can take up free DNA fragments and be genetically altered (transformed) are said to be naturally competent. As will be discussed later, it is possible to force some cells to appear competent by treating them with high concentrations of calcium ions and subjecting them to temperature shocks to increase the permeability of their envelopes (wall plus plasma membrane). This latter situation is part of a laboratory technique referred to as artificial transformation.

Natural transformation has been described with several gram-positive bacteria *(Streptococcus pneumoniae, S. sanguis, Bacillus subtilis, B. cereus, and B. stearothermophilus)* and with species of several gram-negative genera (e.g., *Neisseria, Acinetobacter, Moraxella, Haemophilus,* and *Pseudomonas).* The discovery of transformation involved the bacterium *Streptococcus pneumoniae.* One strain of this species that was used was encapsulated and virulent, and the other strain (of the same species) that was used lacked the genetic information needed to produce a capsule and was avirulent. When dead cells of the virulent strain were mixed with live avirulent cells, live virulent cells were produced. We now know that DNA-containing genes for capsule production were released from the dead cells, and this DNA transformed competent cells in the live, avirulent culture.

Natural competence is affected by the physiologic state of the cells and the composition of the growth medium. For example, in the laboratory, the proportion of competent cells in a population of *S. pneumoniae* rises dramatically during the middle of exponential growth, then falls just as dramatically shortly thereafter. During this brief period when a large number of cells are competent, each competent cell produces and excretes a few molecules of a soluble protein called a competence factor, which induces cells to make about 8 to 10 new proteins. During this period, the outer surface of the competent cells seems to change, so that double-stranded DNA (dsDNA) can bind at specific sites. When this excreted protein is added to noncompetent cells (of the same strain), these cells, too, become competent. Soluble competence factors have only been shown in gram-positive bacteria to date.

Uptake of Donor DNA by Competent Cells. The dsDNA first binds to specific proteins on the surface of competent cells. In the case of the gram-positive bacterium *S. pneumoniae*, there are about 30 to 80 sites per cell, and only dsDNA will bind to these sites. Shortly after binding, one of the strands (of the dsDNA) is degraded by an envelope-bound enzyme. Next, the resulting ssDNA is coated by a single, small, molecular weight polypeptide, and this complex enters the cell by an unknown mechanism.

In the case of the gram-negative *Haemophilus* and *Neisseria* species studied, dsDNA is not degraded to ssDNA before it enters the cell.

Integration of Donor ssDNA into the Chromosome. Once inside the cell, the donor ssDNA from *S. pneumoniae* tries to pair with a similar region on the host cell's chromosome. When a similar region is found (1) one strand of the host's dsDNA is opened up (with an enzyme called an endonuclease), (2) the dsDNA is unwound for a short distance, (3) the opposite end of the host DNA (corresponding to the opposite end of the new donor DNA) is also cut with an endonuclease, (4) the new donor strand is inserted, and (5) DNA ligases fuse the adjacent ends of the donor ssDNA with the adjacent host cell DNA strand. As you might expect, many things can go wrong with this process, and thus the efficiency of natural transformation is usually quite low (from 0.1 to 1.0% of all cells present).

In the case of the gram-negative *Haemophilus* and *Neisseria* species studied, the dsDNA that enters the cell is closely associated with the host cell's chromosome before one strand is degraded. There seem to be no free ssDNA intermediates within the cell prior to incorporation of the donor DNA into the host chromosome. Once again, no single general mechanism appears to account for the way in which the transformed DNA is incorporated into the host chromosome in all bacteria.

Artificial Transformations. Many bacteria (including *E. coli*) appear not to have evolved natural mechanisms for transformation, and attempts to emulate true transformation of open strands of ssDNA or dsDNA into the potential recipient cell's chromosome have generally failed. There seems to be no trouble in getting the linear pieces of ssDNA or dsDNA into the cell, but once inside, these DNA strands seem to be quickly destroyed by the host cell's own

nucleases before they can be integrated into the chromosome.

On the other hand, free, self-replicating forms of covalently closed strands of DNA (like plasmids and viral genomes) can be forced inside normally incompetent cells by subjecting the cells to abnormally high concentrations of calcium ions in the cold, and the frequency of transformants in the survivors is high (about 20%). Apparently these covalently closed circular forms of DNA are not attacked by the recipient cell's intracellular nucleases. The combined calcium and cold-shock treatment for getting DNA into cells seems to be the one most commonly used, but a freeze-thaw technique and treatment of protoplasts with polyethylene glycol have also been successfully used with some bacteria.

The process by which self-replicating forms of DNA are artificially introduced into a cell that would normally not be an appropriate host and the expression of these new genes in the recipient cell are essential to the field now called "genetic engineering." This topic will be more thoroughly explored at the end of this chapter.

Transduction

Transduction is defined as the transfer of host genes between related bacterial strains by bacterial viruses. In terms of the transfer of genetic material, transduction accomplishes the same function as transformation, except that transduction appears to result from errors that sometimes occur during the replication of some bacteriophage. Although most commonly studied in *E. coli*, transduction has been demonstrated in a wide variety of bacteria, and it is believed that it plays an important part in genetic exchange between bacteria in nature.

During the assembly step in phage development, an occasional phage particle becomes filled with host chromosomal DNA or a mixture of both host and phage DNA rather than completely with phage DNA (Fig. 3–11). This aberrant phage is often called a transducing particle. It is a defective phage because it never seems to cause subsequent lysis of the newly infected host. After adsorption of the transducing particle by a new host, the phage DNA or donor-host DNAs or both penetrate the cell envelope. The addition of donor-host DNA to the newly infected host's chromosome and the phenotypic expression of these new genes constitute completion of the transduction event.

Two types of errors in phage development

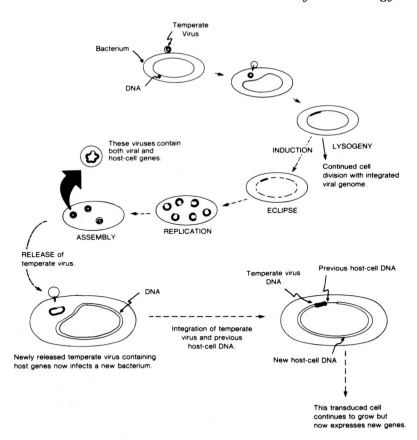

Figure 3–11. Schematic representation of transduction: the transfer of genes from one type of bacterial cell to a similar type by defective temperate bacterial viruses. During virus replication, some adjacent host chromosomal DNA is also replicated. Thus, mature virus particles contain both viral and host genes, and both are integrated upon subsequent infection of a new host. Expression of viral DNA is repressed in the new host, but the newly received bacterial genes may be fully functional.

lead to two types of transduction. The difference between these two types seems to depend upon where the phage genome is integrated into the chromosome of the host.

Specialized Transduction. With specialized transduction, only a few genes are transferred, and they are the same genes each time. Specialized transduction seems to occur only with defective temperate phage and only with those phage whose genomes always integrate into the host cell's chromosome at one specific place (Fig. 3–11). The error occurs when something triggers (induces) the defective prophage to complete the replicative cycle. Normally when this happens, only the prophage is excised from the chromosome that is then replicated. However, during specialized transduction, an error occurs during excision so that part of the adjacent chromosome is also removed, along with part or all of the prophage. Enough prophage DNA must be excised to allow for replication of coat proteins and other requirements for assembly and release of mature phage; otherwise, the replication process will not proceed to completion. On the other hand, the amount of adjacent host-chromosomal material cannot be too large, because there is a

very limited amount of space within the capsid (phage head) for packaged DNA. It is for this reason that only a very few genes are ever transferred during transduction. The more host DNA that is excised the less phage DNA removed, and the greater the chance that replication of mature phage will not occur. However, when mature phage are produced, most contain host gene(s); therefore frequency of transduction is high.

Generalized Transduction. With generalized transduction, almost any gene on the chromosome may be transferred from donor to recipient, but the frequency of transfer is often very low. For example, general transduction frequencies of genes from *Salmonella typhimurium* mediated by phage P22 are usually about one in every 10^5 to 10^9 cells.

Unlike specialized transduction, generalized transduction seems to occur with either temperate or lytic phage. When a population of sensitive bacteria is infected with a phage and the complete replication cycle takes place, the host DNA often breaks down into phage–genome-sized pieces. If some of these chromosomal DNA pieces persist (are not broken down by the cell's own nucleases), then a piece may be incorporated inside a capsid during the assembly step. These defective particles are released, along with the normal phage during lysis of the host. When this lysate is used to infect another population of similar cells, most of this population is infected with normal phage. A very few cells, however, may be infected with these defective (transducing) particles. When that happens, the donor DNA will penetrate the recipient host, and donor DNA may then be inserted into the recipient cell's chromosome. The reason for the low transduction frequencies that occur with generalized transducing phage is probably the low numbers of phage containing host DNA.

When comparing specialized and generalized transduction, the following distinctions seem important. The main requirement for generalized transduction seems to be that all host DNA is not degraded prior to assembling the virus particles, and the mistake made here is in packaging host DNA instead of viral DNA inside a few capsids. In contrast, the mistake made in specialized transduction is in defining the prophage boundaries for excision; some adjacent host DNA is taken out along with part or all of the prophage prior to replication. Hence the new phage will all contain some host cell genes. In addition, the defects that account for specialized transduction are only realized after inducing lysis in a lysogenic culture carrying prophage, whereas generalized transduction may also occur with lytic phage.

From a veterinary standpoint, perhaps the greatest significance of transduction is in the potential use of phage as vehicles for moving animal genes into bacterial cells and the subsequent use of the transduced bacterial cultures for inexpensively producing animal gene products.

Plasmids and Conjugation

Before we can adequately consider conjugation as the third type of recombination event occurring in bacteria, the biology of plasmids must be considered. You may recall that most bacteria have two types of genetic elements (DNA): a chromosome and one or more types of plasmids. Plasmids store genetic information that may (under the right conditions) be phenotypically expressed. However, it is currently believed that plasmids do not carry genes for essential metabolic activities; instead, the plasmid genes are for other more specialized features. For example, plasmids may carry genes for one or more of the following abilities: (1) to mate and serve as a donor for genetic exchange; (2) to be resistant to chemicals, such as heavy metals, that are normally toxic to microorganisms; and (3) to degrade complex organic chemicals, such as aromatic hydrocarbons found in petroleum. Plasmids have veterinary significance, because some contain genes that code for the production of bacterial toxins, and some code for the resistance to various antibiotics.

Plasmid Biology. Plasmids are covalently closed, circular, double-stranded molecules of DNA that probably exist inside the cell in a supercoiled state and seem to be present in essentially all bacteria examined (Fig. 3–12). Plasmids are usually less than one-twentieth the size of the bacterial chromosome, although there is a wide variation in plasmid sizes even within a single bacterial cell. Plasmid DNA replicates in the same way as chromosomal DNA; this involves initiation at a single point and bidirectional replication of each separate strand around the circle. However, plasmid and chromosomal DNA replicate independently of one another, and plasmid DNA is probably under a different type of control. There are usually multiple copies of each plasmid in the bacterial cell, although the copy number seems to depend upon the type of cell and the environment in which it is growing.

Plasmid Transfer by Conjugation. Conjugation between similar bacteria is a mating process that requires cell-to-cell contact and results in transfer of genetic material (DNA) from one cell (the donor) to another cell (the recipient). The genetic material transferred may be a plasmid or part of the donor's chromosome that has been mobilized by a plasmid.

Most of what is currenlty known about conjugation comes from studies of gram-negative bacteria, so the following applies only to this type of bacterial cell.

Cells capable of donating DNA in conjugation carry a plasmid that (in part) codes for the ability to be a donor, and this is called a conjugative plasmid. In gram-negtive (but not gram-positive) bacteria, the conjugative plasmid codes for production of a "sex" pilus and for some other proteins needed for DNA transfer. Although it is not clearly understood, it appears that the distal end of the sex pilus on the donor makes contact with an appropriate recipient cell. The pilus then retracts, pulling the two cells together

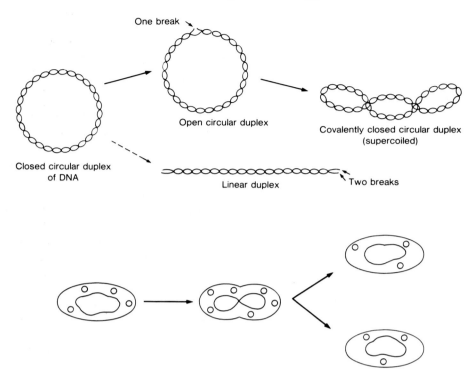

One break

Open circular duplex

Covalently closed circular duplex
(supercoiled)

Closed circular duplex
of DNA

Linear duplex   Two breaks

Multiple copies of plasmids in each cell replicate independent of chromosomal DNA.

Figure 3–12. Molecular architecture, relative size, and copy numbers of bacterial plasmids. Plasmids are covalently closed, circular, double-stranded, and supercoiled molecules of DNA that are about one-twentieth the size of the bacterial chromosome. More than one type of plasmid and several copies of the same plasmids may be present in a single cell.

until a conjugation bridge is formed, through which the DNA can pass between the donor and recipient cells. Although the recipient cell lacks the sex pilus, it must have some sort of specific recognition factor, so that tight bonding may be made with the distal end of the donor's sex pilus.

In order for DNA transfer to occur, DNA synthesis must also occur. Current evidence suggests that this synthesis occurs at or near the conjugation bridge, and that one of the DNA strands inserted into the recipient cell is from the donor and the other is newly made (Fig. 3–13). The "rolling circle" model (devised to explain DNA synthesis in certain phages) seems to best explain how this is done. Initiation may be triggered by cell-to-cell contact, and this may open one strand on the donor's plasmid. As this opened strand (the 5' end) passes through the conjugation bridge, DNA synthesis simultaneously occurs at two places: along the newly unraveled strand, and along the closed complementary strand of the original plasmid. Once the new plasmid is made and fully transferred into the recipient cell, it is covalently closed (circu-

larized) and supercoiled. With this mechanism, the donor cell duplicates its plasmid at the same time transfer occurs, so both the donor and recipient eventually have a complete copy of this plasmid.

Note that conjugative plasmids not only contain genes that allow for conjugation to take place, but they also contain other types of genetic information. Thus, each cell that receives a conjugative plasmid during conjugation not only becomes capable of donating genetic material but it will also receive other genes (such as those that code for antibiotic resistance). This process is so efficient that almost every cell that forms a conjugating pair will acquire new genetic information, and this (along with indiscriminate use of antibiotics) helps to explain how bacterial populations become resistant to antibiotics with such speed. Under proper conditions, the rate of spread of a conjugative plasmid through bacterial culture can be exponential and resemble a bacterial growth curve.

Conjugative transfer of plasmids may occur between two strains of the same species, such as between a chloramphenicol-resistant strain of

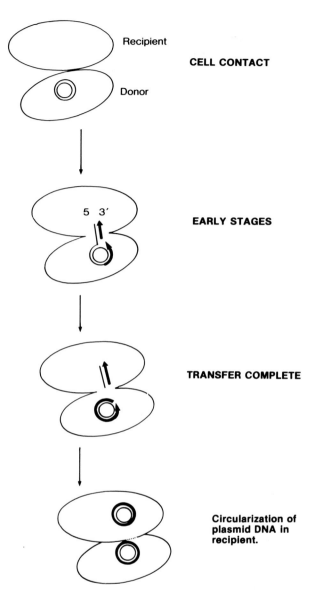

Figure 3–13. Replication and transfer of a plasmid during conjugation. Replication occurs along with transfer, so that conjugation does not leave the donor cell devoid of the transferred plasmid and its genetic material.

E. coli and a chloramphenicol-sensitive strain. Plasmids may also be transferred among different but related bacteria, such as those within the family *Enterobacteriaceae* (from *E. coli* to strains of *Shigella* or *Salmonella).*

Recent studies of conjugation in *Streptococcus faecalis* suggest that conjugation in gram-positive bacteria will prove quite different from that of the well-studied gram-negative bacteria. Conjugation between strains of *S. faecalis* does not require a sex pilus. Instead, potential recipient cells release soluble molecules (called phero-

mones), and these molecules stimulate plasmid-containing cells to produce a substance on their outer surface that allows donor and recipient cells to aggregate. It appears that plasmids are transferred from cell to cell within these aggregates.

Veterinary Significance of Plasmids

Antibiotic Resistance. The emergence of bacteria resistant to several antibiotics is of considerable medical importance and is correlated with the increasing use of antibiotics for the treatment of infectious diseases. There are a variety of plasmids (sometimes called R factors or resistance-transfer factors) that confer multiple antibiotic resistance on the recipient cell. Those most commonly observed carry resistance to four antibiotics (chloramphenicol, streptomycin, the sulfonamides, and tetracycline), but some have fewer or more resistant genes on the plasmid. Plasmids are also known that have resistance to kanamycin, penicillin, and neomycin. Some plasmids also contain genes that allow the bacterium to be resistant to metals like mercury, nickel, and cobalt, and these genes are frequently present on the same plasmids that carry genes for antibiotic resistance. At present, it appears that most R factors are conjugative plasmids, that is, they also carry genes that code for sex-pilus production and other proteins required for conjugation between gram-negative bacteria.

It appears that antibiotic-resistant strains of bacteria studied in the laboratory almost invariably involve mutations within chromosomal DNA. In most cases, resistance produced by mutated chromosomal DNA arises because of a modification in the target of antibiotic action, such as modifications in the cell wall or ribosome that make the mutants resistant to antibiotic attack.

On the other hand, the majority of drug-resistant strains isolated from patients contain drug-resistant plasmids, and these R factors genetically alter the cell in another way. Plasmid-mediated resistance is usually caused by the introduction of new genes that code for the production of new enzymes that inactivate the drug itself. For example, cells having resistance to the aminoglycoside antibiotics (kanamycin, neomycin, streptomycin, and spectinomycin) make an enzyme that chemically modifies the antibiotic (by acetylation, adenylation, or phosphorylation), and the modified drug lacks antibiotic activity. In penicillin resistance, the plasmid codes for the production of penicillinase (a β-lactamase), an enzyme that cleaves the β-lactam ring of the penicillin molecule, thus rendering it inactive. In the case of chloramphenicol resistance, a gene on the plasmid codes for an enzyme that acetylates the antibiotic, thereby destroying its antibacterial activity. Therefore, it can be seen that multiple antibiotic resistance may result from the introduction of a single plasmid.

Toxins and Other Virulence Factors. Work with the gram-negative, enteropathogenic *E. coli* suggests that the ability of pathogenic bacteria both to attach and grow at a specific site in the host and to produce toxins may be carried by genes on a plasmid. Specific recognition and attachment of *E. coli* to the epithelial lining of the intestine require that this bacterium produce a protein on its surface (called "K"). In addition, two toxins (a hemolysin and an enterotoxin) are coded for by plasmid genes. At present it is not clear why these virulence factors are plasmid coded and the others reside on the chromosome, nor is it understood how many other virulence factors are plasmid-related among the gram-negative bacteria.

The common, gram-positive bacterium *Staphylococcus aureus* produces a number of things that add to its virulence, and the production of each is coded for by plasmid genes; these are coagulase, enterotoxin, fibrinolysin, hemolysin, and a yellow pigment. Each of these properties contributes to the evasiveness, invasiveness, and therefore the pathogenicity of *S. aureus*. At the present time, much research is being conducted on the significance of plasmids in determining bacterial virulence.

GENETIC ENGINEERING THROUGH GENE MANIPULATION

Genetic engineering (or biotechnology) refers to the application of basic principles of microbial genetics in the isolation, manipulation, and expression of genetic material. At the present time, there are two rather different ways in which genetically engineered bacteria are used: (1) to increase the quantity of microbial products; and (2) to express inserted genes of animal or plant origin such that the bacterial cell produces a protein normally produced only by an animal or plant cell. The first application of genetic engineering is the oldest in that genetic manipulation has long been used to increase the gene

copy number and therefore to increase the yields of desirable microbial products. In this application, the chromosomes of bacteria are altered so that production of the gene product is no longer tightly regulated by the cell, and this results in a greater rate of gene-product synthesis.

The second use of genetic engineering is more recent and has received more attention in the popular press. In that application, animal or plant genes are excised from the chromosome; these genes are inserted into a bacterial plasmid, and that genetically altered plasmid is placed back into the same bacterial cell so that this cell will now produce a protein that is coded for by the animal or plant genes. Molecules that contain unrelated pieces of DNA (like that "engineered" plasmid) are usually referred to as "recombinant DNA." Hence the phrase "recombinant-DNA technology" is often used in place of "genetic engineering."

What follows is a brief introduction to the second application of genetic engineering and the ways in which genetic engineering may affect the future practicing veterinarian. For a more complete treatment of the basic principles of genetic engineering, the reader is referred to Brock, Smith, and Madigan (1984, Chapter 12).

Plasmids as Cloning Vectors

The microbial geneticist frequently uses the word "clone" to refer to a foreign DNA molecule introduced into a bacterium, and the term "cloning vector" is used to refer to the complete DNA molecule that can bring about the replication of that foreign DNA fragment in the cell. The "host" is the bacterium that contains the genetically reconstructed cloning vector. A good cloning vector must have the following characteristics: (1) it will self-replicate in the host; (2) its DNA can be easily separated from the host and purified; and (3) it must contain regions of the DNA that are not essential for replication and can be removed and replaced with the foreign DNA fragment. In addition, it is very desirable if the cloning vector is a small piece of DNA that is able to enter the cell and replicate to a high copy number (many copies per cell), and if it is stable in the host and gives a high product yield from the foreign gene. To date, the most useful cloning vectors are certain bacterial viruses and plasmids. The following discussion will be limited to the use of plasmids as cloning vectors.

The host for replication of the cloning vector must also be chosen with care. A desirable host is fast-growing, genetically stable, not pathogenic, and able to grow in an inexpensive culture medium. In addition, the desirable host must be transformable, that is, one must be able to make the potential host artificially competent so that it will take up the DNA used as the cloning vector. The methods used to accomplish the insertion of this DNA are the same as discussed in the previous section on transformation.

Optimum expression of the foreign DNA (the clone) on the cloning vector is extremely important. Therefore, the plasmid cloning vector must not only contain the proper foreign genes but it should also have adequate regulatory sequences, so that expression of the foreign genes is under control of the microbiologist. It would be ideal to grow cells to a high population density while the plasmid genes are repressed, then add an inducer to allow maximum expression of the foreign genes. For this reason, regulatory sequences are usually inserted along with and adjacent to the foreign structural genes. For example, constructing plasmid vectors that contain the regulatory components for the *lac* operon (promoter, regulator, and operator) to control synthesis of the foreign DNA is one way to provide a suitable regulatory switch. When this is done, cells are grown in the absence of the inducer, lactose (see Fig. 3–7), so that the switch regulating the adjacent foreign genes is turned off. When the cells reach maximum numbers, the inducer (lactose) is added to start expression of the foreign genes. Production of high levels of several mammalian proteins (e.g., up to 15,000 molecules of human interferon/*E. coli* cell) are achieved using these expression vectors.

Steps in Constructing a Plasmid Cloning Vector

The overall process of constructing a plasmid cloning vector is shown in Figure 3–14. First, a plasmid (preferably one that already has a high copy number) is isolated from a bacterium that will later serve as an acceptable host. Cells are gently lysed, and the plasmid fraction is collected by ultracentrifugation. After separation of the various plasmids by size (molecular weight) and purification of a single plasmid type, this potential cloning vector is ready for gene manipulation.

Second, the plasmid DNA is cut open using a purified, site-specific enzyme called a restriction endonuclease.

Third, the animal or plant gene is precisely described, so that it may be either excised (as shown in Fig. 3–14) or artificially constructed (as is most often the case). If the gene is excised from the chromosome, the same types of restriction endonucleases are used, so that a similarly sized fragment is cut, having ends complementary to those on the cut plasmid. Alternatively, the eucaryotic gene may be artificially constructed in one of at least two ways: (1) the specific mRNA for that protein is isolated and then the enzyme called reverse transcriptase is used to construct a DNA molecule from sequence of bases on mRNA; or, with more difficulty, (2) the desired gene product (protein) is purified, the amino acid sequence determined, an mRNA molecule constructed that will code for synthesis of this protein, and, finally, reverse transcriptase is used to construct the complementary DNA sequence (gene). Regardless of the method used, a gene is either excised from a eucaryotic chromosome or artificially constructed.

Fourth, the broken ends of the foreign DNA are mended to the homologous broken ends of the plasmid DNA with an enzyme called DNA ligase. This creates a recombinant plasmid that is part bacterial and part foreign (eucaryotic) DNA. Note that some time during this process, the regulatory switch, such as that obtained from the *lac* operon, is also added to this recombinant plasmid.

Fifth, host bacteria (usually the same species as that originally contributing the plasmid) are made artificially competent (e.g., by applying excessive calcium ions and temperature-shock treatment), and the DNA is forced into the cells. Unlike the transformation phenomenon, however, it appears that the entire double-stranded DNA molecule is taken in, and there is no subsequent integration into the cell's chromosome. These newly introduced, recombinanat plasmids remain as extrachromosomal self-replicating units and constitute part of the host cell's genomic material.

Sixth, the host is now grown in such a way that the expression of the eucaryotic gene is regulated for maximum expression. Often, "fusion proteins" are made for one (of at least two) reasons: (1) to make the protein more stable inside the cell, which is more resistant to the protein-degrading enzymes normally present inside the bacterial cell; and/or (2) to allow the protein to be exported to the outside, where it can be more easily isolated and purified. Fusion proteins con-

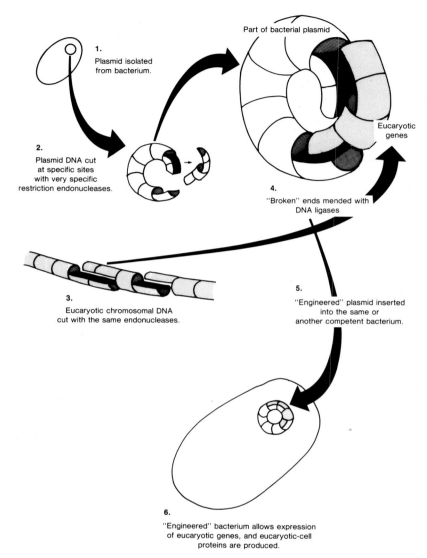

1.
Plasmid isolated
from bacterium.

2.
Plasmid DNA cut
at specific sites
with very specific
restriction endonucleases.

Part of bacterial plasmid

Eucaryotic
genes

4.
"Broken" ends mended with
DNA ligases

3.
Eucaryotic chromosomal DNA
cut with the same endonucleases.

5.
"Engineered" plasmid inserted
into the same or
another competent bacterium.

6.
"Engineered" bacterium allows expression
of eucaryotic genes, and eucaryotic-cell
proteins are produced.

Figure 3–14. Steps in constructing a plasmid cloning vector. This process is commonly used in the field known as genetic engineering.

tain a short, procaryotic, amino-acid sequence at one end of the protein fused to the desired eucaryotic amino-acid sequence at the other. Sometimes the intracellular accumulation of excessive quantities of fusion proteins is toxic to the cell, so additional genes must be added to the engineered plasmid to assure that this eucaryotic gene product also is a secretory protein, in other words, a protein that can get out of the cell and be released into the medium. After the fusion protein is released, the procaryotic portion may be chemically cut away and then the eucaryotic part may be purified and readied for use.

Veterinary Significance of Genetically Engineered Plasmids

The potential application of genetically engineered procaryotic cells for the production of animal proteins is staggering. Not only are these processes much less expensive and time-consuming but also the proteins produced are easier to purify more completely; therefore, when administered to the animal, they cause fewer side reactions than proteins isolated from animal tissue. At present, genetically altered bacterial cells are producing human growth hormone (for treatment of growth defects), human insulin (for the treatment of diabetes), human interferon (an antiviral agent), human serum albumin (for transfusion applications), parathyroid hormone (for calcium regulation), urokinase (for treating blood clotting disorders), and viral proteins (such as coat proteins from cytomegalovirus, hepatitis B virus, influenza virus and foot-and-mouth disease virus for vaccine production).

At present it appears that the most useful veterinary application of genetically altered bacteria will be the production of effective vaccine proteins. Effective vaccines may be made to protect the animal against procaryotic, eucaryotic, or viral pathogens. For simplicity's sake, only virus vaccines will be discussed further.

Virus vaccines for animal use contain either live attenuated or killed virus. In using both types of vaccines, there is the obvious danger that they may contain virus particles that remain virulent. Genetically engineered vaccines contain viral coat (capsid) proteins that serve as antigens to stimulate the immune response. Thus, it is desirable to produce the viral coat protein and use this as the vaccine, so that the potentially dangerous use of live or killed suspensions may be avoided. Safe vaccines composed only of viral coat protein can be made by genetically altered bacteria that have been "engineered" to produce the viral coat protein. Generally, viral DNA is isolated from purified viral suspensions, this DNA is fragmented with endonucleases, the fragments are inserted into an appropriate vector (usually a plasmid) using DNA ligases, and the recombinant plasmid is inserted back into the host bacterium. The purified protein produced by these bacteria is then used as a vaccine without danger of introducing virulent viruses.

In 1981, the U.S. Department of Agriculture announced the first vaccine produced by genetically altered bacteria *(E. coli);* this was the capsid protein for the virus causing foot-and-mouth disease (FMD) of cattle, sheep, hogs, and other animals. Although strict vigilance has prevented an outbreak in the U.S. since 1929, the disease is still a serious problem in Asia, Africa, South America, and southern Europe. The vaccines in use prior to the development of the *E. coli*–produced vaccine presented many problems. For example, the vaccines had to be re-

frigerated, and that presented problems with their use in developing countries. Also, each vaccine protected against only one type of virus. Since the virus readily mutates, the usefulness of any one vaccine was limited. Nevertheless, an estimated 500 million doses were administered annually, which made it the most widely used antiviral vaccine.

From data available in 1981, it appeared that the capsid protein was first made inside the genetically altered bacterial cell as a fusion protein that contained about equal parts of viral and bacterial protein. This fusion protein could be physically removed from the bacterial cell and cleaved by cyanogen bromide. This treatment released a small-molecular weight polypeptide (capsid protein) that protected steers from challenge with FMD virus. The fusion protein was produced in large quantity by the genetically altered *E. coli* (about 10^6 molecules per cell). This meant that one liter of culture medium could produce about 10,000 doses of effective vaccine (purified protein).

Because of the economic advantages of using bacteria to produce pure viral proteins and the safety value of avoiding killed or attenuated viral strains for vaccines, one might logically expect that genetically altered bacterial strains will soon be producing many other vaccines for veterinary use. It is also likely that proteins of animal origin will soon be produced for therapeutic use in domestic animals as is now being done for use with humans.

SOURCES FOR FURTHER READING

Atlas, R.M.: Microbiology, Fundamentals and Applications. New York, Macmillian Publishing Company, 1984.

Birge, E.A.: Bacterial and Bacteriophage Genetics. New York, Springer-Verlag, 1981.

Brock, T.D., Smith, D.W., and Madigan, M.T.: Biology of Microorganisms. 4th Ed. Englewood Cliffs, N.J., Prentice-Hall, 1984.

Hayes, W.: The Genetics of Bacteria and Their Viruses: Studies in Basic Genetics and Molecular Biology. 2nd Ed. Oxford, England, Blackwell Scientific Publications, 1968. (A classic reference.)

Ingraham, J.L., Maaloe, O., and Neidhardt, F.C.: Growth of the Bacterial Cell. Sunderland, Massachusetts, Sinauer Associates, 1983.

Watson, J.D.: Molecular Biology of the Gene. Menlo Park, California, Benjamin/Cummings Publishing Company, 1976.

4

Sources and Transmission of Infectious Agents

The microorganisms causing diseases in animals (including humans) are derived from the following sources:

1. animals (including humans)—by far the most important;
2. inanimate nature—relatively less important.

The various organisms that can cause disease have natural habitats to which they are well adapted. Most organisms that have the potential to cause disease in animals are associated with those animals. Some organisms will usually only grow and multiply in certain host species. Some disease-causing organisms are transmissible from animals to humans and vice versa.

There are a large number of microorganisms living in water, soil, and decaying vegetation. The great majority of these are incapable of causing disease in animals, but there are a few with the capacity to grow and multiply in animal tissue.

ANIMAL SOURCES

The Animal's Own Organisms

All animals have what is called a normal flora (microbiota). It consists of the bacteria, mycoplasmas, viruses, and fungi that live in or upon the normal animal without producing disease. Included in this normal flora are a number of potential pathogens.

When considering the normal flora, it should be kept in mind that the kinds and numbers of bacteria and other organisms present in and upon an animal species vary greatly with different individuals and different circumstances. The intestinal flora of the adult animal differs markedly from that of the young animal. The flora is influenced by nutrition, climate, and geographic location. The technical methods employed to recover pathogenic organisms may give a distorted idea of the kinds and numbers of organisms present. The gram-negative, non-spore-forming bacteria are the most populous in the large intestine, but this fact is often obscured because the methods used in the clinical laboratory do not necessarily support the growth of these bacteria.

The normal floras of the various domestic animal species have not been studied as thoroughly as those of humans and of the mouse. The little information available and the first-hand experience in the veterinary diagnostic laboratory indicate a considerable similarity in the broad sense between the normal flora of humans and mice and that of domestic animals. However, it should be kept in mind that there are marked differences in the flora of the alimentary tract, depending upon whether the animal is predominantly herbivorous, omnivorous, or carnivorous.

While considering the normal flora in general,

it should be kept in mind that it plays an important role in the nutrition of animals, particularly in the herbivores. The normal microbial flora has a protective value in that it tends to exclude other nonresident bacteria, including those that are potentially pathogenic. Disturbances in the normal flora caused by prolonged antibiotic administration may result in overgrowth and infection by various bacteria and fungi such as staphylococci and *Candida albicans*.

Some of the kinds of bacteria that can be expected to occur normally in and upon domestic animals follow.

Mouth, Nasopharynx. Micrococci; *Staphylococcus*; alpha- and beta-hemolytic streptococci, *Bacteroides*; lactobacilli, fusiform bacilli; *Actinomyces*; gram-negative cocci; coliforms and *Proteus* spp.; spirochetes; mycoplasmas; *Pasteurella* spp.; diphtheroids; yeasts, including *Candida albicans*; and *Haemophilus*.

Stomach. In monogastric animals the stomach is sterile or contains fewer than 10^3 organisms per ml. Most of the organisms that enter the stomach with food are killed by the hydrochloric acid or removed by forward peristalsis.

Duodenum, Jejunum, Ileum. Only small numbers of bacteria are present in the duodenum and jejunum of humans. There are small numbers in the ileum, with increasing numbers toward its termination. The same probably applies to most of the domestic animals.

Large Intestine. Fecal streptococci; *Escherichia coli; Klebsiella; Enterobacter; Pseudomonas* spp.; *Proteus* spp.; enterococci; staphylococci; clostridia: *Cl. perfringens, Cl. septicum,* and others; gram-negative anaerobes; spirochetes; and lactobacilli. The gram-negative nonspore-forming bacteria make up more than 90% of the fecal bacteria. One gram of feces contains about 10^{11} bacteria.

Trachea, Bronchi, Lungs. Few if any bacteria and fungi reside permanently in these structures.

Vulva. Diphtheroids; micrococci; coliforms and *Proteus* spp.; enterococci; yeasts; gram-negative anaerobes. The same kinds of organisms and others can be recovered from the prepuce of the male.

Vagina. The numbers and kinds of bacteria vary with the reproductive cycle and age. The cervix and anterior vagina of the healthy mare have few bacteria. Some of the organisms recovered from the vagina are alpha- and beta-hemolytic streptococci; coliforms; *Proteus* spp.;

diphtheroids; lactobacilli; mycoplasmas; and yeasts and fungi.

Skin. By virtue of their habits and environment animals frequently possess a large and varied bacterial and fungal flora on their hair and skin. *Staphylococcus* spp. occur commonly, as do micrococci. Of the many other organisms isolated, it may be difficult to determine which ones make up the resident flora and which ones are "transients."

Milk. Micrococci, staphylococci, nonhemolytic streptococci, mycoplasmas, and diphtheroids, including *Corynebcterium bovis*, are frequently shed from the apparently normal mammary gland. Some reside in the teat canal.

We have mentioned a number of commensal organisms that are potential pathogens. There are also a number of organisms that are not part of the normal flora and that when present in or upon an animal almost always are associated with latent or overt disease. These organisms, for example *Brucella* spp., certain *Mycobacterium* spp., and *Bacillus anthracis*, are sometimes called obligate pathogens.

ANIMALS INCUBATING A DISEASE

The incubation period is that period from the time of infection until clinical signs appear. During this period the animal appears healthy but may be infectious, i.e., capable of discharging disease-producing organisms. Examples are many of the respiratory diseases caused by viruses, pasteurellas, and corynebacteria in which the organisms may be expelled in saliva or droplets. In intestinal diseases pathogenic organisms may be shed in the feces in the incubative stage.

ANIMALS WITH OVERT DISEASE

Ordinarily the largest numbers of organisms are shed when the animal displays clinical signs of disease. The route by which they are shed depends upon the location of the disease. We have mentioned respiratory and intestinal routes of shedding of infectious organisms. They may also be released from the skin in such diseases as dermatomycosis (ringworm) and streptotricosis and via the urine or genital secretions if infections involve these systems. The extent and duration of the shedding of organisms varies with different diseases. In the acute diseases such as anthrax, it is usually short, while in chronic diseases such as tuberculosis, it may be long. Some diseases such as actinomycosis are sporadic in their occurrence and are not considered transmissible. Sporadic endogenous infections (those caused by the animal's own organisms) such as actinomycosis, bacterial endocarditis, and meningitis are often not transmissible to other animals.

CONVALESCENT CARRIER ANIMALS

The causative organisms are usually shed for varying periods after clinical recovery from a disease. In respiratory infections some of the causative organisms—e.g., pasteurellas and mycoplasmas—may be shed by way of droplets during expiration for some time after apparent recovery. Likewise in salmonellosis, the salmonella organisms may be shed for weeks in the feces, although the animal is clinically normal. These animals are referred to as *convalescent carriers,* and the state is often referred to as the *carrier state.* The number of organisms shed will diminish with time, but the period of "excretion" may vary from a week to several months. Not all recovered animals are necessarily shedders. In some diseases such as salmonellosis and fowl cholera, there is a tendency to develop a chronic carrier state. In some severe diseases such as anthrax in cattle, there usually is no convalescent or chronic carrier state.

CONTACT CARRIERS OR SUBCLINICAL INFECTIONS

Animals may acquire pathogenic organisms from other animals with infectious disease without contracting the disease themselves. In most groups of animals exposed to infectious disease there will often be some that acquire the organisms but do not develop clinical disease. The number of such animals depends upon the disease, the virulence of the organism, and the animal's immune state. Such animals are referred to as *contact carriers.* This carrier state may be temporary, lasting only a few days, or chronic, lasting weeks or months. Such contact carriers are seen in diseases such as strangles in horses and erysipelas and salmonellosis in swine. These subclinical carrier states represent a threat to other animals and are a means whereby the disease is perpetuated. Such states can only be detected, sometimes with difficulty, by demonstration of the organisms, usually by culture procedures; this is the case in salmonellosis and Johne's disease. In epizootic bovine infertility it has been necessary to use "test mating" to detect infected or carrier bulls. The suspected bulls are bred to susceptible heifers to see whether or not

they infect them. Some of the more severe diseases such as anthrax and rinderpest of cattle result in very few if any contact carriers.

INANIMATE SOURCES

Organisms such as some species of *Clostridium, Proteus, Klebsiella,* and *Pseudomonas aeruginosa* exist in the free-living state in the soil, where they derive their sustenance from decaying vegetation. Those just mentioned may also inhabit the intestine as commensals and be shed in the feces. Less common free-living organisms such as species of *Acinetobacter, Aeromonas, Chromobacterium,* and *Flavobacterium* on rare occasions will cause disease in humans and animals. However, considering their numbers, most of these organisms cause disease rather infrequently. Most only cause disease under special circumstances. *Pseudomonas aeruginosa* may infect wounds and tissues damaged by burns. *Proteus* can cause urinary tract infections, and *Klebsiella* strains can produce very severe mastitis in cows.

The spores of clostridia gain entrance to wounds and cause such gas gangrene type diseases as blackleg and malignant edema, or tetanus. Other clostridia such as *Cl. botulinum* cause poisoning as a result of the production of a potent exotoxin in contaminated food. In enterotoxemia, *Cl. perfringens,* a widespread soilborne organism, produces its toxin in the small intestine.

A number of ordinarily saprophytic fungi have the capacity to produce disease in animals. They cause such sporadic diseases as sporotrichosis, blastomycosis, and coccidioidomycosis. The occurrence of the last two is dependent upon the geographic distribution of the fungi in the soil.

TRANSMISSION

Infecting agents are most frequently transmitted to new hosts by direct or indirect contact. By the direct process is meant spread by contact with the infecting organisms on the infected host, i.e., contact with discharges on the animal that have emanated from the skin or various body openings. The other means of direct contact is by coitus. In most diseases the indirect process is most often responsible. By this means the organisms shed or excreted by the host are carried in or upon various vehicles such as water, milk, food, litter, air, or dust. Such contaminated inanimate objects as food, water, litter, bedding, mangers, and kennels are referred to collectively as *fomites*. Other indirect means of spread are by contaminated medical, surgical, and dental instruments, syringes, and needles (these may be responsible for equine infectious anemia, and anaplasmosis), speculums, and dressings.

Various arthropods such as ticks, mites, lice, flies, and mosquitoes act as vectors for infectious diseases. Some agents are transmitted in a purely mechanical manner while others are actually inoculated by biting insects, as in tularemia. In several diseases the infecting agent may multiply in the vector, e.g., *Yersinia pestis*, which causes plague, multiplies in the salivary gland of the flea.

Organisms enter the host by one of the following portals of entry:

1. Inhalation and infection via the respiratory tract.
2. Ingestion and infection via the alimentary tract.
3. Inoculation or infection through the skin or mucous membranes by simple contact; injection (e.g., biting insect, contaminated hypodermic syringe or needle); or wound infection.
4. Via the genital tract as a result of coitus. Also by means of contaminated instruments, catheters, and semen from artificial insemination centers.
5. By means of transplacental infection.
6. Via the umbilicus.

Most organisms produce infections only if they enter by way of a particular portal. For example, enteropathogenic *E. coli* gain entrance to the intestine through the upper digestive tract but not through the skin. *Staphylococcus aureus*, on the other hand, readily enters the skin but rarely causes infection as a result of ingestion. Some organisms such as *Brucella* species may enter the host through several portals—the skin and oral or genital tract mucous membranes. The lesions produced by the invading organism may involve tissues and organs remote from the site of entry. Although the mode of infection of the swine erysipelas organism may be ingestion, the lesions are not associated with the alimentary tract.

INFECTION VIA THE RESPIRATORY TRACT

This is the common mode of infection in respiratory diseases, although these infections can also be acquired by direct contact and from fomites. The source of the organisms is generally the secretions of the respiratory tract of another animal. The infections are acquired as a result of the inhalation of contaminated air. The organisms are trapped on the moist mucous membranes of the nasopharynx and lower respiratory tract. This is the way that diseases such as pasteurella pneumonias, viral pneumonias, and tuberculosis are transmitted. The spores of a number of fungi such as *Blastomyces dermatitidis* that infect via the respiratory tract are acquired from the soil by inhalation.

Droplet Infection

Few or no organisms are shed into the air from the nose or mouth in normal breathing. However, large numbers of organisms are expelled during coughing and sneezing. Many of these organisms are derived from the mouth and oropharynx.

In coughing the vast majority of particles emanate from the respiratory tract in the form of droplets. It is estimated that in humans a vigorous cough may release five or six thousand droplets, while a vigorous sneeze may liberate as many as a million droplets.

The majority of the droplets expelled are less than 100 μm in diameter. These evaporate rapidly, leaving *droplet nuclei* suspended in the air for many hours. These consist of dried secretions that may contain organisms. Eventually they fall to the ground or other surroundings, resulting in their contamination. Droplets with a diameter of 100 μm or more have a very short trajectory and fall a very short distance from the host animal.

Of the droplets generated from saliva at the front of the mouth, many do not contain the infecting agent and many are sterile. It should be kept in mind that only a small proportion of the droplet nuclei contain pathogens. However, it often takes only a few organisms to initiate some diseases.

Dust-borne Infections

Many respiratory infections are probably acquired by the following indirect process: (1) the infected animal contaminates itself and its environment with secretions and infected droplets; and (2) the organisms dry on whatever they contaminate to be dispersed into the air subsequenty in the form of dust. The inhalation of these infectious dust particles constitutes an important mode of infection of respiratory diseases. The success of the method depends to a considerable extent on the capacity of the organisms to withstand the effects of drying. This mode of infection is responsible for the transmission of such diseases as psittacosis (transmitted through dried infectious feces) and tuberculosis.

INFECTION BY INGESTION

Organisms causing intestinal diseases gain entrance to the alimentary tract after being swallowed, e.g., salmonellas and enteropathogenic *E. coli. Mycobacterium bovis* may enter by this route and cause disease involving the intestine. The preformed exotoxins of *Clostridium botulinum* and *Staphylococcus aureus* are conveyed to the intestine in food. *Cl. perfringens* organisms giving rise to enterotoxemia may gain entrance to the body by ingestion. A number of infecting agents, such as *Brucella abortus*, enteroviruses, and *Coxiella burnetii*, may enter through the intestinal wall but produce their effects elsewhere. In intestinal disease the feces are the principal source of the pathogens.

Animals may become infected with intestinal pathogens as a result of direct contact with the feces-contaminated host or more commonly by contact with fomites such as contaminated feed, milk, bedding, surroundings (stable, mangers), and water. Because of the habits of animals, with the consequent frequent exposure to feces, intestinal diseases usually spread rapidly through herds and flocks.

INFECTION RESULTING FROM INOCULATION

Contact

Some diseases are spread by agents that can penetrate apparently undamaged skin or mucous membranes. *Brucella abortus, Bacillus anthracis,* and *Francisella tularensis* have this capacity. In animals, spread in this manner is most often by means of fomites such as infected litter and bedding, saddles, milker's hands, and milking machines rather than by direct contact. Included among the diseases that may be spread by these direct and indirect means are skin abscesses, pyoderma, poxvirus diseases, ringworm, the various viral papillomatoses, and dermatophilosis.

Wounds

Many organisms gain entrance to the underlying tissues through breaks in the continuity of skin or mucous membranes. In animals, wounds have numerous causes, including accidents, surgical operations (especially docking and castration), calving, goring, biting, and wounds due to nail punctures and bullets or shot. The sources of organisms that lodge in wounds are various. Tetanus results from the contamination of wounds by spores from the soil or feces. *Staphylococcus aureus* and *Corynebacterium pyogenes*, which are carried in the nasopharynx of many animals, frequently infect wounds. Other soil and fecal-borne organisms that infect wounds, resulting in gas gangrene, are *Cl. septicum* and *Cl. perfringens*. In surgery involving the stomach or intestine, incisions may become infected with such enteric organisms as *E. coli* and *Bacteroides* spp., sometimes leading to peritonitis.

Injection

As mentioned previously, infectious agents may be injected by biting arthropods or mistakenly or carelessly by humans. Diseases such as equine infectious anemia and anaplasmosis, to mention only two, may be transmitted by contaminated hypodermic needles and surgical instruments. These two diseases are also spread by biting insects. The equine viral encephalitides are spread by mosquitoes, and Rocky Mountain spotted fever is initiated by the bite of an infected tick. Tularemia is spread mainly by ticks and plague by fleas. The hog louse appears to be an important disseminator of swine pox virus.

INFECTION VIA THE GENITAL TRACT

Infectious agents may enter the genital tract to set up infections at various times but most frequently after parturition and at estrous. A number of important diseases are transmitted from male to female during coitus, e.g., epizootic bovine infertility, brucellosis, equine vesicular exanthema, and infectious pustular vulvovaginitis. *Corynebacterium renale*, the cause of bovine pyelonephritis, may gain entrance to the urinary tract from the genital tract.

TRANSPLACENTAL INFECTION

The fetuses of several animal species become infected and frequently are stillborn or aborted as a result of transplacental infection. In some diseases, such as brucellosis, *Campylobacter* abortion, and mycotic abortion, the disease process is mostly confined to the placenta, but the organisms can be recovered from the fetal stomach contents and various organs. Lesions within the fetus itself may be minimal. Abortion resulting from *Listeria* infection occurs, and this organism may be recovered from the stomach contents and various organs. The fetus may be profoundly affected by the infecting agent, e.g., a cerebellar hypoplasia may result from infection with the hog cholera virus, and extensive fetal damage occurs in chlamydial abortion of sheep and cattle.

INFECTION VIA THE UMBILICUS

Infection of the newborn may be prenatal—for example, an extension of cervicitis or placentitis—or postnatal—in which the common modes of infection are ingestion, inhalation, or via the umbilicus. The umbilicus frequently becomes infected if the navel is not properly cared for immediately after birth. The young of all the domestic species are prone to infections that start from the umbilicus, but lambs are particularly susceptible. A variety of organisms enter via the umbilicus, e.g., *Erysipelothrix rhusiopathiae*, *Salmonella*, *Klebsiella*, pyogenic streptococci, and *Actinobacillus equuli*.

The disease manifestations are variable, depending upon the virulence of the organism and the resistance of the newborn. First there is bacteremia, which in severe infections may proceed to septicemia and death. However, more often the bacteremia results in organisms being disseminated to organs, lymph nodes, and joints, where disease processes develop. A number of names are applied to what are collectively called the neonatal pyosepticemias. They include navel ill, omphalitis, joint ill, omphalophlebitis, pyemic arthritis, and polyarthritis.

NOSOCOMIAL INFECTIONS

These are hospital-acquired infections. A number of infectious agents may be transmitted within the veterinary hospital or clinic. Latent infections or carrier states may flare up into serious infections as a result of various stresses, and the agents may spread to and threaten other patients. *Salmonella* infections are a major nosocomial problem in many veterinary clinics, particularly the larger ones. These infections can only be prevented and controlled by careful attention to effective sanitation and management practices.

SOURCES FOR FURTHER READING

Beck-Nielsen, S.: Nosocomial (hospital-acquired) infection in veterinary practice. J. Am. Vet. Med. Assoc., *175*:1304, 1979.

Gallis, H.A.: Normal flora and opportunistic infections. *In* Zinsser Microbiology. Edited by W.K. Joklic, H.P. Willet, and D.B. Amos. Norwalk, Connecticut, Appleton-Century-Crofts, 1984.

Halpin, B.: Patterns of Animal Disease. Baltimore, Williams & Wilkins, 1975.

Schwabe, C.W., Preman, H.P., and Franti, C.E.: Epidemiology in Veterinary Practice. Philadelphia, Lea & Febiger, 1977.

Thomas, C.G.A.: Medical Microbiology. 5th Ed. London, Balliere Tindall, 1983.

Youmans, G.P., Paterson, P.Y., and Sommers, H.M.: The Biologic and Clinical Basis of Infectious Diseases. 2nd Ed. Philadelphia, W.B. Saunders Co., 1980.

5

Host-Parasite Relationships

Microorganisms, on the basis of their habitat and mode of living, may be classified as saprophytes or parasites. A small number, such as species of *Candida, Proteus, Klebsiella,* and *Pseudomonas,* can exist as either saprophytes or as parasites (commensals). Some important parasitic states and kinds of pathogens are defined below.

Saprophytism. Organisms in this state live on dead or decaying organic matter. They ordinarily are not parasites of animals, although on occasion they can cause disease. For example, brooder pneumonia is caused by the fungus *Aspergillus fumigatus,* which may be present in large numbers on food or litter. Some of the clostridia live in the soil as well as in the intestine.

Parasitism. This is a general term that denotes a state in which an organism lives on or within another living organism. The parasite does not necessarily harm the host; in fact, the most successful parasites achieve a balance with the host that ensures the survival of both. Among the parasites found on and within domestic animals and humans are bacteria, protozoans, fungi, mycoplasmas, rickettsiae and viruses. A relatively small number of the parasitic microbes have the potential to cause disease.

Some of the terms that are used to describe different parasitic states are given below.

Commensalism. This is a parasitic state in which the organism lives in or upon the host without causing disease. The organism benefits from this relationship, while the host may or may not. Most of the bacteria in the alimentary tract, both aerobic and anaerobic, are commensals.

Symbiosis. This is a state whereby an organism lives in or upon the host in a mutually beneficial relationship. Good examples of symbiosis are the microfloras of the cecum of rabbits and of the rumen of ruminants, which are provided food and shelter while enabling the host to utilize cellulose. Microbial symbiosis is not common in animals, and the term has little use in the discussion of infectious diseases of animals.

Potential Pathogen. This denotes an organism that is ordinarily a commensal, but under certain circumstances, such as the lowering of the host's resistance or an increase in the organism's virulence, can cause disease. For example, *Staphylococcus aureus* may cause bovine mastitis as a result of damage to the udder, and *Pasteurella haemolytica* may cause pneumonia in young cattle fatigued and weakened by shipment and cold.

Opportunistic Pathogen. This term is used by some microbiologists to designate organisms that are generally harmless in their normal habitats but can cause disease when they gain access to other sites or tissues. For example, nonenterotoxin-producing strains of *E. coli* from the intestine causing urinary tract infections have been termed opportunists. The term has also been used for such saprophytic fungi as species of *Penicillium, Aspergillus,* and *Candida,* which can cause infections in the compromised host.

Such species ordinarily have a low potential for causing disease.

Obligate Pathogen. This denotes an organism that almost always causes disease when it encounters animals or humans, e.g., *Brucella abortus, Yersinia pestis, Mycobacterium bovis* and the smallpox virus.

The terms that follow are frequently used in the discussion of infectious diseases.

Pathogenicity. This is the capacity of the organism to produce disease. Variation in this capacity is referred to in terms of virulence.

Virulence. This is a measure of the degree of pathogenicity. For example, pathogenic strains of *Streptococcus equi* may vary in their capacity to produce disease in the horse. All may cause disease, but some may cause more severe disease than others.

Infectivity. This is the capacity of the organism to become established in the tissues of the host. It involves the ability to penetrate the tissues, to survive the host's defenses, and to multiply and disseminate within the animal.

Toxigenicity. This is the capacity of certain organisms to produce exotoxins. For example, there are both toxigenic and nontoxigenic strains of *Clostridium perfringens*; only the former cause disease.

If the host-parasite relationship is kept in balance or equilibrium, no apparent disease results and the infection is asymptomatic. In such diseases as tuberculosis and brucellosis, a delicate equilibrium may be established that is easily upset. Disease results when the parasite cannot be kept in check and a combination of damage done to the host and the host's adaptive reactions results in the phenomenon we recognize as infectious disease.

The two principal determinants of the outcome of the host-parasite relationship are the virulence of the parasite and the resistance of the host. In natural disease the relative significance of each in the development of the disease is difficult to estimate.

For the sake of discussion, it is convenient to treat the roles of the parasite and the host separately.

PATHOGENIC PROPERTIES OF BACTERIA

Bacteria cause disease by two basic mechanisms: (1) invasion of tissues, and (2) production of toxins.

INVASIVENESS

Among the invasive bacteria, there are those that are classed as facultative intracellular parasites and those that are known as extracellular parasites.

Facultative Intracellular Parasites

These parasites are not confined to cells, but they can survive and in some instances multiply in phagocytic cells. These cells may also destroy them and prevent or ultimately eliminate an infection. For example, *Brucella abortus*, and *Mycobacterium bovis* may be eliminated by macrophages in this manner. When a balance is established between the bacterium and the phagocyte, usually macrophages, the bacteria may survive in this intracellular state of relative equilibrium for months or years, as evidenced by *Salmonella, Brucella*, and mycobacteria.

Obligate Intracellular Parasites

The viruses, chlamydia, and rickettsiae are obligate intracellular parasites in that they can only propagate within cells.

Extracellular Parasites

The extracellular organisms damage the tissues while they are outside phagocytes and other cells. They do not have the capacity to survive for long periods in phagocytic cells. When phagocytized, these organisms (e.g., *Klebsiella* and *Pasteurella* spp.) are destroyed.

Antiphagocytic Capsules

These surface structures, principally on extracellular bacteria, consist of hydrophilic gels, usually polysaccharides, that protect the organisms from ingestion by phagocytic cells. Examples are mucoid forms of *Pasteurella multocida, Enterobacter aerogenes*, and *Bacillus anthracis*.

Extracellular Enzymes

Some bacteria produce substances that are not toxic directly but that play an important part in the development of disease:

1. *Coagulase* produced by *Staphylococcus aureus*, which clots fibrin, thus protecting the bacteria.
2. *Hyaluronidases* produced by many bacteria and thought to aid in the spread of organisms by breaking down the ground substance (hyaluronic acid) of tissues.
3. *Collagenase* produced by some strains of

Clostridium perfringens; it aids in the spread of this organism by breaking down the collagen of tissues.

Other extracellular enzymes are streptokinase (a fibrinolysin) and streptodornase (a DNase), produced by streptococci. There are others that will be dealt with under specific pathogens.

Adsorption or Adherence to Surfaces

Although the adsorption of viruses to epithelial cells has been studied extensively, it is only recently that the adsorption and adherence to cell surfaces of pathogenic bacteria with consequent colonization or penetration or both have been investigated. It has been shown that pili of enteropathogenic strains of *Escherichia coli* are involved in adherence and colonization of the mucous membrane of the small intestine. Pili may also be inovlved in the adherence of *Neisseria gonorrhoeae* and *Bordetella spp.* Strains of *Mycoplasma pneumoniae* that have lost their capacity to adhere are also found to have lost their virulence. The adsorption of some bacteria to mucous membranes may be caused by a physicochemical attraction dependent upon certain surface compounds associated with the capsules of virulent organisms. These compounds may be lost on *in vitro* cultivation.

The phenomenon of adherence of bacteria is now receiving a great deal of attention. Its study may have important practical implications, as suggested by the recent development of an *Escherichia coli* pilus vaccine to prevent scours in swine.

General Comments

There is a great variation in the extent of invasiveness of microorganisms. At one end of the scale are the exotoxin producers, such as the tetanus bacillus, which are noninvasive, and at the other end are organisms like *Yersina pestis* and *Bacillus anthracis,* the plague and anthrax bacilli, which are highly invasive. Organisms such as some *Pasteurella spp.,* streptococci, and *Haemophilus spp.* are in-between and have only a moderate capacity to invade.

How do we know that a particular organism is pathogenic? The traditional criteria employed are Koch's postulates: (1) The organism must be regularly isolated from cases of the disease. (2) It must be grown *in vitro* in pure culture. (3) Such a culture should produce the typical disease when inoculated into a susceptible animal species. (4) The same organism must be isolated

from the experimentally induced disease. Although these postulates have been applied to many diseases, they have not been fulfilled for all, e.g., some human viral diseases (because viruses are frequently very host-specific), diseases such as leprosy and Tyzzer's disease (in which the causal agent has not been grown *in vitro*), and diseases associated with stress with a complex etiology such as pneumonic pasteurellosis (shipping fever) of cattle.

TOXIGENICITY

Exotoxins —formed outside cell (bacterial) heat-viable, protein

Most of the weakly or noninvasive bacteria that cause disease produce exotoxins. These are protein substances that are liberated from intact and lysed cells. They vary greatly in their toxicity, from the extremely potent botulinus toxin to the relatively weak toxin of *Corynebacterium pyogenes.* They are almost all antigenic, eliciting specific protective antitoxic antibodies. The various disease-producing clostridia are notable for their production of exotoxins. Some of these toxins can be converted to nontoxic immunizing agents called toxoids by treatment with formalin.

Some of the bacteria other than clostridia that produce exotoxins are enteropathogenic *Escherichia coli, Yersinia pestis,* several *Corynebacterium* species, the highly invasive *Bacillus anthracis,* and *Staphylococcus aureus.* Unlike the endotoxins, the clinical and experimental effects of the different exotoxins vary greatly with each particular bacterial species and are best described in the discussion of the specific diseases.

Endotoxins —present in bacterial cells

Some properties of endotoxins are as follows:
1. They are produced by gram-negative bacteria, both pathogenic and nonpathogenic, species, and they are released during growth and upon lysis.
2. They were originally described as phospholipid-polysaccharide-protein complexes (somatic O antigen). However, their biologic and immunologic properties reside with the lipopolysaccharide portion. The terms endotoxin and lipopolysaccharide are often used synonymously. Their chemical structure is described in Chapter 1.
3. They are a major part of the cell wall of gram-negative bacteria.

4. They are heat-stable, with molecular weights between 100,000 and 900,000.
5. Their toxicity resides in the lipid portion, while their specific antigenic determinants are the sugars that constitute the side chains of the lipopolysaccharide. They do not form toxoids.
6. They are less specific and potent in their cytotoxic effects.
7. They are weak antigens, although they may have an adjuvant effect with other antigens. Potency differs among species.

Although many biologic effects have been ascribed to endotoxins, their role in the pathogenesis of bacterial diseases is poorly understood and largely conjectural. Part of their injurious effect is thought by some investigators to be immunologic in nature. It is suggested that a state of immunologic sensitivity may be involved. It has been noted that germ-free animals are less susceptible to the toxic effects of endotoxins.

Among the effects of endotoxins observed clinically and experimentally are fever, leukopenia, hypoglycemia, hypotension and shock, intravascular coagulation, Shwartzman's reaction, adjuvancy, and activation of complement components leading to acute inflammatory reactions. Endotoxins may have an effect on the clotting system, leading to the kind of intravascular coagulation seen in gram-negative septicemias. Thrombocytopenia with lysis of platelets and the release of histamine, serotonin, and bradykinin may lead to the kind of cardiovascular changes that are seen in endotoxemia, including shock. Endotoxemia occurs in gram-negative bacterial sepsis and hemorrhagic septicemia.

The amount of endotoxin can be determined by the limulus lysate assay. Endotoxin reacts with proteins from horseshoe crab amebocytes to produce a gel. It is a remarkably sensitive test that will detect nanogram amounts of endotoxin.

MECHANISMS OF HOST RESISTANCE

NONSPECIFIC MECHANISMS

The Skin

The skin provides a generally effective barrier. Some microorganisms, such as *Brucella abortus* and *Francisella tularensis*, can penetrate skin. Others enter and cause infections of sweat and sebaceous glands and hair follicles. The glands secrete substances with an acid pH that contain fatty acids and are antibacterial. Young animals are thought to be more susceptible to dermatophytes because they have a lower concentration of fatty acids on the skin than adult animals. Lysozyme, an enzyme that breaks down the cell walls of bacteria, is present on the skin.

Mucous Membrane

Mucus covers the surface of the various tracts of the body. Bacteria are caught by the mucous film and are readily phagocytized. The phagocytes carry the bacteria via lymph channels to the lymph nodes, which act as barriers. The cilia of the respiratory tract are constantly moving bacteria and mucus to the natural orifices. Both mucus and tears contain the protective enzyme lysozyme.

Hair in the nares is protective, as is the cough reflex. Saliva, stomach acid, and proteolytic enzymes have an antibacterial action. The acid pH of the vagina caused by lactobacilli has a limiting and stabilizing influence on the vaginal flora. The normal flora of mucous membranes is a rather stable ecosystem that resists the intrusion of alien bacteria. Disturbance of the flora by antibiotic therapy may allow establishment and multiplication of disease-producing organisms, e.g., staphylococci resulting in staphylococcal enteritis or *Candida albicans* resulting in mycotic gastritis or enteritis.

Phagocytosis

Microorganisms entering organs and tissues such as the lungs, lymphatics, bone marrow, and bloodstream may be engulfed by various phagocytic cells. Among these are the polymorphonuclear leukocytes and the wandering and fixed macrophages of the reticuloendothelial system. Phagocytosis may be nonspecific in the absence of antibody but specific when antibodies to the offending microorganism are available. Phagocytes may kill the engulfed microorganisms or they may survive and in some instances actually multiply in the phagocytic cell (intracellular parasites). The phagocytic vacuole is called the phagosome. Lysosomal granules provide the hydrolytic enzymes, including lysozyme, which aid in the destruction of microorganisms. Macrophages may be specifically activated by immunologically active T-lymphocytic cells.

Reticuloendothelial System

type b phagocyte [handwritten]

This system refers to the macrophages found in blood (monocytes) and the fixed macrophages (histiocytes) found in lymphoid tissue, spleen, liver, bone marrow, and other tissues. They engulf and remove particulate matter and microorganisms from the blood and lymph. Included in the system are the macrophages (Kupffer's cells) lining the blood sinuses of the liver, those lining the lymph sinuses, and histiocytes found in tissues and the alveolar macrophages in the lungs.

Resistance of Tissues

Various constituents of tissues have an inhibitory effect on microorganisms; thus some tissues are more readily invaded than others. The interferon produced by tissues in response to viral infection has antiviral properties.

Most healthy tissues inhibit the multiplication of microorganisms. This resistance can be impaired by depression of the inflammatory response by x-rays, corticosteroids, leukemic disease, and antineoplastic drugs. Injury resulting from foreign bodies, trauma, and disturbances in fluid and electrolyte balance may predispose to infection.

Natural Antibodies

These are immunoglobulins that react with a wide range of organisms and antigens to which the animal has not been exposed or immunized. Low levels are found in germ-free animals. Some examples are ABO blood group system isohemagglutinins and Forssman's antibodies.

Inflammatory Response

Pathogenic microorganisms, like other damaging agents, elicit inflammatory responses of varying kinds and severity. The changes elicited are complex, and some of the phenomena and factors involved are increased vascular permeability, edema, inflammatory exudate, chemotaxis, cellular infiltrates, phagocytosis, various mediators of inflammation, and immunologic reactions. In many inflammatory processes there is a transudation of serum bactericidal factors, including

1. C-reactive proteins: These are β-globulins that react with the group-specific C-carbohydrate of *Streptococcus pneumoniae*. They are encountered in acute infections and other conditions involving fever and

① primary importance [handwritten, vertical]

tissue destruction. They bind to substances from damaged tissues and from microorganisms, activating the complement system.

2. Properdin: This is a complex of serum proteins, including two enzymes that function with certain components of complement in the alternative pathway. It may have antiviral and antibacterial actions.

Inflammation as a process is described in detail by pathologists and immunologists.

Fever

Fever is frequently observed as a manifestation of the inflammatory response. It is the cardinal symptom or sign of infectious disease. Fever results from influences on the thermoregulatory centers in the brain. Two substances that induce fever are endotoxins and *endogenous pyrogen* extracted from normal leukocytes. It is thought that bacteria, viruses, steroids, immune complexes, sensitized T lymphocytes, and endotoxin can stimulate granulocytes and macrophages to release endogenous pyrogen. These are carried in the bloodstream to the thermoregulatory centers in the hypothalamus. The general cell-mediated immune response such as occurs in tuberculosis and brucellosis is also a cause of fever. Fever includes increased heat production and reduced heat loss. There is very little evidence that fever has a beneficial effect on infectious disease.

Fever of Unknown Origin

In cases of fever of unknown origin in animals, the most frequent causes are probably undetected infections and neoplasms. Other causes may be endocrine disturbances and hypersensitivity reactions.

CIRCUMSTANCES AND FACTORS PREDISPOSING TO INFECTION

Stress

The term stress is frequently used to summarize various factors and circumstances that contribute to the development of an infectious disease or diseases. Although there are both mental and physical disturbances that lead to the stress reaction, the latter are probably most important in animals.

Among the more common disturbances leading to stress are fatigue, exposure to extremes of cold and heat, crowding, wounds, transport, change in feed, and weaning. Latent infection such as that caused by *Chlamydia psittaci* in birds may be activated by the stress of transport. A number of physical disturbances contribute to the development of shipping fever (bovine pneumonic pasteurellosis).

If the disturbances are severe enough, a co-ordinated response originating in the cortex and hypothalamus is initiated; this involves either the autonomic nervous system or the pituitary-adrenal axis. Corticosteroids and catechol-amines are released in an effort to counter the deleterious effects of the disturbance. Cortico-steroids in large amounts depress the inflam-matory reaction and have pronounced effects on lymphoid tissues, causing lymphocyte destruc-tion and thymic involution.

Circulatory Disturbances. Such disturbances may be local, causing ischemia or congestion and edema, or general, as occurs in shock. They result in interference with the mobilization and functioning of phagocytic cells. Mechanical ob-struction of the biliary or urinary tracts can have similar effects, thus contributing to infections.

Nutritional Deficiency. There has long been an association between famine and pestilence. Poorly fed animals are most susceptible to a va-riety of infections. Vitamin A deficiency results in the loss of integrity of epithelium. Among the nutritional effects are diminished phagocytic ca-pacity, reduction of the efficiency of the reticu-loendothelial system, weakened antibody re-sponse, lowered production of lysozyme and interferon, undesirable changes in microbial flora, and alterations of the endocrine system.

Extremes of Temperature and Humidity. There is experimental evidence that animals are less resistant to bacterial infections if they are maintained at a low temperature for extended periods. Environmental stresses including cold and intemperate weather no doubt contribute to the occurrence of bovine pneumonic pasteurel-losis (shipping fever). High humidity, with an increase in infectious droplets, may contribute to an increase in respiratory disease in groups of animals. Production of corticosteroids by stressed animals may be anti-inflammatory and immunosuppressive, thus contributing to or ag-gravating the infectious process.

Genetic Effects. There is evidence of genetic resistance to bovine mastitis. Leghorns are more resistant to Marek's disease than some other breeds. Some varieties of rabbits are more re-sistant to myxomatosis as a consequence of the highly susceptible strains having been selected out by the disease. Defects in the immune sys-tem frequently have a genetic basis, e.g., com-bined T and B cell deficiency contributing to fatal adenoviral infections in Arab foals; disseminated histoplasmosis in dogs with thymic hypoplasia; and agammaglobulinemia in humans and ani-mals that are especially prone to bacterial infec-tions.

Chronic Infections. Chronic infections may predispose animals to more severe infection often caused by so-called secondary invaders, e.g., the pasteurellas in shipping fever pneu-monia in cattle. Some viral infections such as influenza may suppress resistance to certain bac-terial infections.

Physical Fatigue. It is widely held that ex-treme fatigue predisposes to infection, presum-ably because it contributes to stress.

Hormonal Imbalance. Diabetics and animals receiving adrenal steroids are known to be ab-normally prone to infections.

Acute Radiation Injury. This injury may result in damage to the bone marrow with consequent granulocytopenia and thus a lowering of the host's resistance.

RESISTANCE AND IMMUNITY

Nonspecific resistance has already been dis-cussed. Immunity (discussed in detail under im-munobiology) is classified as follows:

Immunity $\begin{cases} \text{Natural Immunity} \\ \text{Acquired Immunity} \end{cases}$ $\begin{cases} \text{Passive Immunity} \\ \text{Active Immunity} \end{cases}$

Immunology is of such importance in veteri-nary medicine that it is taught as a separate dis-cipline. The brief outline that follows is provided to emphasize some important immunologic as-pects of infectious diseases.

ACQUIRED IMMUNITY OF INFECTIONS

Humoral Immunity—in blood

This is specific immunity mediated by anti-bodies (immunoglobulins) present in plasma, lymph, and tissue fluids of the body. Some prop-erties of major immunoglobulin classes are sum-marized in Table 5–1. The relative sensitivity of tests used for measuring antibody is given in Table 5–2.

Primary Immune Responses. Antibodies are detectable in one to two weeks after infec-

Table 5–1. Some Properties of Major Human Immunoglobulin Classes*

	IgG	IgM	IgA	IgE
Location	Plasma, tissue and body fluids, lymph	Plasma	Plasma, seromucous secretions, colostrum	Plasma
Function	More persistent than IgM; reaches peak later. Most important antibody in infections.	Produced early and declines early. First line of humoral defense.	Defends surface of mucous membranes	Responsible for anaphylactic reactions and immediate hypersensitivity
Agglutination	+ +	+ + + +	+	—
Precipitation	+ + +	+	+	—
Complement fixation	+ +	+ + + +	—	—
Opsonization	+ +	+ + + +	—	—
Neutralization of toxins	+ + + +	+	+	—

*+ = poor; + + = fair; + + + = good; + + + + = very good.

Table 5–2. Relative Sensitivity of Tests Measuring Antibody*

Test	Approximate Antibody Detectable (μg/ml)
Precipitation	20.0
Immunoelectrophoresis	20.0
Double diffusion in agar gel	1.0
Complement fixation	0.5
Radial immunodiffusion	0.05
Bacterial agglutination	0.01
Hemolysis	0.01
Passive hemagglutination	0.01
Antitoxin neutralization	0.01
Radioimmunoassay, ELISA	0.0005
Virus neutralization	0.00005

*(Reproduced with permission from Hyde, R.M., and Patnode, R.A.: Immunology. Reston, Virginia, Reston Publishing Company, 1978.)

tion. IgM appears first, followed shortly by IgG. IgM lasts for about 15 days; IgG lasts for a much longer period. The primary response does not persist; by the third week, it starts to decline. The peak of the primary response is reached in about two and a half weeks.

Secondary (Anamnestic) Response. This results from the second exposure to the same antigen after the primary response. The antibody response is 10 to 50 times that of the primary response. It is mostly IgG, and it remains high for several months. The animal retains a memory for the antigen, and the secondary response may be obtained months after the primary response.

Antitoxins. Antitoxin (IgG) is specific, neutralizing only one kind of toxin, e.g., tetanus antitoxin will neutralize only tetanus toxin. Antitoxins may be present as a result of natural infection or artificial immunization. Infection may result in a secondary immune response, and if enough antitoxin is provided soon enough, the toxin is neutralized. If there is no immunologic memory, it may be necessary to provide antibody for immediate protection, e.g., as in the use of tetanus antitoxin in the prevention of tetanus following a wound.

Bacterial exotoxins are largely enzymatic in nature. Antibody prevents the enzyme from interacting with its substrate. Antitoxin is most effective against high molecular weight toxins, which cannot reach the active site because the antitoxin blocks them. The lower molecular weight substrate is able to avoid the blocking effect of the antitoxin molecule.

Immunologic Response to Endotoxins. The primary toxicity of endotoxins has been shown in caesarean piglets. Some of the immunologic responses to endotoxins follow.

HYPERSENSITIVITY OF THE IMMEDIATE TYPE. Endotoxins combine with antibodies, and the resulting complexes, together with complement, trigger the kind of reactions ascribed to the primary toxicity of endotoxins, e.g., vasoactive substance release, vascular necrosis, endogenous pyrogen release, and coagulopathy. Lipopolysaccharide and zymosan can activate C3; then proteolytic enzymes released from damaged tissue can release anaphylatoxins from C3 and C5 to initiate acute inflammatory reactions. Immune complexes containing gram-negative organisms may be responsible for some of the lesions seen in diseases such as the pasteurelloses.

HYPERSENSITIVITY OF THE DELAYED TYPE. This may be elicited with endotoxins and result in reactions of the "primary toxicity" type, including fever, vascular necrosis, and inflammatory lesions. Endotoxins have the capacity to transform T lymphocytes.

TOLERANCE. IgM antibodies to endotoxin aid in its uptake and breakdown by macrophages. These antibodies may also prevent disseminated intravascular coagulation.

Opsonization and Phagocytosis. In the absence of exotoxins, antibodies protect by attaching directly to the surface of the microorganism. This encourages phagocytosis by macrophages (monocytes) of the blood, and neutrophils. Antibody probably alters the surface characteristics of the microorganism, making it more susceptible to phagocytosis. When they are present in immune complexes, macrophages have specific receptors with a high affinity for IgG and for the third component of complement.

Cytophilic and opsonizing antibodies provide alternative mechanisms for promoting adherence of bacteria to macrophages. The phagocytic cell may digest the organism in the phagocytic vacuole with digestive enzymes from intracellular lysosomes. Some organisms can resist intracellular digestion, e.g., streptococci (because of the protein M), tubercle bacilli, and capsulated salmonellas. Bacteria may adhere to red cells in the presence of antibody and complement and thus be prepared for phagocytosis. This is called immune adherence.

Cell lysis (IgM) may take place as a result of activation of the complement system, such as occurs in leptospirosis. Localization and immobilization take place by clumping and agglutination (IgM), possibly combined with lysis or phagocytosis or both. Soluble antigens of bacteria may be precipitated by specific precipitins (IgG).

Secretory Antibody. This antibody, IgA, is selectively secreted into saliva, respiratory and intestinal mucous secretions, and colostrum. It is produced locally and has a secretory or transport piece not found in serum IgA. The secretory piece probably makes it relatively resistant to digestion. IgA functions in precipitation, agglutination, and cell lysis, and it probably acts in the gut to prevent adherence. It does not fix complement and is nonopsonizing, but there may be some synergistic action with lysozyme and complement.

Cellular Immunity (Cell-Mediated Immunity)

This form of specific and nonspecific immunity is mediated by small lymphocytes and is transferable by cells (transfer factor) and not serum (antibodies). It is responsible for allograft rejection (graft rejection), delayed hypersensitivity (e.g., tuberculin reaction), and defense against viral infections and mainly against bacteria with an intracellular mode of infection.

Protection against such facultative intracellular parasites as *Salmonella* spp., *Brucella* spp., *Mycobacterium* spp., and *Listeria monocytogenes* is cell-mediated. The following are some important features of cell-mediated immunity vis à vis these intracellular parasites.

1. Bacterial antigen (ribonucleoprotein) is presented to T cells by normal macrophages, resulting in their sensitization.
2. Sensitized T cells activate macrophages, resulting in an increase in lysosomes, which can destroy and eliminate the infecting bacteria.
3. Sensitized T cells produce other lymphokines, resulting in delayed hypersensitivity (type IV hypersensitivity).
4. Intracellular parasites can survive for long periods of time in normal, nonactivated macrophages.
5. Cellular immunity may be specific or nonspecific, depending on the stage of infection. Delayed hypersensitivity is specific.
6. Vaccines consisting of live organisms—particularly those that are facultative intracellular parasites—elicit a considerable cellular immune response, whereas vaccines consisting of dead organisms do not.
7. Many infectious diseases in which cell-mediated immunity plays a major role in the host's resistance are characterized by the formation of granulomas or granulomatous inflammation; however, all granulomas are not immunologic in origin. Granulomas contain large numbers of cells (epithelioid) derived from macrophages. Granulomas serve to wall off and limit infections.

Hypersensitivity Reactions

Some features of the well-known types I, II, III, and IV hypersensitivity reactions are summarized briefly in Table 5–3. Some examples of agents and diseases in which these hypersensitivity reactions have a role are given below.

Type I: Anaphylactic-Type Sensitivity. This type of hypersensitivity is seen most frequently by veterinarians as anaphylactic shock shortly after the parenteral administration of bacterins composed of gram-negative organisms. The local form of type I reactions is probably manifested in some bacterial allergies, e.g., to strep-

Table 5–3. Hypersensitivity Reactions: A Summary*

Type I Anaphylactic-Type Sensitivity	Type II Cytotoxic-Type Hypersensitivity
IgE (reaginic antibody); strong affinity for tissues. Antibody-antigen reaction-release of pharmacologically active substances or mediators, e.g., *histamine* (from granules of mast and other cells); vasodilator, smooth muscle constrictor; wheal and flare response. Serotonin: smooth muscle contraction, vascular permeability vasoconstriction of large vessels. Bradykinin: histamine-like effect. Slow-reacting substance of anaphylaxis: like histamine but slower. Anaphylatoxins (from C3 and C5): formed on fixation of complement; increased vascular permeability; histamine release. Forms ⎱ Systemic: anaphylactic shock ⎰ Local: asthma, hay fever, other allergies Desensitization: small doses of antigen probably induce T suppressor cells.	Cell-associated antigen + antibody (IgM and IgG) + complement = lysis of cell; hemolysis in case of red cells. Clinical entities: (1) Blood transfusion mismatch; blood group antigen involved = intravascular hemolysis. (2) Granulocytopenia. Cytotoxic antibodies to leukocyte antigens resulting from blood transfusions. (3) Sometimes involved in rejection of surgically transplanted organs. (4) Rhesus incompatibility = Rh negative mother sensitized by Rh+ baby; later Rh+ fetus may have hemolytic disease. (5) Autoimmune reactions: antibodies to patient's own cells, e.g., hemolytic anemia in humans. Antibody + cells + complement = cytotoxicity. (6) Some drug reactions: Hapten + cell reacts with antibody = cytotoxicity.
Type III Complex-Mediated Hypersensitivity	Type IV Cell-Mediated (Delayed-type) Hypersensitivity (CMH)
Antibody-antigen union = immune complex. Horse serum → man = serum sickness. Systemic form: antigen excess. Local form (Arthus reaction) resulting from repeated injections of antigen at weekly intervals; antibody excess. Development of antigen-antibody complexes; soluble initially (antigen excess), later insoluble; lodge in vascular bed. Complement fixed = release of mediators from mast cells and platelets, e.g., histamine. Polymorphs present. Inflammation results in vasculitis with hemorrhage and thrombosis.	Mediated by primed lymphocytes. In lesions of the delayed hypersensitivity type, lymphocytes and macrophages are prominent and appear in about 24 hours. Lymphocytes are primed by various antigens, e.g., tubercle bacilli and brucellae. CMH is specific and can be transmitted passively with lymphoid cells (transfer factor). On contact with antigen, the sensitized lymphocyte is activated = blast transformation; migration-inhibiting factor (M.I.F.); chemotaxis (chemotactic for lymphocytes); cytotoxin: blastogenic effect on nonsensitized lymphocytes.

*Immediate hypersensitivity: types I, II, and III.

tococci, staphylococci, and some gram-negative bacteria.

Type II: Cytotoxic-Type Hypersensitivity. This kind of reaction does not appear to have a significant role in infections except when the products of some bacteria are absorbed to red cells, resulting in hemolytic anemia.

Type III: Complex-Mediated Hypersensitivity. It is now realized that immune complexes play an important part in the pathogenesis of a number of diseases, e.g., swine erysipelas, *Haemophilus somnus* infection, leptospirosis, and probably pasteurellosis and many other infections.

Type IV: Cell-Mediated Hypersensitivity. This type of hypersensitivity is important in the pathogenesis of and immunity to facultative intracellular parasites, including the pathogenic mycobacteria and *Brucella* spp.

Type V: Stimulatory Hypersensitivity. Type V hypersensitivity is not involved in infections. The antibody involved reacts with a surface component such as a hormone receptor and thus "switches on" the cell. An example is thyrotoxicosis (Graves' disease), in which the thyroid-

reactivity is caused by a thyroid-stimulating autoantibody.

SOME TERMS USED IN THE DISCUSSION OF INFECTIOUS DISEASES

Disease. Any disturbance of the structure or function of constituents of the animal organism. Some workers make a distinction between infection and disease. Because these terms are mostly used synonymously, such a distinction is not recommended.

Carrier. When this term is used in connection with a microbe, it indicates that it is present on or within an animal, usually as a commensal. There is usually no evidence of disease. A pig may carry *Salmonella cholerasuis* without showing any clinical signs of disease.

Carrier Rate. This denotes the percentage of animals carrying a certain organism. For example, the carrier rate of *Pasteurella multocida* in the mouths of cats may be as high as 60%.

Primary Agent of Disease. A microbial agent that can initiate disease on its own, e.g., *Brucella abortus*.

Secondary Invader. A microbial agent that invades or establishes itself in tissues that have been infected by a primary agent.

Mixed Infections. More than one microbial agent may be associated with a disease, e.g., in shipping fever pneumonia in cattle, a bacterium, a virus, and a mycoplasma may be involved. It may be difficult to determine or estimate the relative importance of each.

Infectivity. The capacity to become established in the tissues of the host.

Invasive. This term is sometimes used to describe an organism's capacity for entering and spreading within tissues.

Natural History of Disease. The usual course of infectious disease from the beginning to the end if there is no treatment.

Latent and Inapparent Infections. Persisting subclinical infections. There is frequently a latent state in tuberculosis.

Zoonosis. A disease or infection of humans acquired from animals.

Epizootic. A disease attacking a large number of animals within a short time span and usually spreading rapidly, e.g., foot-and-mouth disease. Epidemic may be used as a synonym for epizootic.

Enzootic. The habitual presence of an animal disease in a certain geographic area, e.g., swine dysentery in Iowa. The word *endemic* has the same meaning but is usually applied to human beings; however, it may also be used for animals.

Axenic. This term is used to denote animals that have been raised in a germ-free atmosphere and are consequently germ-free. These animals are remarkably susceptible to infectious agents. They have a retarded development of antibody-producing organs and are consequently deficient in immunoglobulins. The absence of normal flora influences the responsiveness of the host to infectious agents.

Gnotobiotic. This term is used to describe animals whose flora and fauna are known because they have previously been defined and established. In order to maintain their gnotobiotic status, they must be kept in isolation to prevent the addition of alien organisms.

Specific Pathogen-Free Animals. Animals that have been derived from stock established from caesarian-delivered animals. Swine thus derived may be maintained free of *Bordetella bronchiseptica*, *Salmonella* species, transmissible gastroenteritis virus, and *Mycoplasma hypopneumoniae*.

Specific Pathogen-Free Flocks. Flocks established from eggs free of known pathogenic agents, includng mycoplasmas. They are used to provide eggs and chickens for research and for the initiation of other similar flocks.

Pathogenicity. The capacity of an infectious agent to cause disease in a susceptible host.

Virulence. The degree of pathogenicity of a microorganism.

Incidence (in Epidemiology). A measurement of only the new cases of a disease occurring during a given period.

Prevalence (in Epidemiology). A measurement of all cases of disease existing at a given time.

epidemiology - the study of the relationships of the various factors determining the frequency + distribution of disease.

SOURCES FOR FURTHER READING

Bitton, G., and Marshall, K.M. (eds.): Adsorption of Microorganisms to Surfaces. New York, John Wiley & Sons, 1980.

Fauci, A.S.: Host-Defense Mechanisms Against Infection. Current Concept Series. Kalamazoo, Michigan, Upjohn Company, 1978.

Herbert, W.J.: Veterinary Immunology. Revised Reprint. London, Blackwell Scientific Publications, 1974.

Mims, C.A.: The Pathogenesis of Infectious Disease. 2nd Ed. New York, Academic Press, 1982.

Roitt, I.: Essential Immunology. 4th Ed. London, Blackwell Scientific Publications, 1980.

Tizzard, I.R.: An Introduction to Veterinary Immunology. 2nd Ed. Philadelphia, W.B. Saunders Company, 1982.

Youmans, G.R., Paterson, P.Y., and Sommers, H.M. (eds.): The Biologic and Clinical Basis of Infectious Diseases. 2nd Ed. Philadelphia, W.B. Saunders Company, 1980.

6

Antimicrobial Drugs

Chemotherapy, a term that originated with Paul Ehrlich, refers to the treatment of infectious diseases by the administration of drugs that are inhibitory or lethal to the infecting agents. An essential requirement of such a drug is a selective toxicity directed at the causative organism rather than the host. Drugs that are highly toxic to both organism and host are obviously unsatisfactory.

Although chemotherapeutic drugs were known before Ehrlich's time, he was the first to deliberately seek new antimicrobial compounds. When he found a compound that showed at least limited activity for an organism, he would synthesize closely related compounds in order to find more effective ones. Organic chemists are still using this approach. After trying many compounds for their activity against the spirochetes of syphilis, in 1907, Ehrlich found that the arsenical compound, arsphenamine, was selectively toxic for *Treponema pallidum*. This was the first of a long series of drugs to be synthesized in the laboratory.

A number of years later, Domagk (1935) showed that the red dye Prontosil was effective in the treatment of streptococcal infections. Later it was shown that its antibacterial activity was due to sulfanilamide derived from Prontosil. The success of this drug stimulated a search for related compounds and resulted in the synthesis of a host of effective compounds of the sulfonamide group.

Although Ehrlich is rightly considered the father of modern chemotherapy, a number of drugs were developed for various diseases prior to his time. Paracelsus (16th century) had used mercury compounds for the treatment of syphilis. By the 19th century the natives of South America had found that quinine was an effective treatment for malaria.

Antibiotics

An antibiotic is defined as an antimicrobial substance produced by a living microorganism. Pasteur and Joubert (1877) first reported that common airborne contaminants had a lethal effect on a culture of *Bacillus anthracis*. Similar observations had been made over the years, and Fleming (1929) observed that a fungus, *Penicillium notatum*, when present on a culture plate, was strongly inhibitory to the growth of staphylococci. In fact, he carried out a crude plate susceptibility test. This discovery was not exploited until 1940, when Chain, Florey, and associates succeeded in obtaining preparations from *Penicillium* that had high antibacterial activity but low toxicity for humans and animals. The remarkable therapeutic efficacy of penicillin against a variety of diseases was soon demonstrated.

After the discovery of penicillin, an extensive search for antibiotics began. The richest source of these drugs was found to be species of *Streptomyces*. Other sources of useful antibiotics have been bacteria, actinomycetes, and certain fungi. Recently some semisynthetic penicillins, e.g., methicillin, ampicillin, carbenicillin, and others, have been derived from naturally produced

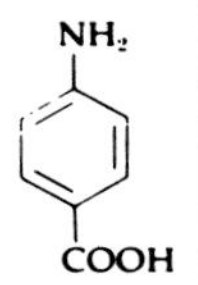

PABA

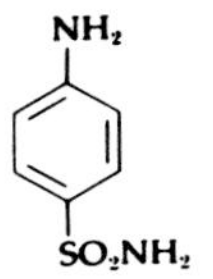

Sulfanilamide

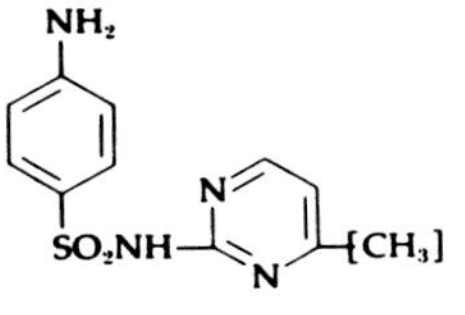

Sulfadiazine

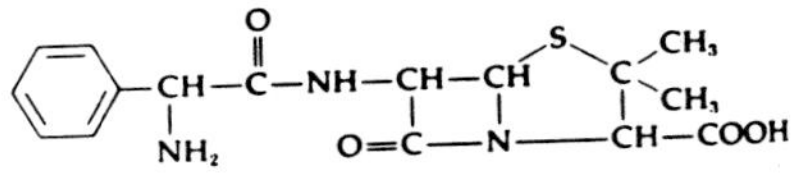

Ampicillin

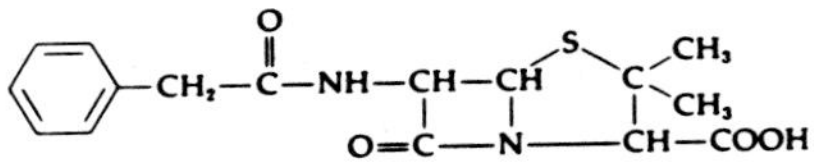

Penicillin G

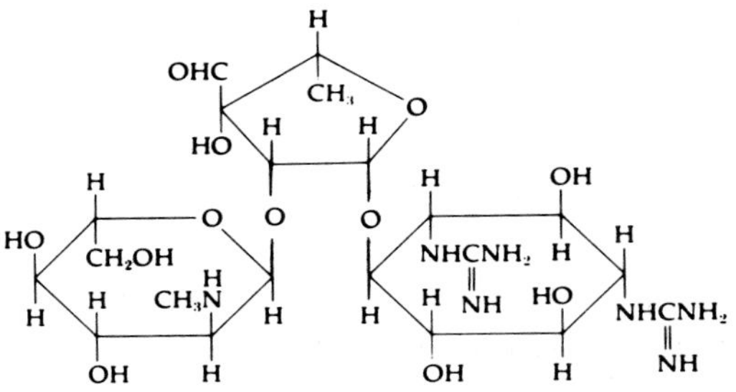

Streptomycin

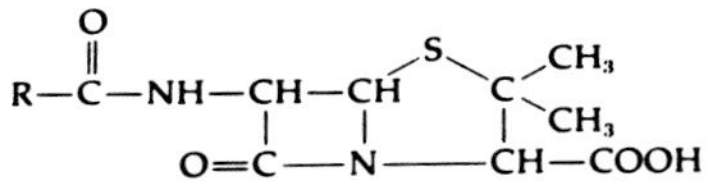

Penicillin nucleus

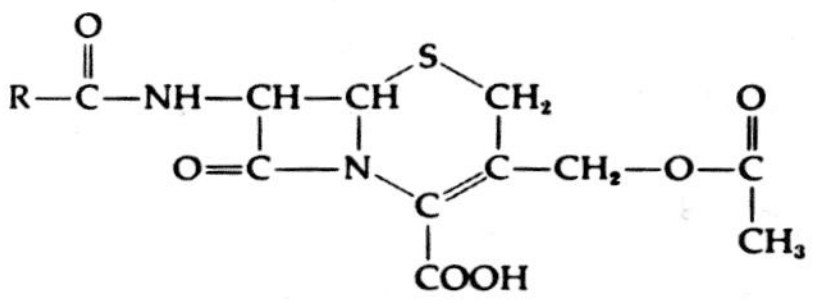

Cephalosporin nucleus

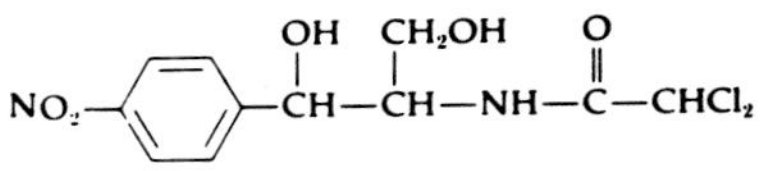

Chloramphenicol

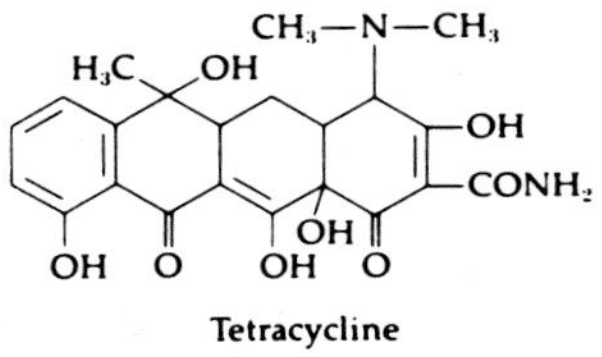

Tetracycline

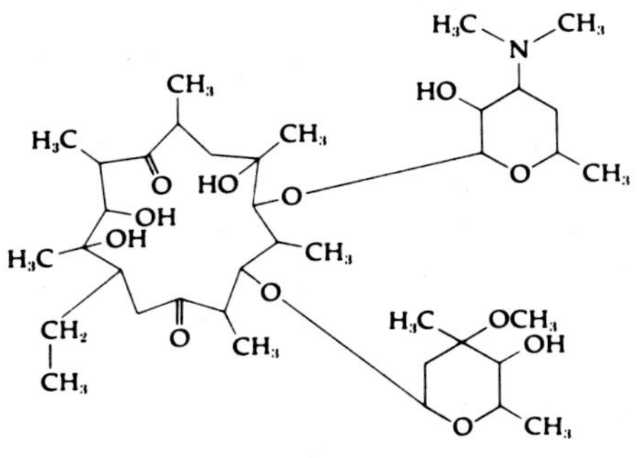

Erythromycin

Figure 6–1. Structures of drugs representing important groups of antimicrobial agents.

6-amino-penicillanic acid. The chemical structure of some important antibiotics is shown in Figure 6–1.

MECHANISM OF ACTION OF ANTIMICROBIAL DRUGS

Antimicrobial drugs are divided into two classes, based upon their general effects on bacterial populations.

1. *Bactericidal* drugs. These have a rapid lethal action. Examples are penicillin, streptomycin, the cephalosporins, polymyxin, and neomycin. In high concentrations erythromycin may be bactericidal.
2. *Bacteriostatic* drugs. These inhibit the growth of organisms. Examples are tetracyclines, sulfonamides, and chloramphenicol.

In practice this classification is not always clear-cut. Most drugs are, in varying degrees, both bactericidal and bacteriostatic. The way in which they act depends upon the drug, its concentration, and factors such as the kind, number, and growth state of the organism. For example, penicillin is strongly bactericidal against rapidly growing organisms but has little effect on organisms in a stationary state. Intracellular bacteria may be dormant in macrophages and thus are not destroyed by antimicrobial drugs.

INHIBITION OF GROWTH BY ANALOGUES

Sulfonamides

Unlike animal cells, for many bacteria para-aminobenzoic acid (PABA) is an essential metabolite in the synthesis of folic acid, which is required in the synthesis of purines. Sulfonamides are structural analogues of PABA and thus can compete with it, resulting in the formation of nonfunctional analogues of folic acid. Some bacteria, like some animal cells, cannot synthesize folic acid but require it for growth. These organisms are not inhibited by sulfonamides.

An excess of PABA will counteract the inhibiting action of sulfonamides, and for this reason PABA may be added to culture media. Another competitive inhibitor of PABA is para-aminosalicylic acid (PAS). It is used in conjunction with isoniazid or streptomycin in the treatment of tuberculosis.

Sulfonamides may be given with trimethoprim (which inhibits bacterial DNA synthesis) or other closely related compounds to produce sequential blocking that results in enhanced activity.

Trimethoprim + sulfadiazine (Tribrissen) has the following spectrum of activity:

Very Susceptible	Susceptible	Moderately Susceptible	Not Susceptible
Escherichia	Staphylococcus	Moraxella	Mycobacterium
Streptococcus	Neisseria	Nocardia	Leptospira
Proteus	Klebsiella	Brucella	Pseudomonas
Salmonella	Fusiformis		Erysipelothrix
Pasteurella	Corynebacterium		
Shigella	Clostridium		
	Bordetella		

INHIBITION OF CELL WALL SYNTHESIS

The peptidoglycan of bacterial cell walls is unique. Thus it is not surprising that a number of antimicrobial drugs that inhibit the synthesis of these glycopeptides are effective clinically. Synthesis of peptidoglycan is inhibited at several points, depending upon the drugs.

Penicillins

Penicillin inhibits the synthesis of cell walls of growing susceptible bacteria. The bacterial protoplasm increases and eventually bursts the cytoplasmic membrane, resulting in lysis and death. If the bacteria are growing in a medium of high osmotic tension, cell wall–deficient forms called protoplasts (gram-positive) or spheroplasts (gram-negative) with intact cytoplasmic membranes are formed. Penicillin inhibits the enzyme responsible for the cross-linking between the layers of peptidoglycan. Although penicillins are most active against the gram-positive organisms, they are also active against a number of gram-negative ones.

Of the different penicillins derived from *Penicillium*, only several are of value in treatment. Two that are widely used are penicillin G (benzylpenicillin), which is administered intramuscularly, and penicillin V (phenoxymethyl penicillin), which is resistant to acid decomposition and can therefore be given orally. Procaine is used in penicillin preparations to delay absorption.

Semisynthetic Penicillins

The origin of semisynthetic penicillins has been referred to previously. They have the important advantage of being resistant to the penicillin-destroying enzyme penicillinase (β-lactamase). Certain penicillins, e.g., cloxacillin and methicillin, can bind the penicillin-destroying enzyme β-lactamase produced by some gram-negative bacteria, e.g., *Pseudomonas aeruginosa.* Thus they can protect simultaneously administered hydrolyzable penicillins such as ampicillin from being destroyed. Ampicillin is acid-resistant and more active against gram-negative bacteria than the natural penicillins, but it is somewhat less active against gram-positive organisms. Carbenicillin has an even broader spectrum of activity against the gram-negative bacteria.

Although remarkably low in toxicity, the penicillins are occasionally allergenic.

Cephalosporins

The original antibiotics in this group were derived from a *Cephalosporium* mold. They have a nucleus that chemically resembles the nucleus of penicillin. Their mode of action is similar to that of penicillin, and they are bactericidal with low toxicity. They have the following characteristics: (1) resistance to penicillinase, (2) they are not as allergenic as penicillin, and (3) they have a broad spectrum of activity and can be used against staphylococci (including penicillin-resistant strains), streptococci—although enterococci are resistant—and a wide range of gram-negative bacteria.

Some of the oral cephalosporins in use are cephradine, cephaloglycin, cephalexin, and cefadroxil. Among the parenteral cephalosporins are cephaloridine, cephalothin, cephapirin, cephradine, cefoxitin, and cefamandole.

Many cephalosporins have been developed, a number of which are not available in the United States. The older cephalosporins (cephalothin, cefazolin, and cephalexin) are referred to as first generation cephalosporins. The more recently developed ones are referred to as second generation (cefoxitin, cefamadole, and cefaclor) and third generation (cefotaxime, cefoperazone, and cefmenoxime).

Cycloserine

This antibiotic recovered from a streptomycete is a structural analogue of D-alanine, and it interferes with the formation of the D-alanine-D-alanine portion of the cell wall pentapeptide. It is bactericidal, producing protoplasts that lyse.

Its antimicrobial spectrum is fairly broad, but its use is limited by its neurotoxic effects.

Bacitracin

Bacitracin is a polypeptide produced by a strain of *Bacillus subtilis.* It interacts with the bacterial cell membrane to prevent the transfer of structural cell wall units. It is bactericidal and acts principally against gram-positive organisms. High toxicity precludes its systemic use, but it is useful for topical application. It is often combined with such drugs as polymyxin and neomycin.

Vancomycin

This antibiotic is derived from a streptomycete. Its mode of action and spectrum of activity are similar to those of bacitracin. Although rather toxic (it may cause nerve deafness, thrombophlebitis, and kidney damage), it is used in emergencies to treat serious staphylococcal infections.

INHIBITION OF PROTEIN SYNTHESIS

Aminoglycosides

All drugs in this group of antibiotics, derived from *Streptomyces* species, have similar structures and modes of action. They bind to the smaller (30S) of the two ribosomal subunits, resulting in the miscoding of proteins and inhibition of peptide elongation.

Streptomycin. This drug is bactericidal and is active against gram-negative bacteria, mycobacteria, and some gram-positive organisms. Resistance to streptomycin is encountered frequently and may be caused by mutation or R factors. It is not absorbed from the gut and normally administered intramuscularly. When combined with tetracycline it is very useful in the treatment of brucellosis and plague.

Streptomycin sulfate has replaced the more toxic dihydrostreptomycin. Prolonged high blood levels of streptomycin can result in severe disturbances of hearing and vestibular function.

Neomycin and Kanamycin. These drugs are closely related structurally and have similar activity and complete cross-resistance. They are stable; both are poorly absorbed from the intestinal tract but readily absorbed if given intramuscularly. Both are excreted in the urine. Kanamycin is less toxic than neomycin and consequently is used systemically.

Both drugs are bactericidal for many gram-negative species. In animals neomycin is used most frequently to treat intestinal infections and bovine mastitis. Neomycin is also used with other drugs in topical preparations.

Both drugs may cause renal damage and nerve deafness.

Gentamicin. Gentamicin resembles neomycin and is mainly active against many gram-negative organisms, including *Pseudomonas aeruginosa*, and some gram-positive species. It is included in topical preparations with other drugs.

It may be nephrotoxic and ototoxic.

Tobramycin. Tobramycin resembles gentamicin chemically and pharmacologically.

Spectinomycin. This drug somewhat resembles the aminoglycosides in structure and site of action. It has been used mainly to treat gram-negative infections.

Amikacin. Amikacin is a derivative of kanamycin and resembles gentamicin. It is active against many gram-negative organisms that are resistant to tobramycin and gentamicin.

Tetracyclines

Drugs in this group are derived from streptomycetes. They act by binding to the 30S ribosomal subunit, causing inhibition of the function of tRNA. They are bacteriostatic and their mode of action is reversible. Trade names of the more common ones are tetracycline = Achromycin; chlortetracycline = Aureomycin; and oxytetracycline = Terramycin.

The tetracyclines are broad-spectrum antibiotics that are active against a wide range of gram-positive and gram-negative organisms, including rickettsiae, chlamydiae, and mycoplasmas. Organisms that are resistant to penicillin are often susceptible to the tetracyclines. Also, they are often of value in treating mixed infections. In animals they may be conveniently administered in feed or water.

Superinfection with *Candida albicans* or *Staphylococcus aureus* can be a complication after treatment with the tetracyclines. Although they are of relatively low toxicity, liver damage has been encountered in pregnant women administered the drugs, and it has been found that they may inhibit the growth of bones and teeth in the fetus and in infants. Long-term administration should be avoided in children and presumably in young animals.

Other drugs in this group are clomocycline, doxycycline, demeclocycline, and minocycline.

The antibacterial activity of drugs of the tetracycline group is similar, but they differ slightly in their rates of absorption and excretion.

Chloramphenicol (Chloromycetin)

This is a broad-spectrum drug derived from a streptomycete. It is bacteriostatic and acts by specifically binding to the larger 50S ribosomal subunit, thus inhibiting protein synthesis. It is a very effective drug in animals, although its use in food-producing animals is restricted in the United States. Because of potential toxicity, its use in humans should be reserved for serious infections such as typhoid fever.

In rare instances, prolonged administration results in severe or even fatal depression of bone marrow function.

Macrolides

Erythromycin, Lincomycin, and Clindamycin. These drugs, which are derived from streptomycetes, inhibit protein synthesis by binding to the 50S ribosomal subunit and are active against a number of gram-positive organisms and several gram-negative organisms that are penicillin-resistant. Clindamycin is useful in the treatment of some anaerobic infections caused by *Bacteroides*. The principal toxic effects encountered with erythromycin and clindamycin are minor gastrointestinal upsets. Erythromycin has been effective in treatment of *Mycoplasma* and *Campylobacter* infections.

Other drugs that closely resemble erythromycin are oleoandomycin and spiramycin.

Tylosin. This drug belongs in the macrolide family of antibiotics. It inhibits protein synthesis by preventing the translocation of the aminoacyl-tRNA on the 50S ribosomal subunit. It displays partial or complete cross-resistance with erythromycin. Tylosin is relatively water-insoluble and is administered in feed to treat intestinal infections (swine dysentery) and systemically for some gram-positive, gram-negative, and mycoplasmal infections, e.g., various pneumonias, chronic respiratory disease of chickens, and infectious sinusitis of turkeys.

IMPAIRMENT OF MEMBRANE FUNCTION

The polypeptide antibiotics polymyxin B and colistin (polymyxin E) are derived from *Bacillus polymyxa*. They damage the membranes of gram-negative species especially, resulting in a loss of osmotic control, with leakage of bacterial components and ultimately death. Polymyxin is poorly absorbed from the intestinal tract and is rather toxic (renal damage). Unlike most other bactericidal drugs, it kills resting as well as multiplying cells. It is reserved for serious infections such as those due to *Pseudomonas*. It is used with other antibiotics in topical preparations.

INHIBITION OF NUCLEIC ACID SYNTHESIS

Nalidixic Acid

This synthetic compound inhibits DNA synthesis without affecting RNA synthesis and is employed mainly for urinary infections caused by gram-negative bacteria.

Rifampin

This is a semisynthetic derivative of the *Streptomyces*-derived antibiotic rifamycin. It inhibits DNA-dependent RNA polymerase activity, which is responsible for the synthesis of cellular RNA. Rifampin is given orally and is active against a wide range of gram-positive and gram-negative bacteria, chlamydiae, and poxviruses. It has been used effectively in combination with other drugs in the treatment of tuberculosis.

Novobiocin

This drug, derived from a streptomycete, is readily absorbed from the intestinal tract, but its effectiveness is limited because of its binding to protein. It is bacteriostatic and acts by inhibiting the synthesis of DNA and teichoic acid at the cell membrane. Although active against gram-positive cocci and some gram-negative organisms *in vitro*, it is only used in combination with other drugs in the treatment of serious staphylococcal infections.

Frequent side-effects, such as impaired renal function, vomiting, and jaundice, are encountered in humans.

ADDITIONAL CHEMOTHERAPEUTIC AGENTS

The Nitrofuran Derivatives

These synthetic compounds are strongly bactericidal *in vitro* for many gram-positive and gram-negative bacteria. Most are very insoluble, and some, such as nitrofurazone, are used in topical preparations and also administered orally for the treatment of enteritis. Nitrofurantoin is absorbed after oral administration and excreted in the urine. In adequate doses it is effective in some urinary infections. This drug and related compounds are bound by blood, thus limiting their value for systemic use. The nitrofurans inhibit a variety of enzyme systems of bacteria but their primary mechanism of action is not known. They are widely used in veterinary practice, and little toxicity is encountered. Those used in animals are listed below.

Nitrofurazone (Furacin). Nitrofurazone is used as a topical agent and by the oral route to treat infectious enteritis in small and large animals.

Nitrofurantoin (Furadantin). This drug is available for intramuscular and oral use. It is absorbed from the intestinal tract and is used mainly to treat gram-negative urinary tract infections.

Furazolidone (Furoxone). Furazolidone is administered in feed and is used widely in poultry to treat salmonellosis, synovitis, and chronic respiratory disease (CRD). It is also used to treat infections caused by enterobacteria in animals, including enteritis of swine. It is not absorbed from the intestinal tract.

Nifuraldezone (Furamazone). This drug is administered orally and used in the treatment of enteritis in calves.

Mandelamine (Methenamine Mandelate)

Like nalidixic acid, this drug is used as a "urinary antiseptic." It is most useful to suppress bacteria in the urine of animals and in humans with chronic urinary tract infections. It requires a urinary pH lower than 5.5 to be effective. At this pH, it is hydrolyzed to ammonia and formaldehyde.

Sodium Arsanilate and Arsanilic Acid

These compounds are used in the treatment of swine dysentery. Their value may result from action against *Treponema hyodysenteriae*.

Ethambutol

This synthetic complex alcohol has tended to replace para-aminosalicylic acid (PAS) in the treatment of tuberculosis. It is active only against mycobacteria, and the mechanism of action is not known.

Isoniazid

This inexpensive, relatively nontoxic compound is very effective in the treatment of tuberculosis. It acts by inhibiting the synthesis of mycolic acids. There is some evidence that it may also be of value in the treatment of nocardial mastitis and actinobacillosis of cattle.

ANTIMYCOTIC AGENTS

These, including the polyene antibiotics such as amphotericin B and nystatin, are discussed in the section on fungal diseases.

SUSCEPTIBILITY TESTS

Two kinds of tests are carried out in the laboratory: the disc susceptibility test and the tube susceptibility procedure.

Disc Susceptibility Test

Resistant strains are now so prevalent that it is recommended that all clinical isolates be tested for susceptibility.

The plate or disc procedure is routinely used in veterinary diagnostic laboratories (Fig. 6–2). It involves the uniform inoculation of a plate containing a suitable medium with a standardized amount of organism of the culture to be tested. Paper discs impregnated with the various antimicrobial drugs are then applied, appropriately spaced with a dispenser. After incubation, usually for 24 hours, the size of the zones of inhibition is estimated or measured, and based upon values that have been established, a culture is reported as being susceptible or resistant. Some laboratories report zones between susceptible and resistant as intermediate.

Most laboratories are now using the Kirby-Bauer procedure, which employs high potency discs and Mueller-Hinton agar in large Petri dishes. The zones of inhibition described as susceptible, intermediate, and resistant relate to blood concentration and therapeutic efficacy in humans. Mueller-Hinton agar is free of para-aminobenzoic acid. If PABA is present in the medium, it will inactivate or inhibit the activity of the sulfonamide disc, thus yielding an erroneous result. PABA should only be used in media for isolation purposes.

Direct susceptibility tests employing clinical material such as pus and urine as inocula are not recommended. The inoculum is not standardized and may contain several different organisms.

Appropriate modifications in the routine Kirby-Bauer procedure are made for fastidious organisms, mycoplasmas, and anaerobes. To grow such organisms as *Haemophilus* species, *Corynebacterium pyogenes*, and some streptococci, blood, serum, and yeast extract may have to be added.

The Tube Susceptibility Test

This procedure is more involved than the disc susceptibility test and is only rarely carried out in veterinary diagnostic laboratories. The aim of the test is to determine the *minimum inhibitory concentration* (MIC) of the drug. This is accomplished by adding a standardized inoculum of organisms (pure culture) to a series of tubes containing increasing concentrations of the drug being tested (Fig. 6–3). After incubation, the results are recorded. The MIC is defined as the highest dilution (i.e., the least amount of the drug) preventing growth. For the drug to be effective clinically, the MIC must be well below the peak blood concentration of the drug expected under normal dosage schemes.

The minimum bactericidal concentration (MBC) can be determined by plating loopfuls from the three successive tubes not showing evidence of growth onto a suitable agar medium. The plate showing no growth indicates the tube with no growth and thus the MBC.

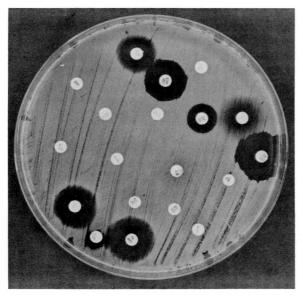

Figure 6–2. Disc susceptibility test. The antimicrobial agents incorporated in the discs diffuse into the agar, inhibiting the bacterial growth (clear zones).

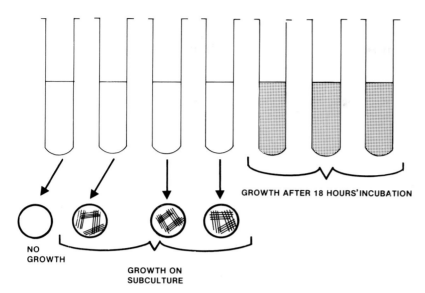

GROWTH AFTER 18 HOURS' INCUBATION

NO GROWTH

GROWTH ON SUBCULTURE

Figure 6–3. Tube susceptibility test for determining the minimum inhibitory concentration (MIC). Those tubes without evidence of growth (turbidity) are plated out to determine the minimum bactericidal concentration (MBC).

MINIMUM INHIBITORY CONCENTRATION = 12.5 µg/ml

MINIMUM BACTERICIDAL CONCENTRATION = 50 µg/ml

MIC's are not commonly conducted in veterinary diagnostic laboratories, but the availability of automated instruments for the performance of MIC's may hasten their use in the larger laboratories.

Serum Bactericidal Test

This is essentially the same as the MIC test except that the drug is present in the patient's serum. This test is rarely carried out in veterinary laboratories. The standardized inoculum of organisms is added to the dilutions of serum. After incubation, the test is read and the *minimum bactericidal concentration* (MBC) is defined as the highest dilution of serum that prevents growth.

DRUG RESISTANCE

Many organisms have the ability to produce mutants that are resistant to most of the drugs they would ordinarily be susceptible to in the wild state. The use of subinhibitory levels of antibiotics contributes to the survival and multiplication of resistant mutants. The amount of resistance and the time it takes to develop depend upon the organism and the drug.

Some organisms, such as *Streptococcus agalactiae* and other pyogenic streptococci, lack the capacity to produce resistant mutants. The development of resistance by *Staphylococcus aureus* in response to penicillin and the tetracyclines is usually slow, occurring in small steps over a considerable period of time and exposure. On the other hand, resistance of the tubercle bacillus to streptomycin may develop to a high level in a single step-wise manner.

Resistance is specific in that an organism will become resistant to a particular antibiotic. Cross-resistance only occurs among closely related drugs such as the different tetracyclines, aminoglycosides, and so forth. Resistance to one drug may be followed by resistance to another drug, and thus strains emerge that are resistant to a number of drugs. Besides this type of chromosomal resistance, multiple drug resistance due to R factors is encountered. This is referred to briefly further on and in detail in the chapter on Bacterial Genetics.

MECHANISMS OF DRUG RESISTANCE

Some of the mechanisms of drug resistance that are known are:

1. Adoption by the organism of an alternative metabolic pathway in order to bypass the inhibited reaction, e.g., those bacteria resistant to sulfonamides adapt to using preformed folic acid.
2. Production of an enzyme that destroys the antibiotic, e.g., penicillinase (β-lactamase)

from *Staphylococcus aureus;* or production of enzymes by some bacteria that inactivate drugs by acetylation, adenylation, or phosphorylation.

3. Change in permeability or decreased uptake of the drug by the cell or some special part of the cell, e.g., such as occurs in tetracyclines and polymyxins.
4. Altered structural target for the drug, e.g., erythromycin-resistant organisms have an altered protein on the 40S subunit of the bacterial ribosome.

DEVELOPMENT OF RESISTANCE DURING TREATMENT

Mutation

Resistant mutants may emerge during treatment. The occurrence and establishment of resistant mutants vary with different drugs. Selection of mutants is favored by underdosage, prolonged administration, and the presence of a "closed" focus of infection such as is found in an abscess.

The drugs are grouped below roughly according to the likelihood that resistant mutants will emerge during treatment.

Frequent: sulfonamides, streptomycin, nalidixic acid, rifamycin.

Moderately frequent: erythromycin.

Infrequent: tetracyclines, penicillin, cephalosporins, chloramphenicol, nitrofurans.

Superinfection

This term is frequently used to describe the infection that develops and is caused by "alien" organisms such as *Candida albicans* as a result of the alteration or suppression of the normal flora by prolonged antibiotic administration. The disturbance of the normal flora in animals does not ordinarily cause more than occasional intestinal upsets and diarrhea. However, prolonged administration of antibiotics affecting gram-negative intestinal organisms may cause a deficiency or diminution in the amounts of vitamin K, biotin, riboflavin, pantothenate, and pyridoxine available to the host. Supplementation with vitamins, particularly vitamin B complex, is used in humans.

The term is also used to describe the replacement of the original infecting agent with a new strain of the same species that is resistant, or a resistant strain of another species. *Pseudomonas* *aeruginosa* and *Acinetobacter* are not infrequently encountered as "replacement" strains.

Infectious Drug Resistance

Transferable multiple drug resistance due to R factors occurs most commonly in members of the Enterobacteriaceae. This type of resistance, i.e., the whole multiple pattern, is transferable among strains of the same species and among strains of different closely related species, e.g., from a *Salmonella* to an *Escherichia coli.* Transfer of this kind can be readily demonstrated *in vitro* and no doubt also occurs *in vivo.* It is now very widespread, and strains are commonly encountered that are resistant to as many as four drugs, e.g., streptomycin, a tetracycline, penicillin, and a sulfonamide. It seems likely that the great increase in infectious drug resistance has resulted from the practice of routinely adding antibiotics to animal feeds.

SUGGESTIONS ON THE USE OF ANTIMICROBIAL DRUGS

The suggestions that follow are based in part on those provided by Thomas.* When selecting and using antimicrobial drugs, the possibility of the emergence of resistant organisms should always be kept in mind.

1. They should not be employed for mild, inconsequential infections. The harm done through possibly selecting out resistant organisms may outweigh the benefit derived from treatment.
2. They should only be used prophylactically for individuals and in contact animals if a real risk of severe infection exists, as, for example, in blackleg in cattle or fowl cholera.
3. One should not be less thorough in surgical asepsis or in the control of cross-infection, because of the availability of many antibiotics.
4. Treatment should be based on a definite clinical and microbiologic diagnosis. Although treatment may have to be started before the laboratory report is received, it should be modified if indicated.
5. The laboratory report is not a directive for treatment. The choice of the best drug to use should be made after considering a

---

*Thomas, C.G.A.: Medical Microbiology. 5th Ed. London, Balliere Tindall, 1983.

Table 6–1. Guide to the Selection of Antimicrobial Drugs in the Absence of Susceptibility Tests

Organism	First-Choice Drugs	Alternative Drugs
Pyogenic streptococci	Penicillin	Ampicillin, erythromycin, cephalosporins
Staphylococcus aureus	Penicillin Synthetic penicillins: methicillin, cloxacillin	Erythromcyin, cephalosporins
Clostridia	Penicillin	Tetracyclines, erythromycin
Erysipelothrix rhusiopathiae	Penicillin	Tetracyclines, erythromycin
Listeria monocytogenes	Penicillin, ampicillin, tetracyclines	Chloramphenicol
Corynebacteria	Penicillin, erythromycin	Tetracyclines, erythromycin
Nocardia asteroides	Sulfadiazine, sulfisoxazole	Tetracyclines, streptomycin
Actinomyces bovis *A. viscosus*	Penicillin, sulfonamides	Erythromycin, tetracyclines
Enterobacteriaceae in general *Escherichia coli* *Salmonella* spp. *Proteus* spp.	Neomycin, tetracyclines, chloramphenicol, ampicillin	Cephalosporins, streptomycin
Pasteurella multocida	Tetracyclines, penicillin	Sulfonamides, erythromycin, ampicillin
Pasteurella haemolytica	Tetracyclines	Sulfonamides, erythromycin, chloramphenicol
Haemophilus spp.	Ampicillin	Tetracyclines, cephalosporins, sulfonamides
Bordetella bronchiseptica	Sulfonamides, erythromycin	Tetracyclines
Pseudomonas aeruginosa	Gentamicin, tobramycin	Carbenicillin
Treponema hyodysenteriae	Tylosin, arsanilic acid, sodium arsanilate	Lincomycin, streptomycin, tetracyclines
Mycoplasmas	Tylosin, tetracyclines, erythromycin	
Campylobacter spp.	Streptomycin with or without penicillin	Tetracyclines
Acinetobacter spp.	Kanamycin	Gentamicin, polymyxin
Bacteroides spp.	Penicillin, clindamycin, chloramphenicol	Tetracyclines, ampicillin
Fusobacterium necrophorum	Penicillin	Tetracyclines, sulfonamides
Actinobacillus equuli *A. lignieresii*	Streptomycin, tetracyclines	Erythromycin
Leptospires	Penicillin, streptomycin	Tetracyclines, erythromycin

Table 6–2. Antimicrobials for Routine Susceptibility Testing*

	Small Animal	Large Animal	Mastitis	Anaerobes
Ampicillin	+†	+	+	+
Carbenicillin				+
Cephalothin	+	+	+	+
Clindamycin (lincomycin)	+	+		+
Chloramphenicol	+	+	+	+
Erythromycin			+	+
Furaltadone			+	
Gentamicin	+	+	+	
Kanamycin			+	
Neomycin	+	+		
Nitrofurantoin	+			
Nitrofurazone		+		
Novobiocin			+	
Oxacillin			+	
Penicillin	+	+	+	+
Polymyxin B	+	+		
Streptomycin		+	+	
Sulfachloropyridazine		+		
Sulfadimethoxine	+			
Trimethoprim + Sulfa	+			
Tetracycline	+	+	+	+

*(From Carter, G.R., Diagnostic Procedures in Veterinary Bacteriology and Mycology. 4th Ed. 1984, p. 392. Reprinted by permission of Charles C Thomas, Publisher, Springfield, Illinois.)
† + = should be tested.

Table 6–3. Group, Action, and Primary Spectrum of Important Antimicrobial Drugs

	Family	Action		Primary Spectrum		
		Static	Cidal	Gram negative	Gram positive	
Ampicillin	Penicillin	−	+	+	+	Inhibit cell wall synthesis
Carbenicillin		−	+	+	−	
Cloxacillin		−	+	−	+	
Methicillin		−	+	−	+	
Nafcillin		−	+	−	+	
Oxacillin		−	+	−	+	
Penicillin G		−	+	−	+	
Gentamicin	Aminoglycoside	−	+	+	−	Inhibition of ribosomal function (protein synthesis)
Kanamycin		−	+	+	+	
Neomycin		−	+	+	+	
Streptomycin		−	+	+	+	
Erythromycin	Macrolide	+	−	−	+	Inhibition of ribosomal function (protein synthesis)
Oleandomycin		+	−	−	+	
Tylosin		+	−	+	+	
Bacitracin	Polypeptide	−	+	−	+	Inhibition of cell wall synthesis; impairment of membrane function
Polymyxin B		−	+	+	−	
Colistin		−	+	+	−	
Vancomycin	Glycopeptide	−	+	−	+	
Cephalothin	Cephalosporin	−	+	+	+	Inhibition of cell wall synthesis
Cephalexin		−	+	+	+	
Cephaloridine		−	+	+	+	
Sulfadiazine	Sulfonamide	+	−	+	+	Competitive inhibition preventing folic acid formation
Sulfamerazine		+	−	+	+	
Sulfadimethoxine (Madribon)		+	−	+	+	
Sulfasoxazole (Gantrisin)		+	−	+	+	
Chloramphenicol		+	−	+	+	Inhibition of ribosomal function
Tetracyclines (Oxy, chloro, etc.)	Tetracycline	+	−	+	+	Inhibits ribosomal function
Rifampin	Rifamycin	+	−	−	+	Interferes with RNA synthesis
Nitrofurantoin	Nitrofurans	−	+	+	+	Mechanism uncertain
Nalidixic acid		+	−	+	−	Inhibits DNA polymerase
Methenamine mandelate		−	+	+	+	Liberates formaldehyde in acid urine
Paraamino salicylic acid		+	−	Mycobacteria		Mechanism uncertain

number of factors. In general it is poor practice to use a broad-spectrum antibiotic if the infecting agent is sensitive to a more specific one. All antimicrobial drugs are potentially toxic and some are actually dangerous, so very serious consideration should be given to their administration.

6. When antimicrobial drugs are administered, they should be given in full therapeutic doses for an adequate period. This will vary with the disease. The period ordinarily should not be less than 3 to 5 days, but in some diseases such as nocardiosis, treatment will have to be continued for weeks. However, because of the danger of superinfection, the use of some drugs such as the tetracyclines should not be unnecessarily prolonged. If there is no response or poor response to treatment, it is possible that a resistant population of organisms has developed. In such cases specimens should be forwarded to the laboratory for additional susceptibility testing. Special attention may have to be given to animals in whom abscesses and mixed infections are involved.

7. In some instances it is advisable to consider the simultaneous use of two drugs. Only

drugs that act synergistically should be given together.

8. As a general rule, only those antimicrobial drugs that are not suitable for systemic use should be used topically or locally. This reduces the likelihood of the development of drug allergy and reserves the use of systemic drugs for serious infections.

9. There are regulations setting various withdrawal times for different microbial drugs prior to slaughter. These vary from 24 hours to 30 days and must be taken into account in the selection of drugs for treatment.

Table 6–1 is provided to assist in the selection of antimicrobial agents in the absence of susceptibility tests. Table 6–2 lists antimicrobials for routine susceptibility testing. Table 6–3 summarizes information on the action and spectrum of major groups of drugs.

COMBINATIONS OF ANTIMICROBIAL AGENTS

In some circumstances, such as the inaccessibility of the infecting agent, mixed infections, and very serious unresponsive infections, it may be advantageous to use a combination of two drugs that act synergistically. The combinations that are generally synergistic consist of pairs of drugs that are bactericidal, e.g., penicillin and streptomycin. Antagonism is usually observed when a bactericidal drug such as penicillin, which kills rapidly multiplying organisms, is used with a bacteriostatic drug such as a tetracycline. Although they are bacteriostatic, the

sulfonamides do not appear to antagonize penicillin, perhaps because their action is slow. Because the bactericidal action of polymyxin is exerted on resting cells as well as on multiplying cells, it is not antagonized by bacteriostatic drugs.

In treating mixed infections with two drugs, it is advisable to select drugs that have rather different spectra of activity, thus broadening the overall antibacterial spectrum. The simultaneous use of two drugs has the following theoretical advantage. Considering the rate of mutation of bacteria to resistance, the probability of an organism's becoming resistant to two antimicrobial drugs being used for treatment is very low. When three drugs are used, as for example in the treatment of tuberculosis, the probability of a mutant's emerging that is resistant to all three drugs is extremely low.

SOURCES FOR FURTHER READING

Balows, A. (ed.): Current Techniques for Antibiotic Susceptibility Testing. Springfield, Il, Charles C Thomas, 1974.

Eisenberg, M.S., Furukawa, C., and Ray, G.G.: Manual of Antimicrobial Therapy and Infectious Diseases. Philadelphia, W.B. Saunders Company, 1980.

Garrod, L.P., Lampert, H.P., and O'Grady, F.: Antibiotic and Chemotherapy. 5th Ed. London, Churchill Livingstone, 1976.

Klastersky, J. (ed.): Clinical Use of Combinations of Antibiotics. New York, John Wiley & Sons, 1975.

Lorian, V. (ed.): Antibiotics in Laboratory Medicine. Baltimore, Williams & Wilkins, 1980.

Pratt, W.B.: Chemotherapy of Infection. New York, Oxford University Press, 1977.

Smith, H.: Antibiotics in Clinical Practice. 3rd Ed. Baltimore, University Park Press, 1977.

Smith, I.M., Donata, S.T., and Rabinovitch, S.: Antibiotics and Infections. Flushing, NJ, Spectrum Publishing, Inc., 1974.

7

Sterilization and Disinfection

Sterilization and disinfection are of great importance to the practicing veterinarian. The sterilization of dressings, surgical instruments, and syringes is a commonplace procedure, as is the disinfection of kennels, infected premises, and contaminated footwear. So that such operations can be carried out effectively, an understanding of the general principles of sterilization, disinfection, and antisepsis is necessary.

Sterilization. This is the process whereby all viable microorganisms are eliminated or destroyed. The criterion of sterilization is the failure of the organisms to grow if a growth-supporting medium is supplied. The limiting requirement of sterilization is destruction of the bacterial spore, the most resistant form of microbial life.

Disinfection. Disinfection involves the destruction of pathogenic organisms associated with inanimate objects, usually by physical or chemical means. All disinfectants are effective against the vegetative forms of organisms but not necessarily against their spores.

Antisepsis. Antisepsis involves the inactivation or destruction by chemical means of microbes associated with the animal. Antiseptics may be bactericidal or bacteriostatic; the former state is irreversible, but the latter is reversible. For ordinary purposes, the terms disinfectant and antiseptic are used synonymously.

PHYSICAL AGENTS

Moist Heat

Heat is used to destroy microorganisms in four different ways.

Boiling

Boiling water or steam (common instrument sterilizer) at 100°C is widely used in veterinary practice for preparing syringes, needles, and instruments for minor surgery. This process kills vegetative forms of microorganisms and viruses in five minutes. Many spores are also killed at 100°C in this same period, but many of the more resistant ones, e.g., those of *Clostridium tetani* and the common *Bacillus* species, can survive boiling for as long as several hours. It is thus apparent that although boiling will kill most pathogenic bacteria, it is not sterilization as the term is defined. If boiling is used, it should be continued for no less than 10 minutes.

Steam Under Pressure (Autoclave)

The most resistant spores are killed by a temperature of 121°C for 15 minutes. This temperature is obtained at sea level by steam at a pressure at 15 lb/in² in excess of atmospheric pressure. The autoclave, which is a metal cylinder designed to contain steam under pressure, is an essential piece of equipment in microbiology laboratories and operating rooms. Many veterinarians have small autoclaves for the sterilization of instruments, dressings, solutions, and surgical packs. In order to obtain a temperature of 121°C, all air must first be blown out. In the large, modern, high-vacuum autoclaves, 98% of the air is removed by a powerful pump. Air is removed in two stages in the downward-displacement autoclaves. Steam is admitted at the top of the chamber and residual air is driven out at the bottom.

The killing power of steam is attributable to the fact that when it condenses on the item being sterilized, it liberates a large amount of latent heat. The shrinkage resulting from condensation—a thin film of moisture on the surface of the load—draws in fresh steam and thus more heat. This proccess continues and the steam penetrates and surrounds the various items, producing a high uniform temperature.

The following points should be kept in mind when using the office autoclave:

1. Air and condensate must be removed for effective sterilization.
2. The required temperature of 121°C must be maintained.
3. All mechanisms such as gauges and timers must be in proper working order.
4. Packs should be properly prepared. They should not be too large nor should the wrappings be impervious. Volumes of fluid should not be too large. The load should be arranged to allow for penetration of steam.
5. The effectiveness of the autoclave can be tested by affixing heat-sensitive tape to the packs being sterilized. Paper strips impregnated with spores of *Bacillus stearothermophilus* can also be used to test the autoclave. If the autoclave is functioning effectively, the spores will be killed.

The high-vacuum autoclaves used in clinics and hospitals should be operated strictly according to directions provided by the manufacturer. Pressures, temperatures, and times of each sterilization cycle must be recorded, and routine checks must be made of temperatures and sterilizing effectiveness.

Steaming (Tyndallization)

This process has largely been replaced by filtration. It involves placing the media or solutions in flowing steam for one hour on each of three successive days. The period between steaming allows the spores to germinate and thus be killed at the next exposure. Tyndallization depends upon the medium or solution's being sufficiently nutritious to promote germination of spores in the intervals between steaming. Bacteriologic media qualify in this respect.

Pasteurization

This process, which involves the heating of milk to the point that all potential human path-

ogens are killed, has greatly reduced the incidence of brucellosis and tuberculosis in humans over the years. The occasional outbreaks of group A (*Streptococcus pyogenes*) streptococcal disease spread by milk have also been eliminated.

In the slow method of pasteurization, milk is held at 63°C for 30 minutes and in the flash method at 72°C for 15 seconds. A few heat-resistant vegetative bacteria (thermophiles) and spores survive. The milk is rapidly cooled after pasteurization to discourage growth of the remaining viable organisms.

RADIATION

Ultraviolet Light

Direct sunlight kills unprotected vegetative organisms fairly rapidly, but spores are resistant. The bactericidal activity of sunlight is due to the ultraviolet portion of the spectrum. Glass is impervious to this radiation. Sunshine is no doubt of great importance in the destruction of pathogenic organisms contaminating fields, pastures, and other areas used by livestock.

Ultraviolet light from mercury lamps is widely used in inoculating hoods, operating theaters, animal quarters, and other areas to reduce airborne infections. Ultraviolet radiation acts by causing errors in the replication of DNA. Its mutagenic activity on living cells is well known.

Ionizing Radiation

This form of radiation has a much higher energy content than ultraviolet light and consequently has a strong disinfectant action. Gamma rays emitted from cobalt-60 are used commercially to sterilize disposable syringes, needles, pipettes, surgical sutures, dressings, bone grafts, plastic arterial prostheses, catheters, plastic Petri dishes, and other heat-sensitive items. Unfortunately when ionizing radiation is used on foods, flavors may be affected, and when it is used on items such as drugs, hormones, and enzymes, potency may be reduced.

FILTRATION

Filtration has been used for decades to sterilize bacteriologic media, serum, injection solutions, and other solutions containing heat-sensitive substances. A pore size of 0.45 μm or less will remove all bacteria from solutions. Of the several different filters that have evolved over the years, the most widely used at present are the sintered glass, the cellulose acetate film (Gelman, Millipore), and the asbestos or Seitz filter. The porosities of these filters range from 0.22 μm to 10 μm. The coarse sizes are used for clarification prior to using the smaller pore sizes. Those filters commonly used to remove bacteria do not hold back viruses or mycoplasmas.

CHEMICAL AGENTS

Chemical agents act more selectively on microorganisms than do the physical agents such as heat and radiation. In this discussion emphasis will be placed upon the antiseptics and disinfectants that are now in current use by veterinarians. The goal should be the selection of the best agent for a particular situation and task.

In assessing an antiseptic or disinfectant, Thomas* has listed the following important considerations:

1. *Organisms killed.* Spores are highly resistant compared with vegetative forms, and only a few disinfectants, e.g., halogens, mercuric chloride, formalin, and ethylene oxide, are effective in the concentrations usually used. Mycobacteria are more resistant than most other vegetative organisms. Phenolic and alcoholic compounds are recommended for this group. Generally speaking viruses are more resistant than vegetative bacteria. Halogens, oxidizing agents, and formalin are active against many viruses. Quaternary compounds and dyes are not.

2. *Organisms inhibited.* Organisms should be killed rather than merely inhibited. The quaternary compounds employed in high dilutions are bacteriostatic rather than bactericidal. Agents such as formaldehyde, ethylene oxide, and chlorine are clearly bactericidal.

3. *Rate of action.* There is a great difference in the rate of action among the various chemical agents. Some act rapidly, while others are completely effective only after some minutes or even hours. Disinfectants have an optimum pH range, and all are more active at higher temperatures. Growing and multiplying cells are more readily poi-

soned than those in a resting or stationary state. All disinfectants are to some extent inhibited in their activity by organic matter such as that found in feces, pus, exudates, discharges, and blood. Mercury salts, halogens, and quaternaries are especially inhibited by organic matter. In the disinfection of premises, stables, and kennels, the power of penetration of dirt, grease, and organic matter is important. Soaps and surface active agents assist penetration.

4. *Side-effects.* Other limiting considerations are toxicity, possession of an irritating vapor, undesirable staining properties, and destructive effects on instruments and fabrics. Antiseptics or disinfectants used on or around animals should be relatively nontoxic to tissues.

5. *Additional considerations.* Disinfectants should be reasonable in price and maintain their potency for long periods of time. They should be soluble in water and stable in aqueous solution.

The Phenol Coefficient

This value expresses the capacity of a disinfectant to kill bacteria when compared with phenol. In the official test a broth culture is diluted 1:10 with different concentrations of the test compound. The end point is the lowest concentration that yields sterile loopful samples after incubation for 10 minutes at 20°C. The compound is generally recommended for use at five times this concentration. For example, a phenol coefficient may be stated to be 40, which means its killing power is 40 times that of phenol. The two organisms used in the official test are *Salmonella typhi* (gram-negative) and *Staphylococcus aureus* (gram-positive).

Although of some value the phenol coefficient does not take into account such considerations as toxicity for tissues, inactivation by organic matter, corrosive properties, and other factors relating to particular situations.

MAJOR GROUPS OF CHEMICAL DISINFECTANTS*

Some of the properties of the common classes of disinfectants are listed in Table 7–1.

---

*Thomas, C.G.A.: Medical Microbiology. 5th Ed. London, Balliere Tindall, 1983.

*Modified from Wilson, M.E., and Mizer, H.E.: Microbiology in Patient Care. 2nd Ed. New York, Macmillan, 1974.

Table 7–1. *Some Properties of the Common Class of Disinfectants**

Disinfectant Class	Quaternary Ammonium Compounds	Phenolics	Sodium Hypochlorite	Iodophors	Glutaraldehyde	Chlorhexidine
Example	Roccal	Staphene	Clorox	Betadine Solution	Cidex	Nolvasan
Property:						
Bactericidal	+ +	+ +	+ +	+ + +	+ + +	+ +
General virucide	−	−	+ + +	+ + +	+ + +	−
Lipophilic or lipophilic-like viruses	+ + +	+ + +	+ + +	+ +	+ + +	+ + +
Sporocidal at room temperature	−	−	−	+	+ +	−
Fungicidal	+ +	+ + +	+ + +	+ + +	+ + +	+ +
Effective in the presence of organic material	+ +	+ + +	+	+ +	+ + +	+ +
Effective in the presence of soaps	−	+ + +	+ +	+ +	+ + +	−
Effective in hard water	+	+ + +	+ +	+ +	+ + +	+ +
Most effective pH range	alkaline	neutral	acid	neutral	alkaline	alkaline

+ + + = High activity; + + = moderate activity; + = slight activity; − = no activity.
*(Adapted from Kowalski, J.J., and Mallmann, W.L.: Is your disinfection practice effective? J. Am. An. Hosp. Assoc., *9:3*, 1973.)

GROUP: SOLUBLE ALCOHOLS

Ethyl (C_2H_5OH),
Isopropyl ($CH_3CHOHCH_3$)

Mode of Action. Protein coagulation and dissolution of membrane lipids.

Dilution. 70–90%.

Recommended for. Thermometers (add 0.2–1% iodine); instruments; skin preparations; hands; spot disinfection.

Advantages. Rapidly bactericidal; tuberculocidal.

Limitations. Not sporicidal; corrodes metals unless reducing agent added (e.g., 2% sodium nitrite); drying to skin (1:200 cetyl alcohol may be used as emollient); bleaches rubber tile.

GROUP: STERILIZING GASES

Ethylene oxide

Mode of Action. Substitution of the cell alkyl groups for labile hydrogen atoms.

Proprietary Products. Carboxide, Cryoxide, Steroxide.

Dilution. Gas; exposure time 4–18 hours.

Recommended for. Blankets, pillows, mattresses; lensed instruments; rubber goods, thermolabile plastics; books; papers.

Advantages. Harmless to most materials; sterilizes.

Limitations. Requires special equipment.

GROUP: DISINFECTANT GAS

Formaldehyde

Mode of Action. Same as ethylene oxide.

Proprietary Product. Bard-Parker Formaldehyde Germicide.

Dilution. Gas, or full-strength solution.

Recommended for. Gas: cabinet and incubator disinfection; solution: transfer forceps, instrument soak.

Advantages. Vapor disinfection of delicate instruments; sporicidal, noncorrosive.

Limitations. Requires long period for effective disinfection; odorous; toxic to skin and mucous membranes.

GROUP: HALOGENS

Chlorines
Iodines

Mode of Action. Inactivate by oxidizing free sulfhydryl groups.

Chlorines. Hypochlorites or hydrochlorous acid derivates (HClO)

Proprietary Products. Hypochlorites such as Clorox, Purex, and other bleaches; HClO: Warexin.

Use Dilution. Hypochlorites: strongest concentration recommended by manufacturers; if dry, mix to thin paste. Warexin used in 1.5% aqueous solution.

Recommended for. Floors, plumbing fixtures; spot disinfection; fabrics not harmed by bleaching; Warexin for dishes but not silverware.

Advantages. Tuberculocidal unless highly diluted (Warexin limited).

Limitations. Bleach fabrics; corrode metals; unstable in hard water; must be freshly prepared; tarnish silver.

Iodines. Tincture or aqueous solution (2 to 5%); iodophors.

Proprietary Products. Wescodyne; Betadine; Iobac; Klenzade; Micro-Klene; Virac.

Dilution. Tincture: full strength. Wescodyne: 75 ppm (90 ml or 3 oz to 5 gal water), or 450 ppm to kill tubercle bacilli; tincture = 10% Wescodyne in 50% ethyl alcohol. Other iodophors: see manufacturer's recommendations.

Recommended for. Tincture: skin preparations; thermometers (see Soluble Alcohols). Wescodyne: thermometers, utensils, rubber goods, dishes; as a tincture, used for spot disinfection, or for single presurgical scrub. Betadine: presurgical skin preparation. Others: many designed for specific purposes, including milking and dairy operations, e.g., Iosan.

Advantages. Iodophors are cleaning and disinfecting; nonstaining; leave residual antibacterial effect; and are tuberculocidal as tinctures. Loss of germicidal activity is indicated by fading color.

Limitations. Tincture of iodine stains and is irritating to tissues. Iodophors are somewhat unstable and are inactivated by hard water; may corrode metals; drying to skin as tinctures.

GROUP: PHENOLICS

Saponated Creosol
Semi-synthetic Phenols
Mode of Action. Protein coagulation. They destroy selective permeability of cell membranes, resulting in leakage of cell constituents.

Proprietary Products. Synthetics: Amphyl, Lysol, O-Syl, Staphene, Vesphene, Tergisyl, Armisol.

Dilution. Creosol, 2% for 30 minutes; 5% if hard water. Amphyl, 0.5 to 1% (also available as spray). Lysol, 1%. O-Syl, 2.5%. Staphene, 0.5 to 2%. Vesphene, 1 to 2%. Tergisyl, 2%.

Recommended for. Creosol: equipment, linen, excreta. Amphyl: instruments. Lysol: laundry rinse for blankets, linens. O-Syl, Staphene, Vesphene: floors, walls, equipment. Tergisyl, Armisol: environmental uses.

Advantages. Not inactivated by organic matter, soap, or hard water (except creosol); residual effect if allowed to dry on surfaces; high detergency.

Limitations. Creosol must be used in soft water and is slow-acting; Lysol and creosol both have odors that may be objectionable.

GROUP: QUATERNARY AMMONIUM COMPOUNDS

Cationic Detergents
Mode of Action. See under Detergents.
Proprietary Products. Zephiran, Roccal, and many others.
Dilution. 1:1000–1:5000 aqueous.
Recommended for. Cleaning and disinfection of instruments, utensils, and rubber goods; also for milking and dairy operations. Instrument soak (except for those with cemented lenses), lacquered catheters, synthetic rubber goods, and aluminum instruments.
Advantages. Bland.
Limitations. Not tuberculocidal; limited viricidal activity; must be diluted with distilled water; is inactivated by protein, soap, and cellulose fibers.

GROUP: SOAP OR DETERGENT ADDITIVES

Anionic Detergents
Because of recent restrictions in use, formulations of products listed may be altered.
Mode of Action. See under Detergents.
Hexachlorophene (G-11). *Tetrachlorosalicylanilide.*
Proprietary Products. Hexachlorophene: Bar soaps—Gamophen. Liquid detergents—Septisol, pHisoHex, Hex-O-San, Surofene. Hand creams—Septisol antiseptic skin cream. Tetrachlorosalicylanilide: Bar soap—Coleo, Dial.
Dilution. Septisol, 2%, pHisoHex, 3%; others as recommended by manufacturer.
Recommended for. Skin disinfection, but note limitations.
Advantages. Good cleansers and have prolonged antibacterial action.
Limitations. Not sporicidal, not tuberculocidal, have slow action; toxic if used continuously and absorbed into the body in increasing quantities (especially through delicate skin of infants); should be rinsed off after use on skin.

ADDITIONAL DISINFECTANTS

Salts. Organic mercury compounds such as mercurochrome and thiomersal are less toxic

8

General Procedures for the Bacteriologic and Mycologic Examination of Clinical Specimens

The term "clinical specimens" denotes those materials, e.g., tissues, blood, urine, skin scrapings, and body fluids, taken from animals for diagnostic purposes. In the diagnosis of microbial diseases it is imperative that such materials reach the diagnostic laboratory with as little change as possible from their original state. The suspension of microbial reproduction is accomplished by maintaining the specimens at refrigerator temperature until they reach the laboratory. On occasion, it may be advisable to freeze specimens.

The diagnostic microbiology laboratory can function most effectively when the correct specimens are selected and properly submitted. Most diagnostic laboratories supply veterinary practitioners with instructions on the selection, packing, and shipment of specimens. The submission form provides space for information on the origin and nature of the specimen, the clinical history, and the disease or diseases suspected.

Just prior to death of the animal and shortly thereafter, a number of intestinal bacteria may invade the host's tissues. The significance of these organisms, some of which are potential pathogens, is difficult to assess when tissues have been taken even a short time after death. Live, sick animals presented for necropsy are usually the best source of specimens. In all instances, the importance of fresh tissues taken as soon as possible after death cannot be overemphasized.

In order to underscore the importance of the correct selection and submission of clinical specimens, some instructions relating to particular diseases are provided.

SPECIMENS FOR BACTERIOLOGIC AND MYCOLOGIC EXAMINATIONS

Preservation and Shipment of Tissues and Organs. Place tissues in plastic bags or leak-proof jars. Portions of intestines should be packed separately. Specimens can be conveniently shipped in a Styrofoam box or ice chest containing a generous amount of ice. Dry ice with plenty of insulation is preferred for longer preservation.

Brains sent for examination should be halved longitudinally. One half is refrigerated or frozen over dry ice and the other is placed in 10% formalin solution for histopathologic examination. Tissues packed in formalin should be not be frozen.

Swabs. Swabs are of value for the submission of infectious material to the laboratory. On conventional cotton swabs many bacteria are susceptible to desiccation during shipment; therefore it is necessary to place the swab in a nonnutritional transport medium. The survival rate of many pathogenic bacteria is markedly increased by good transport media. A number of convenient swab systems utilizing a transport medium are available commercially.

DISEASES REQUIRING SPECIAL CONSIDERATION

Clostridial Infections (Blackleg, Malignant Edema)

Fresh, affected tissue is especially important because clostridia rapidly invade tissues after death. The muscle tissue involved may be difficult to locate.

Enterotoxemia (Clostridia)

Several ounces of fresh intestinal contents are required. This can be submitted in a jar or plastic bag or a section of affected intestine may be tied off and submitted. This material should be dispatched to the laboratory as soon as possible.

Campylobacteriosis (Cattle and Sheep)

To enable isolation and cultivation, semen, fetal stomach, or cervical mucus should reach the laboratory within five hours. If this is not possible, the material should be frozen over dry ice. Failing recovery of live organisms, dead *Campylobacter* can be recognized by negative staining and by a fluorescent antibody (FA) procedure.

Anthrax

Cotton swabs are soaked in exuded blood, or blood is taken from a superficial ear vein. In horses and swine, because the organism may not be present in the blood, swabs should be taken from exudates and the cut surface of hemorrhagic lymph nodes.

Johne's Disease

For the demonstration and culture of *Mycobacterium paratuberculosis*, the most suitable specimens are one or two feet of the terminal sections of the ileum with the ileocecal junction (ileocecal valve) and a similar length of the adjacent cecum, flushed free of intestinal content. Several mesenteric lymph nodes of the ileocecal region should also be included. In the live animal feces are submitted for culture.

Tuberculosis

The directions are those recommended by the Agricultural Research Service, United States Department of Agriculture. The affected tissue and adjacent lymph nodes should be submitted.

If no lesions are observed but there is justification for the mycobacteriologic examination, lymph nodes should be selected to represent the head, thorax, and abdomen.

The tissues should be placed in a 4-oz specimen bottle that has previously been filled with water to dissolve the chloramine-T. A minimum of 10 g of fat-free tissue is required. When infection is discovered by incising a lymph node, that node and one adjacent to it (unincised) should be submitted.

The bottles containing specimens should be placed in a refrigerated polystyrene container and dispatched to the laboratory.

Dermatophytosis (Ringworm)

Scrapings or epilations should be taken at the edge of active lesions. Submit in a cotton-plugged test tube or paper envelope. Saprophytic fungi will frequently proliferate rapidly in a sealed tube because of the moisture.

Anaerobes

Some anaerobes, particularly some of the gram-negative nonspore-formers, are sensitive to oxygen. Special commercial transport systems are available for the submission of materials suspected of containing significant anaerobes. Some laboratories provide screw-cap tubes containing oxygen-free gas for the submission of swabs. Liquid material can be submitted in syringes devoid of air bubbles.

EXAMINATION OF CLINICAL SPECIMENS

The procedures to be followed in processing clinical specimens depend largely upon the disease or organism suspected. Thus an adequate clinical history with suggestions by the veterinarian as to the disease or diseases suspected is extremely important.

The various steps that are followed in the bacteriologic exmination of most specimens are outlined in Figure 8–1. Of particular importance is

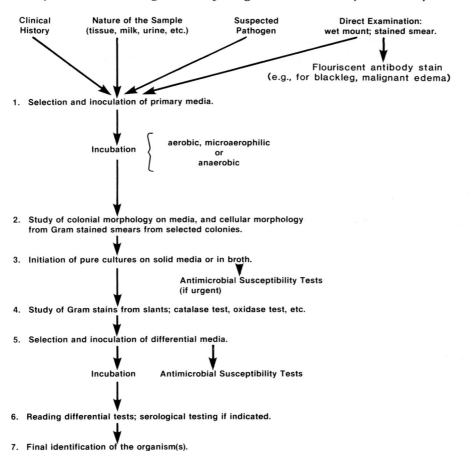

Figure 8–1.   Steps usually followed in the isolation and identification of bacteria from clinical specimens.

the direct microscopic examination of the specimen.

Direct Examination

The materials most frequently submitted for examination are tissues, feces, swabs, milk, urine, pus, discharge, fetal stomach contents, cervical mucus, and skin scrapings. The microbiologist carries out a direct examination for the agent suspected by the veterinarian or veterinary pathologist. These examinations are dealt with in this book under the appropriate pathogen or disease. The examination of stained smears and wet mounts should be routine with most materials. The findings may aid in the selection of appropriate culture media. When indicated, fluorescent antibody procedures are carried out on smears of tissues, fluids, or exudates.

Procedures Followed in Bacteriologic Examinations

The examination of clinical specimens for the purpose of isolating and identifying bacteria and

fungi of possible pathogenic significance is referred to as diagnostic or clinical bacteriology and mycology. This part of veterinary microbiology is traditionally taught in laboratory exercises that accompany the lecture course and thus will only be alluded to briefly here.

The steps listed in Figure 8–1 are followed in the routine processing of specimens. The considerations listed at the top of the chart determine the selection of the primary media. Occasionally a strong presumptive diagnosis can be made on the basis of a direct examination (smear or wet mount), e.g., in actinobacillosis, actinomycosis, blastomycosis, or nocardiosis. The fluorescent antibody procedure is used to identify some organisms in clinical materials, e.g., *Clostridium chauvoei* and *Cl. septicum*, and also in cultures, e.g., *Listeria monocytogenes* and *Francisella tularensis*.

Experienced veterinary microbiologists will first determine the Gram stain reaction and microscopic morphology (e.g., coccus, rod) of the unknown organism. This, along with the history and animal origin, will often suggest the probable genus or family to which the organism belongs. With this knowledge certain differential tests can be carried out to confirm the generic and eventually the species identification. Tables listing the differential characteristics of organisms of veterinary significance are provided in this and other texts.

In urgent cases antimicrobial susceptibility tests may be performed before the organism is finally identified.

The veterinary clinician should interpret the bacteriologic findings. The microbiologist can be of help in this regard by indicating the amount of growth obtained of a particular organism. This may be stated as few colonies, very light growth, moderate or heavy growth, or moderate growth of a pure culture. Interpretation may be particularly difficult if several different organisms are isolated. This illustrates the importance of the veterinary practitioner's having a familiarity with the normal flora, commensals, and pathogens of domestic animals.

SOURCES FOR FURTHER READING

Carter, G.R.: Diagnostic Procedures in Veterinary Bacteriology and Mycology. 4th Ed. Springfield, Illinois, Charles C Thomas, 1984.

Cottral, G.E. (ed.): Manual of Standard Methods for Veterinary Microbiology. Ithaca, NY, Cornell University Press, 1978.

Greene, C.E. (ed).: Clinical Microbiology and Infectious Diseases of the Dog and Cat. Philadelphia, W.B. Saunders Co., 1984.

Part II
BACTERIA

9

Streptococci

Principal Characteristics of the Streptococci

The streptococci are gram-positive, nonmotile (few exceptions), nonspore-forming cocci occurring singly, in pairs, or in chains. They are aerobic, facultatively anaerobic, catalase- and oxidase-negative, and fermentative.

Habitat

The streptococci are widely distributed in nature and as commensals in animals. More than 20 species are listed in *Bergey's Manual of Systematic Bacteriology*. Potentially pathogenic and nonpathogenic species may be present on the skin and on the mucous membranes of the genital tract and the upper respiratory and digestive tracts.

Classification

They can be divided into four principal categories, as shown in Table 9–1.

Another important way in which the streptococci are classified is into Lancefield groups, which are designated by the capital letters A, B, C, etc. This grouping is based upon serologic differences in a carbohydrate substance in the cell wall called component C. The antigenic determinants are amino sugars. A precipitin test is employed using extracts containing component C and specific grouping sera that are usually prepared in rabbits. Other serologic procedures such as latex agglutination, coagglutination, and fluorescent antibody tests can also be used to identify Lancefield groups.

Some of the Lancefield groups may be further divided into types by means of the agglutination test. There are at least 50 types of group A, *Streptococcus pyogenes*, based upon serologic differences in the M protein, as recognized by the agglutination procedure.

There may be more than one species in a group, and species may be identified by their biochemical activities.

Strains are also categorized according to the type of hemolysis:

1. Alpha-hemolysis: partial hemolysis often manifested as a zone of green discoloration around the colony; hemolysis with an inner zone of unhemolyzed cells.
2. Beta-hemolysis: clear, colorless zone due to complete hemolysis.

Table 9–1. Major Categories of Streptococci

	Growth			
Category	MacConkey Agar	45°C	6.5% NaCl	1% Methylene Blue
Pyogenic	−	−	−	−
Viridans	−	+	−	−
Lactic	−	−	−	+
Enterococci	+	+	+	+

3. Gamma-hemolysis: no detectable hemolysis.

MODE OF INFECTION AND TRANSMISSION

Infections may be endogenous or exogenous. In the latter instance they are usually acquired by inhalation or ingestion. Aerosol, direct contact, or fomites are the most common modes of spread.

PYOGENIC INFECTIONS IN GENERAL

The bacteria that most frequently result in the production of pus are the staphylococci, streptococci, and some of the corynebacteria. A pyogenic infection is one characterized by the production of pus. When pyogenic bacteria invade a tissue such as the mucous membrane of the pharynx, they evoke an inflammatory response characterized by vascular dilation and a marked exudation of plasma and neutrophils. In response to chemotaxis the neutrophils move toward the bacteria and engulf many of them. After phagocytosis the bacteria may be digested, but some bacteria are resistant to the lysosomal enzymes and multiply within the neutrophils. Some produce toxins that kill the phagocytic cells, and enzymes liberated from the dead neutrophils bring about partial liquefaction of the dead tissue and phagocytic cells. The liquefied mass becomes visible as thick, usually yellow, pus. The viscous consistency of pus is attributable to a considerable amount of deoxyribonucleoprotein from the nuclei of dead cells.

PATHOGENESIS

A variety of disease processes result from streptococcal infections, and their development depends upon various factors such as portal of entry, animal species, and streptococcal species. Three diseases illustrating somewhat different pathogenesis are strangles of horses, jowl abscesses of swine, and streptococcal arthritis. Although usually localized, streptococcal infections may become septicemic or bacteremic, resulting in death or foci of infection in various locations. As in many microbial diseases, the severity of the infection depends upon the immune status of the animal.

STREPTOCOCCAL METABOLITES

Group A streptococci produce more than 20 extracellular products. No doubt many of these are produced by pyogenic animal streptococci. Some of the better known are listed.

Hyaluronic Acid. Virulence factor that protects some streptococci from phagocytosis.

M Protein. Virulence; type-specific immunity.

Hemolysins. Streptolysins O and S are responsible for beta-hemolysis; each is produced under certain conditions. Antibody to streptolysin O is a good indicator of present or past infection.

Streptokinase (Fibrinolysin). Lysis of fibrin clots.

Lipoteichoic Acid. Responsible for adherence to epithelial cells.

Dnases A, B, C, and D. These extracellular enzymes assist in the production of substrates for growth. Antibody to DNase B is used in the serodiagnosis of group A human infections.

Streptodornase. Deoxyribonuclease that reduces the viscosity of fluid containing DNA. Streptococcal pus may be thin as a result of this enzyme.

Hyaluronidase. There is probably a correlation between the production of this enzyme and virulence, e.g., in streptococcal cellulitis.

Erythrogenic Toxin. Group A; rash in scarlet fever; lysogenic cultures only.

IMPORTANT STREPTOCOCCI

Group A

S. pyogenes. Principal cause of streptococcal disease in humans. May rarely cause bovine mastitis with possible dissemination to humans.

Group B

S. agalactiae. This streptococcus and *Staphylococcus aureus* are the most important and frequent causes of bovine mastitis. *S. agalactiae* is an obligate pathogen that can be eliminated from herds. Five to 20% of women are cervical carriers of group B streptococci that are identical or closely related to *S. agalactiae*. These streptococci may cause septicemia, meningitis, and death in newborn infants.

Group C

S. zooepidemicus. Many infections of animals and occasionally of humans.

S. equi. Strangles and other infections of the horse; genital infections in the mare.

S. equisimilis. Various infections of animals and humans.

S. dysgalactiae. Bovine mastitis; polyarthritis of lambs.

Group D (Enterococci)

Intestinal streptococci, some of which are motile. There are a number of varieties and species.

S. faecalis. Feces of animals and humans. Found in genitourinary and alimentary tracts; not usually pathogenic, although it may cause urinary infections in various animals and endocarditis in chickens.

S. suis. Type 1 = deMoor's group S; type 2 = deMoor's group R. These streptococci produce meningitis, arthritis, bronchopneumonia, and septicemia in young pigs. DeMoor has also identified group T strains from diseases of pigs.

S. equinus. Alimentary tract of the horse.

S. faecium. Same habitat as *S. faecalis*.

S. bovis. Alimentary tract of ruminants.

Group E

This group includes species from milk and a *Streptococcus* that causes jowl abscesses or cervical lymphadenitis of swine.

Group G

Group G streptococci cause infections in cattle, cats, and humans.

S. canis. Various infections in dogs.

Group H

Rare infections in cattle and humans.

Group K

S. salivarius. Commensal in pigs and humans.

Group L

Infections in dogs, cattle, and pigs.

Group M

Infections in dogs.

Group N

S. lactis. Feces of cattle and dairy products.

S. cremonis. Sheep and swine.

Groups O and P

These are occasionally recovered from infections in farm animals.

Group Q

S. avium. Recovered from poultry and other animals.

VIRIDANS GROUP

C substance has not been demonstrated; serologically heterogeneous; alpha-hemolytic; causes endocarditis in humans; urinary infections.

S. uberis. Serologically heterogeneous; causes bovine mastitis; found in the vagina and tonsils of cattle.

S. faecium. Same habitat as *S. faecalis*.

S. bovis. Alimentary tract of ruminants.

ANAEROBIC STREPTOCOCCI OR PEPTOSTREPTOCOCCI

These bacteria are found as commensals in the alimentary and upper respiratory tracts. Because so little effort has been made to isolate anaerobes from infections in animals, their real significance is not known. They may occur alone or in mixed infections, and it seems likely that they will be found as in humans in infections associated with operative procedures or wounds involving the gastrointestinal or genitourinary tract.

SPECIMENS

These vary with the disease. Infectious materials such as pus (strangles), joint fluid (arthritis), milk (mastitis) organs, and blood (septicemia).

DIRECT EXAMINATION

Organisms can be demonstrated in smears stained with Gram stain and in milk with Newman's stain. If the medium in which they are grown is liquid, characteristic chains may be seen.

ISOLATION AND CULTIVATION

The pathogenic strains grow best on serum or blood-enriched media; blood agar is preferred. Colonies are about 1 mm in diameter, round, smooth, glistening, and look like dew drops. Hemolysis may or may not be present, depending on various factors, including the kind of blood used. Colony varieties are mucoid (hyaluronic acid), matt (much M protein, virulent), and glossy (little M protein, low virulence).

IDENTIFICATION

If the streptococci are found to be in the pyogenic group by the tests referred to previously, they are more apt to be of pathogenic significance. Tests for the lactic streptococci are usually only carried out when examining milk samples. Most pyogenic streptococci associated with infections are beta-hemolytic. Some exceptions are listed in Table 9–2. Of help in estimating the significance of an isolate are culture purity, type

Table 9–2. Differential Characteristics of Important Streptococci from Animals*

Species	Group	Hemolysis	Trehalose	Sorbitol	Mannitol	Fermentation: Salicin	Acid Lactose	Raffinose	Inulin	Esculin	Sodium Hippurate†
Str. pyogenes	A	β	+	–	v	(+)‡	+	–	–	–	–
Str. zooepidemicus	C	β	–	+	–	+	+	–	–	–	–
Str. equisimilis	C	β	+	–	–	(+)	v	–	–	–	–
Str. equi	C	β	–	–	–	+	–	–	–	–	–
Str. agalactiae	B	α,β,γ	+	–	–	(+)	+	–	–	–	+
Str. dysgalactiae	C	α,β,γ	+	–	–	–	+	–	–	(–)	–
Str. uberis	D	α,β,γ	+	+	+	+	+	(–)	+	+	+
Str. faecalis	D	α,γ	+	+	+	+	+	(–)	+	+	v
Str. bovis	D	α	v‡	–	v	+	+	+	v	+	–

*(Reproduced from Carter, G.R.: Diagnostic Procedures in Veterinary Bacteriology and Mycology. 3rd Ed. Springfield, Illinois, Charles C Thomas, 1979.)

†Hydrolysis

‡v = variable; ( ) = most strains.

of lesions, and clinical findings. To save time, susceptibility tests may be conducted before precise identification is determined.

Precise identification is based on biochemical reactions and the characteristics listed in Tables 9–2 and 9–3. Lancefield grouping by the precipitin or other tests is not routinely carried out.

The CAMP test may be used for the presumptive recognition of *S. agalactiae*. It involves the completion of the partial hemolysis (beta toxin zone) of *Staphylococcus* when *S. agalactiae* is streaked at right angles to the *Staphylococcus* streak on blood agar. The CAMP test is employed in a medium that contains beta toxin of *Staphylococcus aureus* and is used to screen for *S. agalactiae*. The incorporation of esculin into the medium makes possible the presumptive recognition of *S. agalactiae*, *S. dysgalactiae*, and *S. uberis* (Fig. 9–1).

Edward's medium containing esculin, crystal violet, and thallium acetate is used for the rapid presumptive identification of the important mastitis streptococci. It inhibits gram-negative bacteria and staphylococci.

RESISTANCE

None of the pathogenic streptococci is particularly resistant to the usual chemical disinfectants. Many species will survive for weeks in soil, clothing, bedding, food, stalls, milking machines, and milk containers.

IMMUNITY

Animals infected with streptococci often develop a hypersensitivity of the delayed type. The role of this reaction in streptococcal disease is not known. It has been suggested that immune complexes may be responsible for purpura hemorrhagia in the horse after *Streptococcus equi* infection. Immunity to streptococcal infections is considered to be primarily humoral. Protection is type-specific and considered to depend upon antibodies to M protein.

A *Streptococcus equi* bacterin is available to prevent strangles, and a vaccine consisting of predominantly M protein has been developed to reduce the undesirable reactions that sometimes result from the use of strangles bacterins. A live attenuated strain of group E *Streptococcus* is used to vaccinate pigs against jowl abscesses.

TREATMENT

Penicillin is the preferred drug; resistant pyogenic strains are rare, although there have been some reports of plasmid-mediated resistance to tetracyclines and chloramphenicol. Sulfamerazine and sulfamethazine are useful. Other drugs that may be used are erythromycin, the cephalosporins, lincomycin, and the tetracyclines. Antibiotic resistance is most commonly encountered among the enterococci. It is recommended that all group A throat infections in humans be treated for at least 10 days with therapeutic levels of penicillin to prevent rheumatic fever and glomerular nephritis.

Most viridans streptococci are susceptible to penicillin, but many enterococci are resistant. The latter are usually susceptible to ampicillin.

PUBLIC HEALTH SIGNIFICANCE

S. pyogenes (group A) may infect the bovine udder and be disseminated to humans in milk.

Table 9–3. **Differential Characteristics of Streptococci Recovered from Intramammary Infections**

Organism	Lancefield Group	CAMP test	Hydrolysis of		Acid Produced in Broth Containing		Reduction of 0.1% MBM†
			Esculin*	Sodium Hippurate	Inulin	Raffinose	
Str. agalactiae	B	+	−	+	−	−	−
Str. dysgalactiae	C	−	d	−	−	−	−
Str. uberis	E/Neg‡	−/+	+	+	+	−	−
Enterococci§	D	−	+	d	−/+	−/+	+
Str. bovis	D	−	+	−	d	+	−
Str. species	G	−	+	−	−	−	−

*Tested in Difco tryptose blood agar base containing either 5% defibrinated blood or 5% serum, 0.05% esculin and 0.01% ferric citrate.

†Methylene blue milk.

‡Extracts of some strains of *S. uberis* react with group E antisera but do not induce group E antibodies in rabbits.

§*S. faecalis* and *S. faecium*

d = some strains positive; some negative.

−/+ = most strains negative.

(Reproduced with permission from Microbiological Procedures for Use in the Diagnosis of Bovine Mastitis. Washington, D.C., National Mastitis Council, Inc., 1981.)

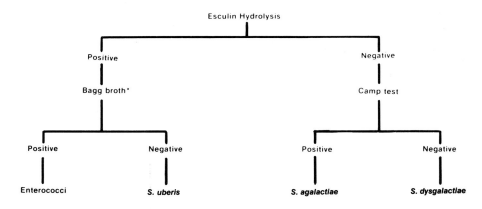

*Buffered azide glucose glycerol broth

Figure 9–1. Presumptive identification of important streptococci from milk samples.

On occasion animal pyogenic streptococci may infect humans. Although women frequently carry group B streptococci, there is no evidence that these bacteria are acquired from milk.

Streptococcus pneumoniae

SYNONYM: *Diplococcus pneumoniae*

This species resembles the other streptococci except that it occurs principally as pairs of cocci rather than as chains. It is made up of many serotypes that are identified on the basis of serologic differences in capsular antigens. They are found as commensals in the upper respiratory tract of humans and less commonly of animals.

PATHOGENICITY

Most of the infections are caused by less than 10 different serotypes. Lobar pneumonia, empyema, sinusitis, and conjunctivitis are among the important diseases *S. pneumoniae* causes in humans. It is an important cause of pneumonia in guinea pigs and has been implicated in respiratory infections in calves, monkeys, rabbits, and rats. There are several reports of bovine mastitis due to pneumococci.

ISOLATION, CULTIVATION, AND IDENTIFICATION

Streptococcus pneumoniae grows well on blood agar. It grows in small round colonies with elevated edges and is alpha-hemolytic. It is gram-positive, and paired cocci are seen in stained smears. It is bile-soluble, and inhibited by optochin; other biochemical tests are used for definitive identification.

IMMUNITY

In humans immunity is considered totally humoral. A vaccine consisting of specific polysaccharides of 14 types is available to protect humans.

SUGGESTED CLINICAL EXAMPLES

An outbreak of strangles in a stable of riding horses.

An outbreak of cervical lymphadenitis in swine.

Multiple streptococcal infections in neonatal pigs.

S. agalactiae mastitis in a dairy herd.

SOURCES FOR FURTHER READING

Anonymous: Microbiological Procedures for Use in the Diagnosis of Bovine Mastitis. 2nd Ed. Washington, D.C., National Mastitis Council, Inc., 1981.

Cullen, G.A.: *Streptococcus uberis*: A review. Vet. Bull., *39:* 155, 1969.

Diebel, R.H.: The group D streptococci. Bact. Rev., *28:*330, 1964.

Krantz, G.E., and Dunne, H.W.: An attempt to classify streptococci isolates from domestic animals. Am. J. Vet. Res., *26:* 951, 1965.

Moeira-Jacob, M.: The streptococci of Lancefield's group E: Biochemical and serological identification of haemolytic strains. J. Gen. Microbiol., *14:*268, 1956.

Patterson, M.J., and Batool-Hafeez, A.E.: Group B streptococci in human disease. Bact. Rev., *40:*774, 1976.

Perch, B., Pederson, K.B., and Henricksen, J.: Serology of capsulated streptococci pathogenic for pigs: New serotypes of *Streptococcus suis.* J. Clin. Microbiol., *17*:993, 1983.

Skinner, F., and Quesnel, L. (eds.): Streptococci. New York, Academic Press, 1978.

Wanamaker, L.W., and Matsen, J.M. (eds.): Streptococci and Streptococcal Diseases. New York, Academic Press, 1972.

Windsor, R.S.: Streptococcal infection in young pigs. *In* The Veterinary Annual. Edited by C.S.G. Grunsell and F.W.G. Hill. Bristol, England, Scientechnica, 1978.

Woolcock, J.B.: Immunology of streptococcal infections. Aust. Vet. J., *49*:85, 1973.

10

Staphylococci

PRINCIPAL CHARACTERISTICS OF *Staphylococci*

Staphylococci are gram-positive cocci occurring in pairs and clusters. They are aerobic and facultatively anaerobic, catalase-positive, oxidase-negative, nonmotile, nonspore-forming, and fermentative.

Three official species are recognized in *Bergey's Manual of Determinative Bacteriology: S. aureus, S. epidermidis,* and *S. saprophyticus.* The principal pathogen of the genus is *S. aureus. S. epidermidis,* a common commensal of the skin, is usually nonpathogenic, but occasionally causes bovine mastitis, abscesses, and low-grade skin infections. *S. saprophyticus* occurs in nature and is usually nonpathogenic but causes some human infections.

A study of staphylococci has disclosed at least six biotypes. Two have been called *S. intermedius* and *S. hyicus.* The former has been implicated in pyoderma and mastitis in the dog. *S. hyicus* subspecies *hyicus* is considered to be the cause of a disease of pigs, exudative epidermitis (greasy pig disease).

Other species, as yet unofficial, are *S. hominis, S. haemolyticus,* and *S. simulans.* Those species of significance in animal diseases are listed in Table 10–1.

The cell wall of *S. aureus* has three major components: peptidoglycan, teichoic acids, and protein A. The chemical composition of these compounds has been useful in the taxonomic differentiation of *Staphylococcus* spp. and *Micrococcus* spp. Protein A makes up the major protein portion of the cell wall and about one third is released into the medium during growth. Protein A is referred to further on.

Micrococci

The micrococci is a large group consisting of many species that resemble the staphylococci morphologically but differ biochemically (see Table 10–1). They are aerobic and are frequently found in soil, water, dust, air, and skin and on articles of daily use. In addition, they are found on dairy utensils and in milk and dairy products. They are recovered frequently from clinical materials but are usually not considered to be pathogenic. They split sugars by oxidation, in contrast to staphylococci, which ferment sugars.

There are other usually non-pathogenic cocci that may be encountered in clinical specimens: *Sarcina:* division in three planes yielding cubical packets; anaerobic; *methanococcus:* anaerobic cocci; *Planococcus:* division in two planes yielding tetrads (motile); *Aerococcus:* division in two planes yielding tetrads (nonmotile).

Staphylococcus aureus

SYNONYM: *Staphylococcus pyogenes*

Habitat

Commensal of the skin and mucous membranes, especially of the upper respiratory and digestive tracts.

Table 10–1. Differential Characteristics of Staphylococci and Micrococci

	S. aureus	S. epidermidis	S. intermedius	S. hyicus ss. hyicus	S. saprophyticus	Micrococci
Coagulase	+	−	+	V	−	−
Hemolysis (beta)	+	V	+	−	−	−
Pigment	+	V	−	−	V	V
Maltose	A[2]	A	V	−	A	−
PAB	+[3]	+	+	−	NT[4]	NT
Mannitol	A	−	V	−	V	
DNase	+	−	V	+	−	−
Novobiocin	S[5]	S	S	S	R[6]	S
Glucose (O–F)	F[7]	F	F	F	−	O[8]

+, 90% or more strains positive; −, 90% of strains negative.

[1], variable reactions; [2], acid; [3], purple agar base (acid production); [4], not tested; [5], susceptible; [6], resistant; [7], fermentation; [8], oxidation.

Staphylococcal Metabolites

Some of the substances thought to be involved in the production of staphylococcal infections are listed below. For the most part their effects have been demonstrated experimentally in rabbits and mice.

Leukocidin: kills leukocytes, antigenic, nonhemolytic, associated with alpha and delta toxins.

Dermonecrotoxin: necrotizing; associated with alpha toxin.

Lethal Toxin: rapidly lethal for mice and rabbits; associated with alpha and beta hemolysins.

Hemolysins (Hemotoxins): All are antigenically distinct. Erythrocytes from various animal species differ in susceptibility. Alpha hemolysin: inner clear zone; beta hemolysin: outer partial zone; gamma hemolysin and delta hemolysin: poorly characterized. Double zone hemolysis on blood agar is characteristic of many strains of *S. aureus.*

Exfoliative Toxin (Exfoliatin): Some strains of *S. aureus* produce a soluble protein that induces exfoliation or intraepidermal separation in newborn mice after parenteral inoculation. Skin changes in staphylococcal epidermal infections in humans, especially children, are attributed to this toxin.

Enterotoxins: About one third of coagulase-positive strains of *S. aureus* produce enterotoxins. There are six antigenically distinct types, which are coded by plasmids. A favorable milieu is required for their production such as custards, raw milk, cream, ice cream, meat gravy, fish, cheese, or oysters. Clinical signs are nausea, abdominal cramps, and diarrhea in four hours. In contrast, *Salmonella* food poisoning takes effect in 24 to 48 hours. The test for toxin is an agar gel precipitin test with specific antisera. The toxin is thermostable (100°C for 15 min).

Coagulase: Clotting of plasma; its role in virulence has been questioned.

Clumping Factor: This factor, which is not related to free coagulase of the test-tube test, can be demonstrated in a slide test that was erroneously referred to as the "slide coagulase test." Its significance is not known.

Staphylokinase: A weak fibrinolysin.

Nuclease: Most cultures of *S. aureus* produce a thermostable DNase. Its role in disease is not clear.

Hyaluronidase: "Spreading factor" that may be involved in virulence.

Lipase: Lipase-positive strains tend to cause abscesses of the skin and subcutis; lipase destroys protective fatty acids on skin. Staphylococci causing generalized infections are usually lipase-negative.

Protein A: It is present as a surface component on most strains of virulent *S. aureus.* It has the unique ability to bind to the Fc region of IgG and thus may have a role in pathogenesis. The useful serologic procedure, coagglutination, depends upon protein A. When specific IgG antibody is added to staphylococci possessing protein A followed by homologous antigen, coagglutination is produced.

Distribution and Transmission

Endogenous infections are probably most frequent but exogenous infections also occur. Transmission is usually by direct contact or by fomites.

Pathogenesis

Strains of this widespread commensal have the capacity to invade tissues, producing abscesses, pustules, various other pyogenic infections, and on occasion bacteremia and septicemia. Some of the metabolites referred to earlier are no doubt involved in the development of these infections. Virulent *S. aureus* can survive but not multiply in polymorphonuclear leukoyctes.

Pathogenicity

Botryomycosis: infrequent chronic granulomatous lesions involving the udder of the mare, cow, and sow and the spermatic cord of horses. Suppurative wound infections and septicemia in all animals. Pyoderma, especially of dogs (more commonly *S. intermedius*) and horses. Pyemia in lambs, especially tick-bite wounds.

Mastitis in the cow, sow, and ewe. Staphylococcal bovine mastitis, which can be acute but most frequently is chronic and subclinical; this diagnosis is of great economic importance. Gangrenous mastitis due to alpha-toxin is seen in postparturient cows.

Various infections of the skin of many animals; subcutaneous abscesses.

Staphylococcal arthritis and septicemia in turkeys.

Urinary infections in humans and animals.

Staphylococcal enterocolitis, seen principally in humans after prolonged antibiotic therapy, e.g., after intestinal surgery.

Impetigo: sow's udder; piglets from biting.

Humans: osteomyelitis, sinusitis, mastitis, tonsillitis, and impetigo. Nosocomial infections. Food poisoning.

Specimens

Pus, usually provided on swabs; affected tissue; milk samples.

Isolation, Cultivation, and Identification

Staphylococci grow well on common laboratory media. Selective media are available, e.g., mannitol salt agar. Blood agar is generally preferred. Colonies appear in 24 hours and are up to 4 mm in diameter, round, smooth, and glistening; they may have "gold" pigmentation. Double zone hemolysis is especially characteristic, although not with *S. epidermidis*.

Smears disclose clumps of gram-positive cocci. Presumptive identification is made on the basis of the double zone of hemolysis and cultural and morphologic features. Definitive identification is based upon coagulase production and the other characteristics listed in Table 10–1. Staphylococci are sensitive to lysostaphin while micrococci are not.

Antigenic Nature and Serology

Antigenic structure is complex and heterogeneous. Polysaccharide A and protein A are group-specific antigens.

Some strains of *S. aureus* can be identified by their susceptibility to one or several staphylococcal phages, e.g., strain 80/81 (penicillin-resistant) is susceptible to lysis by phages 80 to 81; this variety has been important in human nosocomial infections. Phage typing is of value in the study of the epidemiology of staphylococcal infections. There are a number of phage types. Animal staphylococci are usually different types than human strains.

A number of phage culture lysates are used in the typing procedure. A single drop of each lysate is added to a plate confluently inoculated with the organism to be tested, it is incubated overnight at 30°C, and then observed for zones of lysis. The pattern of lysis indicates the type. Sources of error include the fact that staphylococci may be lysogenic for the phages used and that some harbor as many as five different temperate phages.

Resistance

Organisms are susceptible to common disinfectants. Pus is protective, and organisms remain viable in dried pus for weeks. This is an important consideration in clinics.

Unlike many other vegetative bacterial forms, some staphylococci can survive a temperature of 60° C for 30 minutes.

Immunity

Strains of *S. aureus* possessing capsular and certain surface antigens are most immunogenic. Bacterins and toxoids are employed. They are considered to be of questionable value in the prevention of bovine mastitis. Autogenous bacterins have given variable results.

Hypersensitivity to staphylococci probably plays a role in aggravating infections; thus the need to desensitize dogs with pyoderma when using an autogenous bacterin. Immunity is both cell-mediated and humoral; the latter is antibacterial as well as antitoxic.

Treatment

It is advisable to conduct antimicrobial susceptibility tests on isolates considered significant. Penicillin is the drug of choice if strains are susceptible. Penicillin-resistant strains 80/81 of human origin have been found in cattle and dogs; resistance is attributable to penicillinase (beta-lactamase), an enzyme that hydrolyzes the beta-lactam ring of penicillin. Plasmid-based penicillin resistance may be transferred by transduction. New synthetic (penicillinase-resistant) penicillins are of value, e.g., methicillin, oxacillin, and nafcillin. Tetracyclines, bacitracin, nitrofurans, and erythromycin may be effective. Trimethoprim-sulfamethoxazole, vancomycin, first generation cephalosporins, and clindamycin have been effective against *S. aureus* infections. Surgical drainage may be indicated.

Public Health Significance

Human beings may become infected with *S. aureus, S. hyicus,* and possibly other staphylococci of animal origin.

SUGGESTED CLINICAL EXAMPLES

Pyoderma in a dog.
Pyoderma in a horse.
A staphylococcal urinary infection in a dog.
Staphylococcal mastitis in a dairy herd.

SOURCES FOR FURTHER READING

Biberstein, E.L., et al.: Antimicrobial sensitivity patterns in *Staphylococcus aureus* from animals. J. Am. Vet. Med. Assoc., 164:1183, 1974.

Cohen, J.O. (ed.): The Staphylococci. New York, John Wiley, 1972.

Devriese, L.A., et al.: *Staphylococcus hyicus* (Sompolinsky 1953) comb. nov. and *Staphylococcus hyicus* subsp. *Chromogenes* subsp. nov. Int. J. Syst. Bact., 28:482, 1978.

Easmon, C.S.F., and Adlam, C. (eds.): Staphylococci and Staphylococcal Infections. Vols. 1 and 2. Orlando, Florida, Academic Press, Inc., 1984.

Feltham, R.K.A.: A taxonomic study of the Micrococcaceae. J. Appl. Bacteriol., 47:243, 1979.

Kloss, W.E., and Schliefer, K.H.: Simplified scheme for routine identification of human *Staphylococcus* species. J. Clin. Microbiol., 1:82, 1975.

Lacey, R.W.: Genetic basis, epidemiology and future significance of antibiotic resistance in *Staphylococcus aureus:* A review. J. Clin. Pathol., 26:899, 1973.

Madoff, M.A.: The staphylococci: Ecological perspectives. Ann. N.Y. Acad. Sci., 128:122, 1965.

Markham, N.P., and Markham, J.G.: Staphylococci in man and animals. Distribution and characteristics of strains. J. Comp. Pathol., 76:49, 1966.

Musher, D.M., and Mackenzie, S.O.: Infections due to *Staphylococcus aureus.* Medicine, 56:383, 1977.

Wentworth, B.B.: Bacteriophage typing of the staphylococci. Bacteriol. Rev., 27:253, 1963.

White, S.D., et al.: Occurrence of *Staphylococcus aureus* on the clinically normal canine hair coat. Am. J. Vet. Res., 44:332, 1983.

Yortis, W.W. (ed.). Recent advances in staphylococcal research. Ann. N.Y. Acad. Sci., 236:1, 1974.

11

Corynebacteria

Principal Characteristics of the Corynebacteria

The corynebacteria are gram-positive, small, pleomorphic rods. They are nonmotile (except for some plant pathogens) and nonspore-forming. Most are aerobic or facultatively anaerobic, catalase-positive (except *Corynebacterium pyogenes)*, and fermentative.

Historical

C. diphtheriae was shown to be the cause of human diphtheria by Löffler in 1884.

General

Members of this genus other than *C. diphtheriae* are commonly called "diphtheroids." The genus *Corynebacterium* is closely related to the genera *Mycobacterium* and *Nocardia* according to chemical and serologic similarities in their principal cell wall antigens. Some of the pathogenic species may be reclassified. The name *Rhodococcus equi* has been proposed for *C. equi*. More than 30 species have been identified, of which about a third are parasitic on humans and animals. Some that occur in animals are commensals that have not been identified as to species. Nonpathogenic diphtheroids are frequently recovered from clinical specimens.

C. diphtheriae strains may produce a potent toxin that has been studied extensively. The capacity to produce toxin depends upon the infection of the bacteria by a temperate phage. The toxin is only produced when the concentration of iron in the medium is low.

The cell wall of some species is weaker at the ends, resulting in a club-like shape. During division the daughter cells can remain attached on one side, resulting in L and V arrangements that are referred to as "Chinese letters" in groups. The corynebacteria have a wide variety of colonial types, and they can be superficially confused with *Actinomyces* spp. (Table 11–1).

Habitat

Commensals on skin and mucous membranes of the genital and upper respiratory tracts, e.g., *C. pyogenes* may be recovered from the nasal passages and tonsils of normal swine; *C. renale* has has been recovered from the apparently normal male and female bovine genital tract. *C. equi* is present as a commensal in the intestine of many horses; it will survive for long periods in the manure and litter in stables. Some nonpathogenic strains are widely distributed in nature.

Mode of Infection and Transmission

This may vary with the different pathogenic species (Table 11–2).

Pathogenesis

Little is known about the manner in which these organisms produce disease. *C. pseudotuberculosis* and *C. pyogenes* produce relatively weak exotoxins. Abscesses frequently result from *C. pyogenes* and *C. equi* infections; they are usually confined to one organ or locale but they can also be disseminated. *C. pseudotuberculosis* is a facultative intracellular parasite. Adherence of

Table 11–1. *Differentiation of Some Important Corynebacteria*

Species	Catalase	Hemolysis	Gelatinase	Nitrate Reduction	Urease	Acid Production Glucose	Maltose	Lactose	Sucrose
C. pyogenes	−	β	+	−	−	+	+	+	−
C. haemolyticum	weak +	β	+	−	−	slow +	+	+	+
C. pseudotuberculosis	+	V	V	V	V	+	V	V	V
C. renale	+	−	−	V	rapid +	+	V	V	−
C. equi¹	+	−	−	+	V	−	−	−	−
C. suis (anaerobic)	−	−	−	−	+	V	+	−	−
C. bovis	+	−	−	−	−	−	−	−	−
C. kutscheri	+	α or −	−	+	V	+	+	−	+
C. diphtheriae	+	V	−	+	−	+	+	−	−

+ = 90% or more positive.
− = 90% or more negative.
V = variable.
¹ = mucoid colonies with pink pigment

Table 11–2. *Summary of Some Important Features of Major Animal Corynebacteria*

	C. pyogenes (Pyobacillosis)	C. pseudotuberculosis (C. ovis)	C. renale	C. equi
Mode of Infection	Exogenous or endogenous; inhalation; contact.	Contact. Shearing wounds, other wounds. Possibly ingestion.	From bull? Contact with infectious urine. Endogenous/exogenous.	Contact, inhalation. Endogenous or exogenous.
Pathogenicity	Exotoxin produced; relatively weak. Very important pyogenic organism of cattle and swine. Cattle, sheep, swine: chronic abscessing mastitis, suppurative pneumonia, arthritis, abscesses, umbilical infections, infections of wounds and surgical incisions.	Exotoxin produced; resembles diphtheria toxin but much weaker. Equidae: ulcerative lymphangitis. Pectoral abscesses in horses. Sheep: caseous lymphadenitis; usually a low-grade infection. Purulent arthritis of lambs.	Exotoxin has not been demonstrated. Pyelonephritis in cows and heifers; cystitis. Swine: kidney abscesses.	Exotoxin has not been demonstrated. Bronchopneumonia with abscesses in foals. Simulates tuberculosis in the cervical and pharyngeal lymph nodes of swine. Infrequently causes metritis and abortion in mares. Enteritis in neonatal foals.
Specimens	Pus or affected tissue or organ, preferably from early infections.			
Isolation and Cultivation	Can be demonstrated but only tentatively identified as corynebacteria in stained smears from clinical material. All grow on blood agar and can be readily seen after 48 hours of aerobic incubation.			
	Colonies: pinpoint, smooth, glistening, strep-like. With age they become opaque and dry. A large colony type of *C. pyogenes* has been described. Resembles *C. haemolyticum*.	Young colonies resemble *C. pyogenes* but rapidly become more opaque, dry, crumbly, 3–4 mm in diameter; chromogenic: cream to orange.	Young colonies resemble *C. pyogenes* but rapidly become more opaque and ivory-colored. Usually they are moist first and later become dry and granular.	Large, moist, creamy-white colonies that later become salmon-colored and tend to coalesce.
Morphology and Staining	Gram-positive; very pleomorphic; may appear as coccoid, straight, or slightly curved rods with swollen ends; single, paired, or short chains; palisade arrangement; metachromatic granules.			
Identification	See Table 11–1			

C renale may be facilitated by the presence of pili.

Immunity

Cell-mediated immunity is probably important in some of the infections, e.g., those caused by *C. equi* and *C. pseudotuberculosis*. It seems likely that with these two organisms, humoral immunity is both antibacterial and antitoxic. Immunization is not practiced to any extent. *C. pyogenes* is included in mixed bacterins, the value of which has not been demonstrated. Autogenous bacterins have been employed to prevent *C. equi*, *C. pyogenes*, and *C. pseudotuberculosis* infections, but their value is questionable. Toxoids have not been shown to be of value in preventing infections produced by *C. pyogenes* or *C. pseudotuberculosis*. The antigenic nature of the animal corynebacteria has received little attention. *C. pyogenes* is thought to be serologically homogeneous, but *C. equi* is antigenically heterogeneous.

Resistance

Corynebacteria are susceptible to common disinfectants. *C. equi* is very resistant to drying and will persist in the soil and stable litter for months. Pus is protective.

Treatment

C. pyogenes, C. pseudotuberculosis, and *C. equi* are susceptible to a number of antibiotics *in vitro,* but because of the suppurative processes, including abscesses, treatment is not usually satisfactory. The drugs most commonly tried are penicillin, sulfonamides, and tetracyclines.

There are reports of successful treatment of *C. renale* infections with large doses of penicillin, although remissions are frequent. Treatment is unsatisfactory in advanced cases. Effectiveness of treatment should be monitored by urine culture.

Other Species

C. diphtheriae. This species is a cause of diphtheria in humans; there are three varieties. It does not cause disease in animals. It produces a potent exotoxin.

C. bovis. A commensal frequently recovered from cow's milk considered to be nonpathogenic.

C. kutscheri (C. murium). Resembles *C. pseudotuberculosis* but can be distinguished biochemically. Causes caseous and tuberculosis-like focal lesions in the lungs and other organs of mice and rats.

C. minutissimum. Found in docking wounds in lambs; inflammation of interdigital spaces ("scold"); and scabs on brisket. A superficial infection of the axillary and pubic regions in humans called erythrasma (scaly plaques).

C. suis. An anaerobic diphtheroid that produces a disease in sows similar to that produced in cows by *C. renale,* viz., pyelonephritis. It can be recovered from semen of some boars.

C. parvum (now renamed *Propionibacterium parvum*). A nonpathogenic anaerobe used for its adjuvant properties in tumor therapy.

C. haemolyticum. Resembles the large colony variety of *C. pyogenes*; causes infrequent infections in humans.

Public Health Significance

C. pyogenes and *C. equi* have only rarely caused infections in humans.

SUGGESTED CLINICAL EXAMPLES

A case of bovine mastitis due to *C. pyogenes.*

An outbreak of enzootic pneumonia in calves in which *C. pyogenes* is a secondary invader.

Cases of caseous lymphadenitis in goats.

A case of pyelonephritis in a cow due to *C. renale.*

A case of pyelonephritis in a sow due to *C. suis.*

Cases of suppurative pneumonia in foals due to *C. equi.*

C. kutscheri infections in a rat colony.

SOURCES FOR FURTHER READING

Myers, J.L.: Caseous lymphadenitis in goats and sheep: A review of diagnosis, pathogenesis and immunity. J. Am. Vet. Med. Assoc., 171:1251, 1977.

Barton, M.D., and Hughes, K.L.: Corynebacterium equi: A review. Vet. Bull., 50:65, 1980.

Benham, C.L., Seaman, A., and Woodbine, M.: Corynebacterium pseudotuberculosis and its role in diseases of animals. Vet. Bull., 32:645, 1962.

Crutchley, M.J., Seaman, A., and Woodbine, M.: Microbiological aspects of Corynebacterium renale. Vet. Rev. Annot., 7:1, 1961.

Duckett, S.M., Seaman, A., and Woodbine, M.: The bacteriology of Corynebacterium bovis. Vet. Bull., 33:67, 1963.

Elissalde, G.S., and Renshaw, H.W.: Corynebacterium equi: An interhost review with emphasis on the foal. Comp. Immunol. Microbiol. Infect. Dis., 3:433, 1980.

Giddens, W.E., Jr., Keahey, K.K., Carter, G.R., and Whitehair, C.K.: Pneumonia in rats due to infection with Corynebacterium kutscheri. Pathol. Vet., 5:227, 1968.

Knight, H.D.: Corynebacterial infections in the horse: Problems of prevention. J. Am. Vet. Med. Assoc., 155:446, 1969.

Pijoan, C., Lastra, A., and Leman, A.: Isolation of Corynebacterium suis from the prepuce of boars. J. Am. Vet. Med. Assoc., 183:428, 1984.

Purdom, M.R., Seaman, A., and Woodbine, M.: The bacteriology and antibiotic sensitivity of Corynebacterium pyogenes. Vet. Rev. Annot., 4:55, 1985.

12

Listeria

PRINCIPAL CHARACTERISTICS OF *Listeria*

They are small, motile, gram-positive rods that are catalase-positive, oxidase-negative, aerobic and facultatively anaerobic, fermentative, and nonspore-forming.

Listeria monocytogenes

Historical

The organism was first recovered from guinea pigs and rabbits showing hepatic necrosis by Murray, Webb, and Swann in 1926.

Habitat

Listeria monocytogenes has been recovered from the soil. It has been found in the feces (many enteric carriers), genital secretions, and nasal mucus of apparently healthy animals, and in silage. Organisms multiply when pH of silage rises above 5.5.

Mode of Infection

The modes of infection of the neural and visceral forms are considered to be different. In the neural form infection is via branches of the trigeminal nerve or probably via the eye, nose, and oropharynx; in the visceral form ingestion is the mode of infection. Most infections are thought to be exogenous.

Pathogenesis

The neural form of the disease is seen most frequently in ruminants. The visceral form is seen most in monogastric animals, and spread appears to be hematogenous after ingestion. Organisms are intracellular in both forms. As with other intracellular bacteria, there is a granulomatous reaction leading to focal areas of necrosis in the liver in this disease. A toxin has not been demonstrated but a monocytosis-producing agent (a glyceride) has been extracted from organisms, although monocytosis is not a regular feature of the natural disease.

Virulence appears to be dependent upon a hemolysin and a lipolytic antigen. A lipopolysaccharide-like substance that is highly toxic for rabbits is found on the surface of organisms.

Pathogenicity

The disease is referred to as listeriosis or listerellosis, and the neural form is sometimes called "circling disease."

The neural form of the disease is most common in ruminants. It is seen in cattle and sheep in winter and early spring particularly; all ages are susceptible. Epizootics occur in feedlots. The occurrence of the disease has been associated with feeding of silage. CNS signs include unilateral ataxia and meningitis. Microabscesses are found, principally involving the brain stem.

Keratoconjunctivitis and ophthalmitis have been described in cattle and sheep.

Abortions occur in cows and ewes, but without the neural manifestations of the disease. The organism can be recovered from the aborted fetus and uterus.

The neural form of the disease occurs in the horse, but it is infrequent.

In chickens and turkeys, it usually takes an epidemic form. Necrotic foci of the liver and myocardium are seen.

A visceral form of the disease with liver necrosis is seen in the rabbit, guinea pig, chinchilla, and other species. Several cases of neural listeriosis have been encountered in the dog.

Specimens

Neural form: pons and medulla.
Visceral form: portions of affected organs.
Abortion: fetus and fetal membranes.

Isolation and Cultivation

It is frequently difficult to recover the organism from the brain in neural listeriosis, presumably because the organisms are intracellular and present in small numbers. Ground brain stored at refrigerator temperature ("cold enrichment") should be recultured for up to 12 weeks before it is discarded as negative if no growth is obtained initially. The organism is able to grow at refrigerator temperatures; thus the value of cold enrichment. It is more difficult to recover from the bovine brain, in which the numbers are fewer than in the sheep and goat brain. Cultural procedures may be indicated by the finding of microscopic lesions characteristic of listeriosis in the brain or brain stem.

The organism grows well on ordinary media but is routinely isolated on blood agar. Five to 10% carbon dioxide stimulates primary growth. Smooth colonies are approximately 2 mm in diameter, round, entire, glistening and bluish by transmitted light; narrow zones of beta-hemolysis are evident.

Small, gram-positive rods occurring singly, in pairs, or in short chains are seen in stained smears. Morphologically they may resemble some diphtheroids and streptococci. A characteristic tumbling motility is noted at room temperature.

Identification

The organism somewhat resembles *Erysipelothrix rhusiopathiae*. Three important distinguishing features of *L. monocytogenes* are (a) it is catalase-positive; (b) it is motile at room temperature; and (c) experimental infections in guinea pigs are fatal. See Table 12–1 for additional data.

A polyvalent fluorescent labeled globulin is available for the identification of *L. monocyto-*

genes. It is most satisfactorily employed with organisms from cultures.

Bergey's manual describes three additional species of *Listeria*: *L. denitrificans* (habitat not known), *L grayi* (from chinchilla), and *L. murrayi* (from vegetation and soil). These three are not beta-hemolytic nor are they pathogenic for mice, possibly except for *L. denitrificans*. The Anton test in rabbits is negative with the three species, and their potential for causing disease is probably very low. These species differ quite markedly in antigenic composition from. *L. monocytogenes* and may ultimately be included in a different genus.

Experimental Animals. Mice, rabbits, and guinea pigs are susceptible. A keratoconjunctivitis (Anton test) is produced within 24 hours after the instillation of organisms into the eyes of guinea pigs and rabbits.

Antigenic Nature and Serology

On the basis of somatic (O) and flagellar (H) antigens, four principal serologic groups and 11 serotypes have been identified. They bear no relation to the host species or the clinical syndrome from which they were recovered. Serotype 4b is the predominant strain in Canada and the United States. Most infections are caused by three serotypes: 1/2a, 1/2b, and 4b.

Resistance

Pasteurization (62°C for 30 min; 71.6°C for 15 to 30 sec) destroys *L. monocytogenes*. It is remarkably resistant to drying, can survive for months in food, straw, and shavings, and is susceptible to common disinfectants.

Immunity

Immunization has not yet been found to be of value. Autogenous bacterins have given inconclusive results. Studies in experimental animals indicate that much of the immunity in listeriosis is cell-mediated. In view of this, live, attenuated vaccines might be of value.

Public Health Significance

In humans, *L. monocytogenes* causes meningoencephalitis, meningitis, and encephalitis; uterine infections with abortion, still births, and a neonatal septicemic form called granulomatosis infantiseptica; valvular endocarditis; and septicemia. The possible sources for human infections are soil, animals, and human carriers. Infections are frequently associated with the use

Table 12–1.   **Differentiation of Listeria *and* Erysipelothrix**

	Motility	Beta-Hemolysis	Catalase	Nitrate Reduction	Guinea Pig Inoculation	Anton Test	Glucose	Mannitol
L. monocytogenes	+ (25°C)	+	+	−	Death 3–4 days	+	+	−
E. rhusiopathiae	−	−	−	−	Resistant	−	−	−
L. denitrificans	+	−	+	+	Resistant	−	+	−
L. grayi	+	−	+	−	Resistant	−	+	+
L. murrayi	+	−	+	+	Resistant	−	+	+

of corticosteroids, radiation therapy, and other underlying diseases.

Several cases of bovine mastitis due to this organism have been reported. Unpasteurized cow's milk yielding the organism is a potential source of human infections. There may be human genital and enteric carriers.

Treatment

Treatment is usually of little value, particularly in sheep and goats after neurologic signs are seen. The drugs of choice are chloramphenicol and the tetracycline antibiotics, given at maximum dosage. Cephalosporins are not recommended because of their limited penetration of the meninges. Penicillin or ampicillin along with an aminoglycoside is frequently used in human immunosuppressed patients. Treatment may be of some use in cattle, but there may be relapses. Sulfonamides, penicillin, and tetracyclines may be used prophylactically.

SUGGESTED CLINICAL EXAMPLES

An outbreak of listeriosis in feedlot cattle.

An outbreak of listeriosis in sheep on corn silage.

A case of listeriosis in a horse.

A case of listeriosis in a dog.

An outbreak of listeriosis in turkeys.

SOURCES FOR FURTHER READING

Busch, L.A.: Human listeriosis in the United States. J. Infect. Dis., *123*:328, 1971.

Gray, M.L., and Killinger, A.H.: *Listeria monocytogenes* and *Listeria* infections. Bacteriol. Rev., *30*:309, 1966.

Jones, S.M., and Woodbine, M.: Microbiological aspects of *Listeria monocytogenes* with special reference to listeriosis in animals. Vet. Rev. Annot., *7*:39, 1961.

Killinger, A.H., and Mansfield, M.E.: Epizootiology of listeric infection in sheep. J. Am. Vet. Med. Assoc., *157*:1318, 1970.

Ladds, P.W., Dennis, S.M., and Njoku, C.O.: Pathology of listeric infection in domestic animals. Vet. Bull., *44*:67, 1974.

Nieman, R.E., and Lorber, B.: Listeriosis in adults: A changing pattern. Report of eight cases and review of the literature, 1968–1978. Rev. Infect. Dis., *2*:207, 1980.

Seelinger, H.P.R.: *Listeriosis.* 2nd Ed. New York, Hafner, 1961.

Wilkinson, B.J., and Jones, D.: A numerical taxonomic survey of *Listeria* and related bacteria. J. Gen. Microbiol., *98*:399, 1977.

Woodbine, M. (ed.): Problems of Listeriosis. Proc. 6th Int. Symp., Leicester, England. Leicester University Press, 1976.

13

Erysipelothrix

Erysipelothrix rhusiopathiae

SYNONYM: *Erysipelothrix insidiosa*

Principal Characteristics

Erysipelothrix rhusiopathiae is a small, nonmotile, gram-positive rod. It is nonspore-forming, catalase-negative, facultatively anaerobic, and fermentative.

Historical

The organism was first described adequately by Löffler in 1886 and first recovered in the United States in 1892.

Habitat

Erysipelothrix is found in the tonsils and on the mucous membranes of normal swine and some other animals. It may also be present in the slime on the bodies of fresh and salt-water fish and crustacea. The organism lives and multiplies during the warm months in alkaline soil throughout the world.

Mode of Infection and Transmission

Erysipelas is worldwide in distribution and is acquired by direct contact with infected pigs and fomites. The mode of infection is thought to be by ingestion. The organism occurs in the surface slime of fresh and salt water fish and consequently may be transmitted in fish meal.

Pathogenesis and Pathogenicity

Toxins have not been demonstrated. Hyaluronidase and neuraminidase are produced by some strains and may be related to virulence.

The organisms regularly invade the bloodstream, and the type of disease that develops probably depends to a considerable extent on the immune status of the individual.

Swine. Pigs are most susceptible in the 3 to 18 months' age range. Erysipelas is enzootic and of considerable economic significance in certain regions. Several forms of the disease are seen, including the acute form, the skin or urticarial form, the arthritic form, and the cardiac form (endocarditis). These various forms may occur separately, in a sequence, or together. In the acute septicemic form, the course is short and the mortality is high. Reddish or purple rhomboidal blotches, scabs, and sloughing are seen in the skin form. Lesions are probably due to thrombus formation follwing Arthus-type reactions (immune complexes). The arthritic form is usually seen in older pigs; it is characterized by a marked periarticular fibrosis due in part to an allergic reaction.

Sheep. Post-dipping lameness in sheep: a laminitis resulting from an extension of a focal cutaneous infection in the region of the hoof. Nonsuppurative polyarthritis is seen in lambs. The organisms gain entry via the unhealed navel and wounds. This form of the disease may also be seen in calves.

Fowl. Turkeys, chickens, geese, and many other avian species are susceptible. Erysipelas is an important economic disease of growing turkeys. The acute disease is characterized by septicemia, and the organism may be recovered from all tissues.

126

Dogs. A number of cases of valvular endocarditis have been reported in dogs. The organism may be recovered in blood cultures.

Marine Mammals. Serious and fatal infections are encountered in cetaceans (dolphins, porpoises) and pinnipeds (sea lions, walruses).

Specimens

Acute or Septicemic Form: Blood and blood smears from live animals and liver, spleen, and coronary blood of necropsied animals.

Chronic Form: Affected tissues, e.g., heart, skin, and joint fluid. The organism may be difficult to obtain from advanced skin and joint lesions.

Isolation and Cultivation

Erysipelothrix rhusiopathiae grows readily on media enriched with serum or blood. Five to 10% CO_2 stimulates growth.

Two kinds of colonies are seen: smooth colonies are small, smooth and round, while rough colonies are larger, with irregular borders. The latter are obtained more frequently from chronic infections. Growth is very light after 24 hours' incubation but readily apparent after 48 hours. Alpha (greenish) hemolysis is usually seen around young colonies.

Gram-stained smears from smooth colonies reveal slender gram-positive rods resembling those of *Listeria* species. Smears from rough colonies disclose highly pleomorphic and filamentous forms. Characteristic organisms can be demonstrated from the blood and tissues of infected animals.

Identification

This organism most closely resembles *Listeria* species. Important features that differentiate it from *Listeria* are: *E. rhusiopathiae* is nonmotile and catalase-negative. Guinea pigs are resistant to infection. See also Table 12–1.

Experimental Animals. Mice are susceptible to infection, usually dying within four days after intraperitoneal inoculation. Pigs can be infected by applying virulent organisms to scarified skin.

Antigenic Nature and Serology

Employing agglutination procedures, groups or types designated A, B, and N have been identified on the basis of differences in somatic antigens. Type A strains were the principal cause of the acute disease in swine, while types B and N were associated with the chronic disease. Some workers have used numbers rather than letters to designate serologic varieties. The various serologic varieties are closely related immunologically. Serologic tests are of little value in diagnosis.

Resistance

The organism is remarkably resistant for a nonspore-former. It survives drying at room temperature for several months. Moist organisms will survive for years; one broth culture remained viable for 17 years. The organism survived boiling for two hours in pork six inches thick. It survives for long periods in smoked and unsmoked meats and in cadavers. Disinfectants, except for phenolic compounds, are quite effective against it.

Immunity

Immunity is mainly humoral. The formation of immune complexes and the occurrence of hypersensitivity reactions are responsible in part for some of the lesions seen.

Passive. Hyperimmune antierysipelas serum is no longer widely used. It is prepared in horses and cattle. It may be used during an outbreak therapeutically and to protect in-contact pigs. Protection is of short duration.

Active. (a) Avirulent living vaccines are fairly widely employed. One of these is administered orally. (b) Bacterins consisting of formalin-killed cultures adsorbed on alumina gels are widely employed, but immunity is of rather short duration.

Treatment

Penicillin is the drug of choice; it may be combined with antiserum. Erythromycin is used in human patients who are allergic to penicillin.

Public Health Significance

Erysipeloid is usually an occupational disease of veterinarians, packing house workers, butchers, and fish handlers. The organism usually enters via the skin (intact or broken) and after 1 to 5 days' incubation there is an erythematous swelling at the site of entry. Infection is usually localized and most frequently involves the hand. The course is usually about three weeks; there are occasionally more severe systemic complications. Several cases of valvular endocarditis have been reported.

SUGGESTED CLINICAL EXAMPLES

An outbreak of swine erysipelas in which several forms of the disease are seen.

An outbreak of erysipelas in turkeys.

An outbreak of post-dipping lameness in sheep.

An outbreak of nonsuppurative polyarthritis of lambs.

A case of erysipeloid in a veterinary practitioner.

SOURCES FOR FURTHER READING

Doyle, T.M.: Can swine erysipelas be eradicated? Epidemiological and immunological aspects. Vet. Rev. Annot., *6*:95, 1960.

Gledhill, A.W.: Swine erysipelas. *In* Diseases Due to Bacteria, vol. 2. Edited by A.W. Stableforth and I.A. Galloway. London, Butterworths Scientific Publications, 1959.

Goudswaard, J., Hartman, E.G., Janmatt, A., and Huisman, G.H.: *Erysipelothrix rhusiopathiae* strain 7, a causative agent of endocarditis and arthritis in the dog. Tijdschr. Diergeneeskd., *98*:416, 1973.

Grieco, M., and Sheldon, C.: *Erysipelothrix rhusiopathiae.* Ann. N.Y. Acad. Sci., *174*:523, 1970.

Jones, T.D.: Aspects of the epidemiology and control of *Erysipelas insidiosa* polyarthritis of lambs. *In* The Veterinary Annual. Edited by C.S.G. Grunsell and F.W.B. Hill. Bristol, Scientechnica, 1978.

Rosenwald, A.S., and Corstvet, R.E.: Erysipelas. *In* Diseases of Poultry. 8th Ed. Edited by M.S. Hofstad. Ames, Iowa State University Press, 1984.

Simerkoff,M.S., and Rahal, J.J., Jr.: Acute and subacute endocarditis due to *Erysipelothrix rhusiopathiae.* Am. J. Med. Sci., *266*:53, 1973.

Sneath, P.H.A., Abbott, J.D., and Cunecliffe, A.C. The bacteriology of erysipeloid. Br. Med. J., 2:1063, 1951.

Timoney, J.F., Jr., and Berman, D.T. *Erysipelothrix* arthritis in swine. bacteriologic and immunologic aspects. Am. J. Vet. Res., *31*:1411, 1970.

Wood, R.L.: Survival of *Erysipelothrix rhusiopathiae* in soil under various environmental conditions. Cornell Vet., *63*:390, 1973.

Wood, R.L., and Harrington, R., Jr.: Serotypes of *Erysipelothrix rhusiopathiae* isolated from swine and from soil and manure of swine pens in the United States. Am. J. Vet. Res., *39*:1833. 1978.

14

Clostridia

PRINCIPAL CHARACTERISTICS

Clostridia are large, gram-positive (young cultures) rods. Most are motile (*C. perfringens* is an exception), anaerobic (some are facultatively microaerophilic), spore-forming, fermentative, and catalase-negative.

HISTORICAL

Bollinger (1875) is usually given credit for first describing a pathogenic *Clostridium*, viz., *C. chauvoei*. Other species were also described quite early, but *C. haemolyticum* was not characterized until 1926 by Vawter.

GENERAL

Bergey's Manual of Determinative Bacteriology groups the clostridia as follows.
I. Spores subterminal
   A. Gelatin not hydrolyzed—group I (none associated with disease in animals)
   B. Gelatin hydrolyzed—group II
      C. sordellii
      C. botulinum
      C. novyi
      C. perfringens
      C. haemolyticum
      C. chauvoei
      C. septicum
II. Spores terminal
   A. Gelatin not hydrolyzed—Group III (none associated with disease in animals)
   B. Gelatin hydrolyzed—group IV
      C. tetani

III. Species with special growth requirements—group V (none associated with disease in animals).

HABITAT

Clostridia are free-living saprophytes distributed widely in the soil. Some species are more prevalent in some geographic areas. A number of species commonly occur in the intestinal tract. Of the large number of species (>60), only a few cause disease.

MODE OF INFECTION

Ingestion. Blackleg (cattle), botulism (food), enterotoxemia, bacillary hemoglobinuria, and black disease are caused by ingestion.
Wounds. *C. chauvoei* (sheep), *C. septicum, C. tetani*, and other gas gangrene organisms infect wounds.

MORPHOLOGY

The disease-producing clostridia are motile (except for *C. perfringens*) and nonencapsulated. They are relatively large rods with rounded ends occurring singly, in short chains, or as long filaments. Endospores may be located centrally, subterminally, or terminally.

CULTIVATION

Most grow well on blood agar, in cooked meat medium, and in thioglycolate broth in an atmosphere devoid of oxygen. Colonies are 1 to 3 mm in diameter, round or slightly irregular, slightly raised, granular, and transparent or translucent with fine filamentous margins. Special media are employed for toxin production.

RESISTANCE

The endospores of clostridia are very resistant to physical influences and disinfectants. In this respect they are similar to the spores produced by *Bacillus anthracis*, e.g., it may require 30 minutes of boiling to kill the spores of *C. botulinum*; 121°C in an autoclave for 20 minutes is lethal.

Clostridium chauvoei

Synonym. *Clostridium feseri.*

Disease. *C. chauvoei* causes blackleg.

Occurrence. *C. chauvoei* is widespread, but is more prevalent in certain geographic areas. It is found in the intestine and in normal tissues of some animals, including the livers of some apparently normal dogs and cattle. It is not as common in the soil as some other clostridia.

Toxins
1. Alpha toxin: hemolysin, necrotoxin.
2. Beta toxin: deoxyribonuclease.
3. Gamma toxin: hyaluronidase.
4. Delta toxin: hemolysin.

Pathogenesis. In blackleg, *C. chauvoei* is thought to enter the animal by ingestion or to be endogenous. The pathogen is carried by the blood to damaged muscle tissue, where it multiplies if conditions are anaerobic. *C. chauvoei* may enter wounds along with other organisms. The mixed infection and necrotic tissue provide an anaerobic milieu for *C. chauvoei*, which multiplies and produces its exotoxin and other metabolites. Bacteremia usually occurs late in the disease.

Pathogenicity. Blackleg in ruminants: cattle (4 months to 2 years)—ingestion; may be endogenous; sheep and goats—wounds. The lesion is not always easy to find; dry, dark, gas bubbles and rancid odor. There may be a bacteremia.

Immunity. Formalinized whole-broth cultures are used to produce life-long immunity. Protection is both antibacterial and antitoxic. Recovery from disease renders animals immune for life. There is a double bacterin that contains *C. chauvoei* and *C. septicum*. Some products contain *C. novyi* type A or *C. sordellii* or both.

C. chauvoei is antigenically heterogeneous, although there is considerable cross-protection among strains.

Clostridium septicum

Disease. *C. septicum* causes malignant edema.

Occurrence. It occurs worldwide and is found in the intestine and soil.

Toxins
1. Alpha toxin: lethal, necrotizng, and hemolytic
2. Beta toxin: a deoxyribonuclease.
3. Gamma toxin: hyaluronidase.
4. Delta toxin: a hemolyzing and necrotizing factor.

Pathogenicity. The pathogenesis of *C. septicum* infection is similar to that of gangrene caused by *C. chauvoei*.

It affects horses, cattle, sheep, pigs, and occasionally other animals in the form of malignant edema or gas gangrene. The common portals of entry are wounds and compound fractures. There is a large expanding swelling involving skeletal muscles that on pressure pits, is gelatinous, red, and has little gas.

In sheep the disease braxy is associated with eating frozen succulent feed. It produces necrotic lesions and hemorrhagic edema of the abomasal and duodenal walls. It is a European disease, although several cases have been reported in the United States.

In chickens it produces gangrenous dermatitis.

Immunity. *C. septicum* is included in some multiple component bacterins. The species is antigenically heterogeneous.

Clostridium haemolyticum

Synonym. *Clostridium novyi*, type D.

Disease. *C. haemolyticum* causes bacillary hemoglobinuria.

Occurrence. *C. haemolyticum* is probably worldwide wherever liver flukes occur. In the United States it is found predominantly in the mountain valleys of Nevada, Montana, and several other western states as well as along the Gulf of Mexico. Apparently it is not abundant in either the intestine or soil. Subclincial infections may occur in some animals, and these may serve as carriers that shed organisms via the intestinal tract.

Toxins. Toxins include lecithinase C, which is lethal, necrotizing, and in addition causes hemolysis of erythrocytes *in vitro* as well as *in vivo*. Other minor toxins are produced.

Pathogenicity. Infection with *C. haemolyticum* is limited to cattle and sheep, in which it causes bacillary hemoglobinuria or "red water." The mode of infection is by ingestion, with the organism probably reaching the liver hematogenously. Liver flukes result in infarction of branches of the portal vein. The organism can germinate and grow in the damaged anaerobic tissue, where it produces its toxin. The infarct is usually 5 to 20 cm in diameter. The disease does not appear in areas where conditions are not favorable for the flukes or the snails.

Death is apparently brought about by lysis of erythrocytes by the toxin, and the animal perishes of anoxia. The disease appears to be produced by a single enzyme, lecithinase, acting upon a single substrate, the lecithoprotein complex of the surface of the erythrocyte.

Immunity and control. The disease may be controlled by elimination of liver flukes through destruction of the carrier snails.

Formalized whole-broth cultures are used to produce an active immunity. Immunity is considered to be more antibacterial than antitoxic and is of relatively short duration. Animals at risk should be vaccinated every six months.

Strains are antigenically homogeneous.

Clostridium novyi

Synonym. *Clostridium oedematiens.*

There are two types: Type A—Gas gangrene: worldwide in man, cattle, and sheep; big head in rams. Type B—Black disease: It has been reported in Oregon, Colorado, Montana; worldwide.

Occurrence. Worldwide where liver flukes occur. It has been identified in sheep in Colorado and Montana.

Toxins. A number of exotoxins are produced, including ones with lethal and necrotizing properties. The two types differ antigenically and with respect to their toxins. Serum protection tests in animals will distinguish them.

Pathogenicity. Type A, which causes gas gangrene, is found in mixed infections with *C. chauvoei, C. septicum,* or *C. sordellii.* It is also seen in "big head," a disease of rams characterized by a marked swelling of the head and neck that is edematous in nature. Damage caused by butting allows entrance of the organism into the subcutis of the head.

Type B causes black disease or infectious necrotic hepatitis in sheep (and occasionally cattle). The mode of infection is oral, with the organism being carried to the liver via the blood. This is a localized infection of the liver, initiated by local tissue destruction resulting from the migration of young liver flukes. Toxin is produced in the local lesion and absorbed into the circulating blood, eventually producing death. Recovery is rare. Intense congestion of the blood vessels of the skin may result in blackening of the pelt. Cutaneous edema due to impairment of the heart may be present; it is usually sterile.

Immunity and control. Elimination of liver flukes by destruction of snails is required.

Formalinized bacterin and toxoid are of value. Type A is included in some bacterins for the prevention of gas gangrene infections.

Clostridium perfringens

Synonym. *Clostridium welchii.*
Disease. *C. perfringens* causes enterotoxemia.
Occurrence. *C. perfringens*, type A, is probably more widespread than any other potentially pathogenic bacterium. It is present in air, soil, dust, and manure and in water of lakes, streams, and rivers. It has been isolated from vegetables, milk, cheese, canned food, fresh meat, shellfish, and mollusks. It is constantly present in the intestinal contents of humans and animals and in their environment. Types B, C, D, and E strains are found less commonly in the intestinal tracts of animals.

Toxins. *C. perfringens* produces a number of exotoxins and enzymes that have important roles in the production of the various disease manifestations. The species is divided into types A to F on the basis of immunologic differences in the toxins, as determined by protection tests in animals. The alpha toxin referred to below is the principal lethal toxin. Among the substances produced are lethal, necrotizing toxins, hemolysins, collagenase, hyaluronidase, and deoxyribonuclease.

Some of the more important toxins and enzymes are listed.

ALPHA. This is the principal lethal toxin produced in varying amounts by all types of *C. perfringens*. In addition to being lethal, hemolytic, and necrotizing, it possesses the ability to split lecithin or lecithin-protein complexes.

BETA. This toxin is produced by strains of types B, C, and F. In addition to its lethal properties, it is responsible for inflammation of the intestine and the partial loss of the mucosa. These properties are associated with the types causing enteritis in cattle, sheep, and humans.

EPSILON. Epsilon toxin is produced by strains

of types B and D as a protoxin that is only slightly if at all toxic. The protoxin is then converted to toxin by proteolytic enzymes such as trypsin and pepsin as well as those produced by the microorganism itself (kappa and lambda). This toxin is necrotizing and highly lethal.

THETA. Theta is a lethal, hemolytic, necrotizing toxin produced by strains of types A, B, C, D, and E.

IOTA. This toxin is produced only by type E strains. Like epsilon it is formed as a protoxin and is subsequently activated by proteolytic digestion.

KAPPA. Kappa is a proteolytic enzyme that breaks down collagen. This toxin is the one principally responsible for the softening and "pulping" of affected muscles.

LAMBDA. Lambda is a proteolytic enzyme produced by strains of types B and E and by some strains of type D. It differs from kappa in that it is without activity on native collagen, but it does attack gelatin, casein, and hemoglobin.

MU. Mu has the property of hydrolyzing hyaluronic acid.

Pathogenicity

TYPE A. Most widespread of types; nontoxigenic *C. perfringens* are designated type A. Wound infection; gas gangrene and food poisoning in man (diarrhea: 6 to 24 hours after eating meat; not serious); these strains are especially heat resistant.

TYPE B. Type B causes dysentery in newborn lambs, which is primarily an enterotoxemia with marked enteritis and extensive ulceration. It does not occur in the United States or Australia.

TYPE C. Type C produces struck, an acute intoxication in adult sheep in England and Wales and hemorrhagic enteritis in neonatal calves, lambs, and young pigs. It is also responsible for enteritis necroticans, a serious disease of humans.

TYPE D. Type D causes enterotoxemia, "overeating disease," or "pulpy kidney" disease in sheep of all ages but particularly in feedlot sheep. It is a problem in lambs in feedlots. It is a true toxemia with little evidence of enteritis. Epsilon toxin is apparently produced in the upper intestine and the protoxin is activated by tryptic enzymes.

TYPE E. Type E is found in uncommon enterotoxemia (dysentery) of lambs and calves.

Immunity and Control. Good management and feeding practices are important in prevention.

Immunity is primarily antitoxic rather than antibacterial. Immunization is practiced principally in sheep. Formalinized whole-broth cultures prepared from strains of type C and type D are used to produce an active immunity. Immunity may not last for more than 6 to 12 months unless booster injections are given.

In addition, antitoxins derived from horses that have been hyperimmunized against toxins produced by types B, C, and D *C. perfringens* are available. Passive immunization is protective for no longer than 2 to 3 weeks.

Toxoids and bacterins are used to protect against types B, C, and D enterotoxemia of lambs. Ewes are given two doses of toxoid 6 weeks before lambing. Lambs may be immunized with bacterin or toxoid during the first week of life if ewes were not immunized and prior to entering feedlots.

C. perfringens antigens are sometimes included in multivalent clostridial bacterins.

Clostridium tetani

Occurrence. Spores of *C. tetani* are found throughout the world. It may be part of the normal flora of the soil, especially in the eastern part of the United States; it is less common west of the Mississippi River. It has frequently been isolated from the intestinal tract. As is sometimes thought, it is not more common in horse manure. However, the horse is more subject to hoof injuries and quite susceptible to tetanus.

Toxins. Three toxic substances are produced: a hemolysin (tetanolysin), a potent lethal toxin (tetanospasmin or neurotoxin), and nonspasmogenic toxin. The former is responsible for areas of hemolysis around colonies on blood agar plates, while neurotoxin is responsible for the characteristic signs of tetanus.

Neurotoxin (tetanospasmin), which is a protein, is highly toxic when injected parenterally; however, it is harmless if administered by mouth. Animals vary in their susceptibility to the toxin; horses and humans are the most susceptible. One milligram of pure toxin contains at least one million mouse lethal doses.

Toxin is elaborated at the site of infection and passes directly to major nerves and then to the spinal cord; it may also travel via blood and lymph. Once in the cord, it ascends to the medulla. The toxin acts at the inhibitory synapse, where it blocks the normal function of the inhibitory transmitter.

Little is known about nonspasmogenic toxin.

Pathogenesis and Pathogenicity. Spores usually germinate in dirty and neglected wounds with some necrosis (lowered oxidation reduction potential); infection is usually mixed. Toxin is elaborated at the wound site after spores germinate. Docking and castration wounds, umbilical infections (tetanus neonatorum), parturition (puerperal tetanus), dehorning, and ringing are among the circumstances that can contribute to tetanus.

Humans and horses are most susceptible, followed by pigs. Cattle and sheep are next; it is rare in dogs, and cats and poultry are resistant.

Immunity. Immunity can be considered almost totally antitoxic.

Toxoid is of value and is widely used in horses. Antitoxins are employed prophylactically but are of questionable value therapeutically. Recovery from tetanus does not necessarily confer permanent immunity.

Treatment. If indicated, surgical debridement of the wound or probable site of infection should be carried out. Antitoxin and penicillin are administered for prophylaxis. Toxoid may be administered at another site. Mortality may be as high as 50% in generalized tetanus in humans and horses.

Clostridium botulinum

Occurrence. Spores of *Clostridium botulinum* are frequently encountered in the soil. Ordinarily it does not take up residence in the intestine; however, some cases of infant botulism have occurred in which the toxin has been produced in the stomach or intestine. The type of *C. botulinum* may vary from one geographic area to another.

Toxins. Like other clostridial toxins, the exotoxins of *C. botulinum* are heat-labile proteins (100°C for 10 minutes).

Seven types of neurotoxin (A, B, C, D, E, F, and G) have been identified on the basis of antigenic differences. The toxins have been purified and are the most potent toxic substances known. One milligram of neurotoxin contains more than 20 million mouse lethal doses.

The toxins that are usually produced in foods are absorbed from the intestinal tract. Unlike most other toxins, they are resistant to peptic and tryptic digestion. After absorption, the toxin is transported to susceptible neurons via the bloodstream. It appears to be specifically directed to the peripheral nerves and is without effect on other body cells. It does not abolish conduction in the motor nerves but rather prevents the passage of impulses from the nerve to the muscle. The action may be concerned with inhibition of the release of acetylcholine. There is no evidence that the toxin affects the nerve cells of the brain. Paralysis is ascending, and death is caused by circulatory failure and respiratory paralysis, a result of the action of the toxin on motor nerves.

Pathogenicity. The principal media for the production of botulinus toxins are various spoiled foods, e.g., canned vegetables, meat, and fish. The toxin may also be produced in animal carcasses that dogs, chickens, and other animals may eat. Botulism in mink (types A, B, and C) has been traced to spoiled meat, including whale meat.

Type C botulism has occurred in chickens ("limberneck") and wild fowl, particularly water fowl that have eaten rotting vegetation. Forage (spoiled hay, silage) poisoning of horses has been claimed to be type C botulism.

Type D botulism causes "lamziekte" or "loin disease" in cattle with pica (phosphorus deficiency) in South Africa and Texas. The toxin is produced in bones of dead animals as a result of the growth of *C. botulinum* in carcasses.

Types A, B, E, and F have been reported most commonly in humans.

Wound and infant botulism occasionally occur in humans. In the latter, the toxin is produced in the gastrointestinal tract.

Many clinical diagnoses of botulism are not confirmed in the laboratory.

Immunity. As in tetanus, immunity is almost totally antitoxic. Immunization is not widely practiced in the United States; toxoids have been used principally in cattle and mink, with success in some parts of the world. Bivalent or trivalent antitoxins are available for prophylactic use; they are of questionable value after clinical signs have appeared.

Control. This involves the avoidance of spoiled or otherwise suspicious food. Cooking at 100°C for 10 minutes destroys the toxin.

OTHER CLOSTRIDIA

C. spiroforme. This organism is considered the cause of antibiotic-associated diarrhea and colitis in rabbits.

C. bubalorum. This clostridium is closely related to *C. novyi* type B and has been associated with osteomyelitis in buffaloes in Indonesia.

C. sordellii (bifermentans). *C. sordellii* causes gas gangrene and enterotoxemia in cattle.

C. colinum. This species is the cause of an acute or chronic ulcerative enteritis of quail.

C. difficile. *C. difficile* is responsible for pseudomembranous colitis in humans on prolonged antibiotic regimens.

C. sporogenes. This is a nonpathogen that occurs occasionally along with other bacteria in clostridial gas gangrene.

LABORATORY DIAGNOSIS

GAS GANGRENE (ANAEROBIC MYOSITIS)–TYPE DISEASES

Specimens. Should be from affected muscles and should be fresh. Because clostridia of the type that cause gas gangrene invade tissues from the intestine shortly after death, isolation or demonstration of these organisms is not always significant. This is especially so with *C. septicum* and *C. perfringens*.

C. chauvoei. Isolation and identification. Animal inoculation: guinea pigs die within 48 hours, while rabbits are resistant. There is a reliable direct fluorescent antibody (FA) procedure for identification of organisms in tissues or cultures.

C. septicum. Isolation and identification. Animal inoculation: lethal for guinea pigs; rabbits are susceptible. Long chains of filaments are seen in impression smears from the tissues of guinea pigs and rabbits. An FA procedure is available similar to that for *C. chauvoei*.

Other clostridia that occasionally cause gas gangrene, such as *C. novyi*, type A (FA available), *C. sordellii*, and *C. perfringens*, type A, are isolated and identified by conventional procedures.

Table 14–1. Neutralization Reactions between **Clostridium perfringens** *Toxins and Antitoxins*

Type	Major Lethal Toxins	Antitoxins				
		A	B	C	D	E
A	Alpha	+*	+	+	+	+
B	Alpha, beta, epsilon	–†	+	+	–	–
C	Alpha, beta	–	+	+	–	–
D	Alpha, epsilon	–	+	–	+	–
E	Alpha, iota	–	–	–	–	+

* + = toxin neutralized, mice protected.
† – = no neutralization, mice die.

BACILLARY HEMOGLOBINURIA AND BLACK DISEASE

Specimens. These should be taken from affected liver tissue.

C. haemolyticum. Isolation and identification. An FA procedure is available, but it does not distinguish between types. This species is also difficult to isolate.

CLOSTRIDIAL ENTEROTOXEMIA

Specimens. Fresh, small intestinal contents. Refrigerate.

C. perfringens. In cases of enterotoxemia, large numbers of large gram-positive organisms will usually be seen in smears from the smalll intestine.

First determine if the intestinal content is toxic for mice intravenously. If it is, mice are injected with mixtures of intestinal contents and *C. perfringens* type sera. The tests may also be carried out in the skin of guinea pigs. The type of *C. perfringens* involved is determined by the protection pattern observed (Table 14–1).

Isolation and identification can also be carried out. All toxigenic strains of *C. perfringens* produce the lethal alpha toxin (lecithinase C), which can be identified by the Nagler reaction. The latter is an opalescence shown in a special medium, produced by the neutralization of the toxin by antitoxin. The type is determined by animal protection tests using toxin produced (if toxic) in a broth culture. Not all strains are toxigenic. *C. perfringens* produces few spores unless grown on special media and is nonmotile. Although characteristic, stormy fermentation in milk is not specific for *C. perfringens*.

TETANUS

Specimens. Material from wound site.

C. tetani. Diagnosis is usually based on clinical signs. Organisms cannot always be demonstrated. Not all cultures of *C. tetani* are toxin producers. Characteristic "drumstick" spores (terminal) are produced. Swarming is seen in cultures.

BOTULISM

Specimens. Suspected food, meat, forage, and serum.

C. botulinum. Extracts of food or forage are inoculated into guinea pigs or mice to determine whether or not toxin is present. If this material is toxic, protection tests are carried out using the

Table 14–2. Differentiation of Important Clostridia

	Spores	Egg Yolk Agar		Milk	Gelatin Hydrolysis	Indole	Fermentation				Principal Fermentation Products
		Lecithinase	Lipase				Glucose	Maltose	Lactose	Sucrose	
C. perfringens	ST	+	–	S	+	=	+	+	+	+	A, B
C. chauvoei	ST	–	–	C	+	–	+	+	+	+	A, B
C. septicum	ST	–	–	C	+	–	+	+	+	–	A, B
C. novyi, A	ST	+	+	CG	+	–	+	+	–	–	A, P, B, V
C. novyi, B	ST	+	–	V	+	V	+	+	–	–	A, P, B, V
C. haemolyticum	ST	–	–	AC	+	V+	+	–	–	–	A, P, B, V
C. sordellii	ST	+	–	CD	+	+	+	+	–	–	A, F, P, 1B, 1V, 1C
C. bifermentans	ST	+	–	CD	+	+	+	+	–	–	A, F, P, 1B, 1V, 1C
C. sporogenes	ST	–	+	D	+	–	+	+	–	–	A, P, 1B, 1V, V, 1C
C. histolyticum	ST	–	–	CD	+	–	–	–	–	–	A
C. botulinum:											
Group 1	ST	–	+	(C)(D)	+	–	+	+	–	–	A, P, 1B, B, 1V, V, 1C
Group 2	ST	–	+	(C)	+	–	+	+	–	–	A, B
Group 3	ST	V	+	(C)(D)	+	–	+	V	–	–	A, P, B
C. tetani	T	–	–	V	+	V	–	–	–	–	A, P, B

A = Acetic acid
A = Acid
B = Butyric
C = Curd
D = Digestion

F = Formic
G = Gas
IB = Isobutyric
IC = Isocaproic
IV = Isovaleric

P = Proprionic
S = Stormy fermentation
ST = Subterminal
T = Terminal
V = Valeric
( ) = Variable

extract and type antitoxins in guinea pigs or mice to determine the type involved. Food is fed to the species involved. The organism can often be recovered from food and typed.

IDENTIFICATION OF CLOSTRIDIA IN GENERAL

The determination of the metabolic end products produced in glucose broth by gas chromatography is helpful in the final identification of some species. Criteria of the kind listed in Table 14–2 are also used.

TREATMENT

Penicillin and broad-spectrum antibiotics are effective if given very early in the gas gangrene diseases and bacillary hemoglobinuria. In blackleg it is advisable to treat all cattle of a susceptible age in a group or herd. Treatment is of little value in the enterotoxemias and black disease.

SUGGESTED CLINICAL EXAMPLES

An outbreak of blackleg in feeder cattle.

A case of malignant edema in the horse.

An outbreak of gas gangrene in sheep caused by *C. novyi*, type A.

An outbreak of black disease in sheep.

An outbreak of gas gangrene of cattle due to mixed clostridial infections.

Outbreaks of hemorrhagic enteritis in calves, lambs, or pigs produced by *C. perfringens*, type C.

An outbreak of "overeating disease" in lambs due to *C. perfringens*, type D.

A case of tetanus in the horse.

Botulism in mink.

Botulism in wild ducks.

An outbreak of "loin disease" in cattle.

SOURCES FOR FURTHER READING

Abbitt, B., et al.: Catastrophic losses in a dairy herd attributed to type D botulism. J. Am. Vet. Med. Assoc., *185*: 798, 1984.

Batty, I., and Walker, P.D.: Differentiation of *Clostridium septicum* and *Clostridium chauvoei* by the use of fluorescent labelled antibodies. J. Pathol. Bacteriol., *85*:517, 1963.

Borriello, S.P., and Carman, R.J.: Association of iota-like toxin and *Clostridium spiroforme* with both spontaneous and antibiotic-associated diarrhea and colitis in rabbits. J. Clin. Microbiol., *17*:414, 1983.

Holdeman, L.V., and Moore, W.E.C.: Anaerobic Laboratory Manual. 4th Ed. Anaerobe Laboratory, Blacksburg, Virginia Polytechnic Institute and State University, 1977.

Laird, W.J., et al.: Plasmid associated toxigenicity of *Clostridium tetani*. J. Infect. Dis., *142*:623, 1980.

Lamana, C., and Sakaguchi, G.: Botulinal toxins and the problem of nomenclature of simple toxins. Bacteriol. Rev., *35*:242, 1971.

MacLennan, J.D.: The histotoxic clostridial infections of man. Bacteriol. Rev., *26*:177, 1962.

Oakley, C.L., and Warrack, G.H.: Routine typing of *Clostridium welchii*. J. Hyg., *51*:102, 1953.

Roberts, T.A., Keymer, I.F., Borland, E.D., and Smith, G.R.: Botulism in birds and mammals in Great Britain. Vet. Rec., *91*:11, 1972.

Smith, L.D.S.: The Pathogenic Anaerobic Bacteria. 2nd Ed. Springfield, Il., Charles C Thomas, 1975.

Sterne, M., and Battey, I.: Pathogenic Clostridia. London, Butterworths, 1975.

Sterne, M., and Warrock, G.H.: The types of *Clostridium perfringens*. J. Pathol. Bacteriol., *88*:279, 1964.

Sutter, V.L., Vargo, V.L., and Finegold, S.M.: Wadsworth Anaerobic Bacteriology Manual. 3rd Ed. St. Louis, Mosby, 1980.

Weinstein, L.: Tetanus. N. Engl. J. Med., *289*:1293, 1973.

15

Bacillus

PRINCIPAL CHARACTERISTICS

Species of the genus *Bacillus* are gram-positive (old cultures decolorize easily) large rods. They are also aerobic (some are facultative anaerobes), spore-forming, mostly catalase-positive, and fermentative or respiratory or both. Some do not attack sugars and most are motile.

There are a large number of species. They are ubiquitous, occurring widely in the soil, air, dust, and water. They are among the most common laboratory contaminants. If clinical specimens such as bovine milk samples are not collected carefully, they are often contaminated with *Bacillus* species.

Bacillus anthracis is the only important pathogen of animals and humans in the genus. Occasional infections have been attributed to *B. cereus*, but animal disease caused by other species is rare.

Bacillus anthracis

HISTORICAL

Discovery of the bacillus that causes anthrax is credited to Davaine and Rayer (1863–1868). Koch fulfilled his postulates with *B. anthracis* in 1876–1877.

DISTRIBUTION

B. anthracis is found worldwide, in areas where anthrax spores are located. Anthrax organisms sporulate with greater frequency in low-lying marshy areas. Apparently vegetative forms grow poorly if at all in the soil. Some regions of the Mississippi and Missouri river valleys harbor spores and flooding disseminates them. Animals may become infected from contaminated bone meal, oil cake, and tankage. Humans become infected from animal fibers (e.g., toothbrushes), wool, hides, and infected animals.

MODE OF INFECTION

The microorganism is transmitted by ingestion, inhalation, wounds, scratches, and through the unbroken skin.

PATHOGENESIS

In the past death was attributed to the plugging of capillaries by the bacilli. Neither endotoxin nor exotoxin had been demonstrated. However, it was apparent that animals died of toxemia, and recently exotoxin was demonstrated in the plasma of dead or dying animals.

The anthrax toxin is a complex consisting of three protein components, I, II, and III. Component I is the edema factor, component II the protective antigen, and component III is the lethal factor. Components I and II cause edema with low mortality; however, when component III is included, there is maximum lethality. Only encapsulated, toxigenic strains are virulent. The unique capsular polypeptide is antiphagocytic but does not elicit protective antibodies.

The spores usually enter through the skin or mucous membranes and germinate at the site of entry. In the septicemic form, the vegetative bacilli spread via the lymphatics to the bloodstream. In the more localized form, as seen in swine, the infection may principally involve the lymph nodes of the head and neck.

PATHOGENICITY

The organism is generally classed as an obligate pathogen. Per-acute, acute, chronic, and cutaneous forms of the disease are seen. The more acute infections occur in cattle, sheep, horses, and mules. The cutaneous form is occasionally seen in horses and cattle when wounds or abrasions become infected.

Swine. The disease results in acute pharyngitis with extensive swelling and hemorrhage of the throat region. It is infrequent in other animals.

Dogs and Cats. A rare infection resembling that seen in swine.

Humans. The forms seen in humans are pulmonary anthrax, malignant carbuncle or pustule (>90% of cases), and intestinal anthrax.

DIRECT EXAMINATION

To prevent sporulation, diseased animals should not be opened. Cremation or deep burial (at least 6 feet) in lime is recommended for disposal.

Smears from tissues or blood are made and stained with Gram's or Giemsa or Wright's stain; the capsule stains a reddish-mauve. The finding of large, square-ended, gram-positive rods suggests the possibility of anthrax. It should be kept in mind that clostridial organisms are frequently found in the blood and tissues shortly after death. They can be eliminated in the differential diagnosis by the fact that they are not capsulated and because they fail to grow aerobically.

SPECIMENS

Septicemic form (cattle, sheep, horses, and possibly other species): swabs from exuded blood or blood taken by syringe. Blood smears may also be submitted.

Localized form (swine): swabs from the cut surface of hemorrhagic lymph nodes or fluid aspirated from affected lymph nodes is preferred.

ISOLATION AND CULTIVATION

If tissues are submitted, a composite suspension is prepared with a Ten Broeck grinder or mortar and pestle using sterile physiologic saline or broth as a diluent.

The organism grows well on all laboratory media. Guinea pigs and mice are inoculated from suspensions or blood and usually begin to die within 24 hours; large capsulated rods can be demonstrated in smears from the spleen and blood.

Colonies appear in 24 hours. They look rough, flat, gray, and usually are nonhemolytic. Some are called Medusa-head or "judge's wig" type colonies; the wavy edge of the colony resembles a tangled mass of curly hair. There are rough, smooth, and mucoid colonies; the rough variant is the most virulent.

Other *Bacillus* species resemble *B. anthracis*, especially *B. cereus*.

IDENTIFICATION

This may be based on the following:
1. Pathogenic for guinea pigs and mice.
2. Characteristic colony morphology; gram-positive rods; spore-formers. Spores are centrally located.
3. Nonmotile and aerobic. Other "anthracoids" are motile.
4. Virulent cultures are encapsulated; square ends.

B. anthracis may be distinguished from *B. cereus* as follows:

B. anthracis	B. cereus
Nonmotile	Motile
Salicin: slow or not at all	Rapid
Methylene blue reduction: slow	Rapid
Gelatin liquefaction: slow	Rapid
Slight or no hemolysis	Hemolytic
Penicillin-susceptible (some exceptions)	Not susceptible
Virulent strains: encapsulated	Not encapsulated

String of Pearls Test. This test produces characteristic growth showing cell wall impairment in a medium containing penicillin.

Bacteriophage. A preparation of specific phage (gamma phage) is added to a diffusely inoculated plate of suspected *Bacillus anthracis* culture. Only *B. anthracis* is lysed.

Fluorescent antibody may be used to presumptively identify *B. anthracis*.

See Table 15–1 for the identification of some species of *Bacillus*.

ANTIGENIC NATURE AND SEROLOGY

Srains appear to be closely related antigenically.

Table 15–1. *Differentiation of Some Species of* **Bacillus**

Species	Motile	Gelatin	Nitrites	Citrate	Urease	Glucose*	Arabinose*	Mannitol*
B. anthracis	−	+	+	+	−	+	−	−
B. subtilis	+	+	+	+	V	+	+	+
B. pumilis	+	+	−	+	−	+	+	+
B. coagulans	+	−	V	−	−	+	V	V
B. firmus	+	+	+	−	−	−	−	−
B. lentus	+	−	−	−	+	−	−	−
B. megaterium	+	+	−	+	V	+	+	+
B. cereus (and var. mycoides)	V	+	+	+	V	+	−	−
B. thuringiensis	+	+	+	−	V	+	−	−
B. stearothermophilus	+	+	+	−	V	+	V	−

*Because of ammonia production from peptones, peptone-free media must be used for the testing of carbohydrate utilization.

RESISTANCE

The endospores of *B. anthracis* are considerably more resistant to physical influences and chemical disinfectants than are vegetative cells. They may survive at least 22 years in dried cultures; they remain viable in soil for many years; and freezing temperatures have little if any effect on them. However, they are destroyed by boiling for 10 minutes and by exposure to dry heat at 140°C for 3 hours. When used, most chemical disinfectants must be employed in high concentrations over long periods of time. Spores are destroyed by lye in 8 hours; by 5% phenol in 2 days; by 10 to 20% formalin in 10 minutes; and by autoclaving at 121°C for 15 minutes. Mercuric chloride 1:1000 added to heat-fixed smears kills in 5 minutes.

TREATMENT

It is recommended that sick animals be treated and that well animals be immunized. The organism is susceptible to penicillin, tetracyclines, erythromycin, and chloramphenicol; the first two are commonly used. Treatment is effective in the malignant pustule-type infection but not usually in pulmonary anthrax in humans.

IMMUNITY

Protective immunity is thought to be largely antitoxic.

Active immunity can be produced in a number of ways:

1. Attenuated spore vaccine: Pasteur strain grown to sporulate. Rarely used now.
2. Avirulent spore vaccine: Sterne's noncapsulated strain gives good protection and has largely replaced Pasteur's spore vaccine. It is used in the spring in enzootic areas.
3. Bacterins: they are not as effective as the first two vaccines but are used in uncontaminated areas. Immunity is of short duration. They are not used in North America.

Because toxin production by *B. anthracis* is dependent on a plasmid, a vaccine consisting of purified protective antigen may result from recombinant DNA technology.

CONTROL

In most states it is required that all suspected cases of anthrax be reported to government veterinary officials.

PUBLIC HEALTH SIGNIFICANCE

There is need for great care in performing necropsies on animals, particularly if there is a likelihood that death was caused by anthrax.

OTHER *Bacillus* SPECIES

Bacillus cereus has been incriminated as a cause of gangrenous bovine mastitis and abortion in cows. In humans it has been implicated in food poisoning, especially after the consumption of fried rice that has been stored.

Bacillus subtilis is claimed to occasionally cause conjunctivitis and iridocyclitis in human beings.

Bacillus licheniformis has been implicated as a cause of bovine abortions in a number of herds.

SUGGESTED CLINICAL EXAMPLES

Outbreaks of anthrax in horses, cattle, sheep, and swine. Outbreaks may involve more than one animal species.

A case of anthrax in humans.

SOURCES FOR FURTHER READING

Fish, D.C., and Lincoln, R.E.: Biochemical and biophysical characterization of anthrax toxin. Fed. Proc., 26:1534, 1967.

Fox, M.D., et al.: Anthrax in Louisiana, 1971: Epizootiologic study. J. Am. Vet. Med. Assoc., *163*:446, 1973.

Fox, M.D., et al.: An epizootiologic study of anthrax in Falls County, Texas. J. Am. Vet. Med. Assoc., *170*:327, 1977.

Kaufmann, A.F., Fox, M.D., and Kalb, R.C.: Anthrax in Louisiana, 1971. An evaluation of the Sterne strain anthrax vaccine. J. Am. Vet. Med. Assoc., *163*:442, 1971.

Lincoln, R.J., Walker, J.S., Klein, F., and Haines, B.W.: Anthrax. Adv. Vet. Sci., *9*:327, 1964.

Mikesell, P., et al.: Plasmids, Pasteur, and anthrax. Am. Soc. Microbiol. News., *49*:320, 1983.

Sterne, M.: Anthrax. *In* Infectious Diseases of Animals: Diseases Due to Bacteria. Edited by A.W. Stableforth and I.A. Galloway. London, Butterworths Scientific Publications, 1959.

Sterne, M.: Distribution and economic importance of anthrax. Fed. Proc., *26*:1493, 1967.

Van Ess, G.B.: Ecology of anthrax. Science, *172*:1303, 1971.

Whitford, H.W.: Factors affecting the laboratory diagnosis of anthrax. J. Am. Vet. Med. Assoc., *173*:1467, 1978.

Wohlgemuth, K., Bicknell, E.J., and Kirkbride, C.A.: Abortion in cattle associated with *Bacillus cereus*. J. Am. Vet. Med. Assoc., *161*:1688, 1972.

16

Nonspore-forming Anaerobic Bacteria

The nonsporulating anaerobic bacteria constitute a large group of ill-defined organisms that exist in nature and are present in large numbers, particularly in the intestinal tract of animals.

Many reports dealing with various infections in humans indicate that necrotic and suppurative processes frequently yield nonspore-forming anaerobic bacteria, either alone or with aerobic bacteria. There is now considerable evidence that such is also the case with certain animal infections.

The lack of knowledge of the extent and importance of infections in animals caused by these anaerobes is mostly because they are difficult and expensive to isolate (for example, because of oxygen sensitivity) and identify, and also because the infections are usually sporadic rather than multiple in occurrence. Improved procedures and techniques for the isolation and identification of members of this group have spurred much interest in this neglected area of veterinary bacteriology.

It should always be kept in mind that isolation of such organisms does not necessarily mean they are of pathogenic significance, any more than does the isolation of aerobic organisms necessarily mean they are significant.

Most of the disease-producing nonspore-forming, anaerobic, gram-negative bacteria causing disease in humans and animals are in the family Bacteroidaceae. There are a large number of species in this family and not all are pathogenic. Several of the more important and better-known species are listed here, as are some of the anaerobic gram-positive bacteria occasionally recovered from clinical specimens and infectious processes.

FAMILY BACTEROIDACEAE

As mentioned previously, there are a large number of species in this group. Only several of the better-known species are mentioned here. All are gram-negative rods that occur in the feces of some animals and humans.

Bacteroides

B. fragilis. This rod is isolated from the feces of humans and animals; it is the most important of this group in humans.

B. melaninogenicus. *B. melaninogenicus* causes infections in humans and animals.

B. serpens. This species causes infections in humans.

B. nodosus. *B. nodosus* is responsible for contagious foot rot in sheep.

B. pneumosintes. This organism causes infections in humans.

B. corrodens (ureolyticus). *B. corrodens* causes infections in humans and animals.

Fusobacterium

F. necrophorum. This species produces many infections in animals and in humans.

F. nucleatum. *F. nucleatum* causes infections in humans and animals.

GRAM-POSITIVE ANAEROBIC COCCI

There are a number of genera. Several species of *Peptococcus* (cocci) and *Peptostreptococcus* (an-

141

aerobic streptococci) have been associated with infrequent infections in humans and animals. Their pathogenic significance is not always clear.

NONSPORE-FORMING GRAM-POSITIVE RODS

Species of *Eubacterium* and *Propionibacterium* are occasionally recovered from clinical specimens, but they are not thought to have pathogenic significance. Both occur widely in the feces of humans and animals.

HABITAT

Many of these anaerobes are commensals on mucous membranes of the upper respiratory, genital, and alimentary tracts of animals. They make up more than 90% of the bacteria of the intestinal tract, and they are predominant in the large bowel and in the rumen flora, where they have a vital role in digestion. There are many species, a number of which have probably not yet been identified.

INFECTIONS IN WHICH NONSPORE-FORMING ANAEROBES MAY BE INVOLVED

These organisms frequently invade tissues that are damaged and in which some necrosis provides a favorable anaerobic milieu for their growth. They may also be secondary to other primary infections. They are frequently recovered from

1. Necrotic, gangrenous (often with clostridia), and suppurative processes. They may be foul-smelling.
2. Abscesses in the lung, liver, and brain; pyometritis; infrequently cystitis and urinary tract infections; some postsurgical abscesses; septicemias and bacteremias; foot rot of cattle and sheep; cellulitis; periodontal abscesses; gutteral pouch infection; chronic sinusitis; and suppurative mastitis and osteomyelitis.

METHODS FOR THE ISOLATION AND CULTIVATION OF ANAEROBES

1. Anaerobic jars: Brewer, Torbal, and GasPak systems. These use catalysts to eliminate oxygen.
2. Anaerobic roll tube technique (Hungate method) using prereduced media. Air is excluded by means of "gasing" the media lined tubes.
3. Glove box technique using prereduced media. Oxygen is excluded from the glove box. All operations are carried out in the glove box.
4. Media containing reducing agents, e.g., cooked meat media and thioglycolate broth.

Of utmost importance is the exclusion of oxygen from clinical specimens and cultures. Thus special precautions must be taken in submitting specimens. Special anaerobic transport systems are available. Fluid material can be submitted in a syringe, and some laboratories provide special tubes with oxygen excluded.

Reference may have to be made to detailed differential tables for the precise identification of many species.

Fusobacterium necrophorum

Synonym. *Sphaerophorus necrophorus.*

Distribution and Mode of Infection. Distribution is worldwide. *F. necrophorum* is a commensal in the alimentary tract and on mucous membranes. Infections are endogenous.

Pathogenesis and Pathogenicity. *F. necrophorum* invades and multiplies in the anaerobic environment provided by damaged tissue. It is frequently a secondary invader. Infections are characterized by a necrotic process and are frequently mixed (e.g., liver abscesses in cattle, where it is often found with *Corynebacterium pyogenes*). Lesions are thought to be due in part to necrotizing endotoxin.

F. necrophorum may be isolated from numerous infections initiated by a variety of wounds and injuries in all domestic animals. It is a common secondary invader in necrotic stomatitis, pharyngitis, and enteritis. Enteritis is seen most commonly in swine. The general term used for *F. necrophorum* infections is necrobacillosis.

Some of the better-known diseases with which *F. necrophorum* is associated in various animals follow.

HORSE. It is usually involved in the infectious process called "thrush," involving the frog of the horse.

CATTLE. It is associated with calf diphtheria and is found in necrotic foci in the mouth, larynx, and trachea. It is also seen in necrotic laryngitis in feeder cattle. It has been suggested that the primary cause of these two diseases is *Haemophilus somnus*. *F. necrophorum* has also been implicated in liver abscesses and foot rot.

SHEEP. It is a frequent secondary invader in lip and leg ulcerations (primary cause is the ulcerative dermatosis virus). In combination with

Corynebcterium pyogenes, it causes foot abscess (ovine interdigital dermatitis).

PORCINE. It is considered the principal cause of "bull nose" resulting from the injury caused by "ringing" boars. It is a secondary invader in swine dysentery.

FOWL. It is involved in avian diphtheria, the primary cause of which is the fowl pox virus.

Specimens. Affected tissue; pus from abscesses. Specimens should be cultured immediately, or precautions must be taken to prevent exposure to oxygen. Material can be conveniently collected and submitted in a syringe.

Direct Examination. Gram-stained smears of affected tissues reveal gram-negtive rods of variable length with long characteristically beaded filaments.

Isolation and Cultivation. The organism is a strict anaerobe and grows best on enriched media. Several days of incubation are required. Many strains produce some L-forms on initial isolation. L-forms are cell wall–deficient forms that resemble mycoplasmas in some respects.

Colonies are small, smooth, convex, and whitish-yellow in color, with a narrow zone of alpha- or beta-hemolysis. Initially cultures may be very pleomorphic; short rods, long filaments, and "moniliform" bodies may be seen.

F. necrophorum can occasionally be recovered in pure culture from bovine liver abscesses. Pus or caseous material is taken aseptically by syringe or pipette and inoculated into previously heated thioglycolate broth.

Identification. Definitive identification is made on the basis of differential characteristics of the kind listed in Table 16–1.

Treatment. Surgical measures should be taken when indicated. Sulfonamides, penicillin, tetracyclines, and erythromycin have been effective against *F. necrophorum*. Susceptibility tests should be carried out. The aminoglycosides are ineffective.

Bacteroides nodosus

Synonym. *Fusiformis nodosus.*

General. This organism is a large, gram-negative, nonmotile, anaerobic rod. It is the primary cause of contagious foot rot of sheep. *F. necrophorum* is a common secondary invader and *Treponema penortha*, although present, is not pathogenic. *B. nodosus* can cause infections of the foot in goats, pigs, and cattle. Virulence appears to be associated with the production of proteolytic enzymes resulting in the breakdown of keratin.

The disease is aggravated by moist environmental conditions.

Direct Examination. Contagious foot rot of sheep can be diagnosed by the demonstration of the characteristic organism in gram-stained smears from typical lesions. Smears are made from material taken well down in the lesion after the horn has been pared away. The rods of *B. nodosus* may be straight or slightly curved and vary from 0.6 to 1.2 cm in length. They do not form spores and are gram-negative. When stained with Löffler's methylene blue, one, two, or more red-staining granules can be seen at either end or along the rod.

T. penortha can be seen in large numbers in positive smears as slender filaments displaying loose, irregular curves. The organism is gram-negative and stains faintly compared with *B. nodosus*.

Isolation and Cultivation. Foot rot can be readily diagnosed by demonstration of the characteristic organisms in smears from typical lesions, and the rather elaborate cultural procedures are not usually carried out.

Treatment and Control. Formalin or copper sulfate foot baths; 10% tincture of chloromycetin. The organism does not survive for longer than 2 weeks in pastures. Systemic use of penicillin and streptomycin is of value when accompanied by other control measures.

An oil-adjuvant *Bacteroides nodosus* bacterin has been shown to be useful in prevention.

Bacteroides melaninogenicus Group

The three former subspecies of this group have become the following species: *B. melaninogenicus*, *B. denticola*, and *B. loescheii*. The former species has been found in a considerable number of specimens from suppurative processes in cattle, sheep, dogs, and cats. It is frequently associated with *Fusobacterium necrophorum* in foot rot of cattle.

Bacteroides fragilis Group

This group formerly was made up of five subspecies, each of which has now been given species status. *B. fragilis* is the most common anaerobe causing infections in humans. It is encountered occasionally in various anaerobic infections in domestic animals.

TREATMENT OF INFECTIONS CAUSED BY GRAM-NEGATIVE ANAEROBES

Antimicrobial susceptibility tests should be carried out, because antibiotic resistance and

Table 16–1. *Differentiation of Some Important Gram-Negative, Nonspore-forming Anaerobes*

Test	Organism			
	Fusobacterium necrophorum	*Bacteroides corrodens*	*Bacteroides fragilis*	*Bacteroides melaninogenicus*
Motility	−	−	−	−
Nitrate	+	(+)	−	(−)
Gelatinase	−	−	−	+
Glucose	A	−	A	A
Lactose	−	−	A	−
Maltose	(A)*	−	A	V
Sucrose	−	−	A	V
Mannitol	−	−	−	−
Salicin	−	−	V	(−)
Indole	+	−	−	+
Organic acids detected by GLC†	A, P, B	A	A, P	A, others (Variable)

*( ) = Most strains.
{ †GLC = Gas liquid chromatography.
Acids: A = acetic acid; B = butyric acid; P = propionic acid.
Note: *B. melaninogenicus* produces black pigment on blood agar after 5 days. *B. melaninogenicus* ss. *asaccharolyticus* does not ferment any of the above carbohydrates.

beta-lactamase production by some *Bacteroides* strains have been reported. If the organism is susceptible, penicillin is recommended. Other useful drugs are chloramphenicol and clindamycin. Carbenicillin and the related drug, ticarcillin, as well as cefoxitin (a cephalosporin), have been used in humans.

SUGGESTED CLINICAL EXAMPLES

Multiple cases of foot rot in cattle.

An outbreak of contagious foot rot of sheep.

A brain abscess in a dog caused by *Bacteroides*.

Postoperative sepsis in a dog caused by *Bacteroides*.

A pulmonary abscess in a cat due to *Bacteroides melaninogenicus*.

SOURCES FOR FURTHER READING

Beveridge, W.I.B.: Foot rot of sheep: Its epidemiology and control. Bull. Off. Int. Epizoot., *59*:1537, 1963.

Berg, J.N., and Loan, R.W.: *Fusobacterium necrophorum* and *Bacteroides melaninogenicus* as etiologic agents of foot rot in cattle. Am. J. Vet. Res., 36:1115, 1973.

Berg, J.N., Fales, W.H., and Scanlon, C.M.: Occurrence of anaerobic bacteria in diseases of the dog and cat. Am. J. Vet. Res., 40:876, 1979.

Berkhoff, G.A., and Redenbarger, J.L.: Isolation and identification of anaerobes in the veterinary diagnostic laboratory. Am. J. Vet. Res., 38:1069, 1977.

Biberstein, E.L., Knight, H.D., and England, K.: *Bacteroides melaninogenicus* in diseases of domestic animals. J. Am. Vet. Med. Assoc., *153*:1045, 1968.

Holdeman, L.V., and Moore, W.E.C.: Anaerobic Laboratory Manual. 4th Ed. Anaerobe Laboratory, Blacksburg, Virginia Polytechnic Institute and State University, 1977.

Prescott, J.F.: Identification of some anaerobic bacteria in nonspecific anaerobic infections in animals. Can. J. Comp. Med., 43:194, 1979.

Prescott, J.F., and Chirino-Trejo, M.: Non-sporeforming anaerobic bacteria. *In* Diagnostic Procedures in Veterinary Bacteriology and Mycology. Edited by G.R. Carter. 4th Ed. Springfield, Ill. Charles C Thomas, 1984.

Roberts, D.S., Graham, N.P.H., Egerton, J.R., and Parsonson, I.M.: Infective bulbar necrosis (head-abscess) of sheep, a mixed infection with *Fusiformis necrophorus* and *Corynebacterium pyogenes*. J. Comp. Pathol., 78:1 1968.

Simon, P.C., and Stovell, P.L.: Diseases of animals associated with *Sphaerophorus necrophorus*. Characteristics of the organism—a review. Vet Bull., *39*:311, 1969.

Smith, L.D.S.: The Pathogenic Anaerobic Bacteria. 2nd Ed. Springfield, Ill., Charles C Thomas, 1975.

17

Enterobacteriaceae

PRINCIPAL CHARACTERISTICS

Enterobacteria are gram-negative, aerobic, and facultatively anaerobic medium-sized rods. They are oxidase-negative, catalase-positive (there are some exceptions), nonspore-forming, fermentative (often with gas), and usually motile.

gm ⊖
rods
kidase ⊖
tdase ⊕
n-spore
ment-dex
u. motile
(ability to adjust to certain situations)

CLASSIFICATION

Different classifications are used. The grouping used in Table 17–1 is based on that proposed by the Centers for Disease Control.

HABITAT

The enterobacteria are worldwide in distribution. There are both potentially pathogenic and nonpathogenic species. Many of the enterobacteria are part of the normal flora of the intestinal tract.

Some species are free-living, occurring in soil and water. Fecal contamination of water is indicated by the presence of *E. coli. Klebsiella* (including *K. pneumoniae*), *Enterobacter*, and *Citrobacter* species have been recovered from vegetable produce and wood products.

MODE OF INFECTION AND TRANSMISSION

This is almost always by ingestion. Fomites are especially important. Some infections are endogenous.

PATHOGENICITY

Clinical manifestations and pathologic changes may be due partly to endotoxins. The enterotoxins of *E. coli* are important in diarrheal diseases. Salmonellae and shigellae are frankly pathogenic. Other species such as *Proteus, Serratia*, and *Enterobacter* are opportunists that produce disease under certain circumstances, e.g., trauma to tissues (mastitis), debilitation, wounds, and malnutrition.

Escherichia

E. coli is recovered from a wide variety of infections in many animal species. It may be a primary or secondary agent. Nursing and young animals are particularly susceptible, and urinary tract infections are frequent.

From the standpoint of disease, two principal categories of *E. coli* are recognized: the opportunists and the enteropathogenic (enterotoxigenic, ETEC) or enterotoxin-producing strains. The enteropathogenic cultures are represented by different serotypes; certain serotypes show a host preference and are encountered more frequently in certain diseases.

Some strains have a unique invasive potential based on their ability to penetrate the intestinal mucosa. There may be lymphatic involvement and not infrequently a terminal septicemia. This type of *E. coli* infection is seen in calves, young pigs, lambs, foals, and occasionally in cows with mastitis.

Colonization of the small intestine by enterotoxigenic strains of *E. coli* is dependent upon certain pili. Two enterotoxins, one heat-stable (ST) and one heat-labile (LT), are produced by enterotoxigenic strains of *E. coli;* not all cultures

Table 17–1. Classifications of Enterobacteria

Tribe	Genus	Species
I. Escherichieae	*Escherichia*	coli
	Shigella	dysenteriae
		flexneri
		boydii
		sonnei
II. Edwardsielleae	*Edwardsiella*	tarda
III. Salmonelleae	*Salmonella*	choleraesuis
		typhi
		enteritidis
	Arizona	hindshawii
	Citrobacter	freundii
		diversus
		amalonaticus
IV. Klebsielleae	*Klebsiella*	pneumoniae
		oxytoca
		ozaenae
		rhinoscleromatis
	Enterobacter	aerogenes
		cloacae
		agglomerans
		sakazakii
		gergoviae
	Hafnia	alvei
	Serratia	marcescens
		liquefaciens
		rubidaea
V. Proteeae	*Proteus*	mirabilis
		vulgaris
	Morganella	morganii
	Providencia	alcalifaciens
		stuartii
		rettgeri
VI. Yersinieae	*Yersinia*	pestis
		pseudotuberculosis
		enterocolitica
		intermedia
		fredriksenii
		ruckeri
VII. Erwinieae	*Erwinia*	
	Pectobacterium	

will produce both of these plasmid-based enterotoxins. The action of one or the other can be demonstrated in ligated intestinal segments, certain cell cultures, and suckling mice. The enterotoxin producers do not ordinarily invade, but their enterotoxin is adsorbed to epithelial cells. The LT stimulates adenylcyclase, resulting in conversion of ATP to cyclic AMP. The latter induces the excretion of Cl⁻ and inhibits the adsorption of Na⁺, causing great fluid losses. The two enterotoxins can be differentiated on the basis of their ability and their toxic, immunologic, physical, and chemical characteristics. Some of the properties of the two different enterotoxins are given in Table 17–2.

The letter K ordinarily stands for the surface or envelope antigen of enterobacteria (discussed further on). In the case of K88 and K99 cultures of ETEC, these terms represent different pilus antigens. K88 cultures of ETEC are associated with diarrhea in swine and K99 cultures of ETEC with diarrhea in calves.

As a general rule, the acute infections of neonatal animals chracterized by bacteremia or septicemia are caused by invasive strains of *E. coli*, while the diarrheal infections are due to enterotoxin-producing strains (enteropathogenic or enterotoxigenic). The invasive strains give a positive Sereny test (see further on).

Colibacillosis is a general term that denotes an *E. coli* infection characterized by one or more of the following: diarrhea, enteritis, septicemia, or bacteremia. Rota and corona viruses may be involved as well as *E. coli*.

Cattle. Infection with *E. coli* takes the form of neonatal calf scours or diarrhea occurring during the first three weeks of life; dehydration due to enterotoxin(s); colisepticemia with a course as short as 48 hours; or mastitis.

Swine. It produces diarrhea in pigs a few days old and marked dehydration due to enterotoxin(s). Hemorrhagic gastroenteritis and edema disease may occur one to two weeks after weaning. The edema of edema disease has been attributed to vasotoxin.

Edwardsiella

Edwardsiella tarda is recovered occasionally from the intestinal tract of animals and humans. A small number of opportunistic infections have been reported in human beings and animals.

Enterobacter

Strains of this group, *Klebsiella*, and *E. coli* are referred to as coliforms.

Strains of *Enterobacter* are only occasionally incriminated in animal disease. The most common infection they produce is bovine mastitis.

Klebsiella

Klebsiella strains have been recovered from various animal infections: pneumonia and suppurative infections in foals; cervicitis and metritis in mares; mastitis in cows; wound infections; urinary infections, particularly in dogs; and septicemia and pneumonia in the dog. Most of the strains recovered from clinical specimens are *K. pneumoniae*.

Table 17–2. *Some Properties of the Two Enterotoxins of* Escherichia coli

	Heat-Stable (ST)	Heat-Labile (LT)
Calves	Most cases	Few cases
Pigs	Most cases	Most cases
Molecule	Very small; peptide	Large; protein
Heat stability	Resists 121°C/15 min	Destroyed by 60°C/30 min
Antigenicity	Negative	Positive
Antibody neutralization	Generally negative	Positive
Onset time and duration (Ligated rabbit ileal loop)	Rapid and short	Slow and long
Adenyl cyclase activation	No	Yes
Guanylate cyclase activation	Yes	No
Tissue culture assay	Negative	Positive
Suckling mouse assay	Positive	Negative

Arizona

Infections in animals, except in reptiles, chicks, and turkey poults, are rare. Two serotypes of *A. hinshawi* (7:1,7,8 and 7:1,2,6) cause chronic intestinal disease in chicks and turkey poults. The infections are egg-transmitted.

Providencia

Species of this genus rarely cause animal infections.

Proteus

Proteus mirabilis has been implicated in a variety of sporadic infections of dogs, cattle, and fowl. Cystitis and urinary infections are the most common, particularly in dogs. On occasion *Proteus* species are thought to be involved in diarrhea in young minks, lambs, calves, goats, and puppies.

Serratia

The one species of significance in infections is *S. marcescens*, which may produce a red pigment. It is responsible for infrequent cases of bovine mastitis and other uncommon sporadic infections.

Salmonella

Infection is by the oral route. Unlike the other enteric bacteria, except for *Yersinia*, the salmonellae are frequently facultative intracellular parasites. The invasive strains are taken up by macrophages, and spread is via the lymphatic system. Three principal forms of salmonellosis are described as occurring in humans: enteric fevers, septicemia, and gastroenteritis. The forms seen in animals are principally septicemia, acute enteritis, subacute enteritis, and chronic enteritis. An asymptomatic carrier state is common.

More than 1,000 species (actually different serotypes) have been identified, all of which are potentially pathogenic, causing sporadic infections as well as outbreaks of frequently fatal disease.

Recently the *Salmonella* have been reclassified as three distinct species on the basis of biochemical differences (Table 17–3): *S. choleraesuis, S. typhi,* and *S. enteritidis.* The latter species includes many serotypes and all the species listed below except for *S. typhi* and *S. choleraesuis.* Thus in the new classification all of the species except *S. choleraesuis* and *S. typhi* are identified as *S. enteritidis,* followed by the original species name, e.g., *S. newport* becomes *S. enteritidis* sero *newport.* The older classification is used below.

Some important diseases caused by the *Salmonella* appear in Table 17–4.

Serotypes within a group have a common O antigenic determinant. There are additional groups, but most clinical isolates from humans and animals are found in groups A through O.

Shigella

Members of this group are not important as causes of disease in domestic animals. All species cause dysentery in humans and other primates. Unlike the salmonellae, they do not cause systemic disease.

Yersinia

This genus was created for bacteria that were formerly called *Pasteurella pestis, P. pseudotuberculosis,* and other closely related bacteria. They are true enterobacteria and did not belong in the genus *Pasteurella. Y. pestis* is the cause of plague; *Y. pseudotuberculosis, Y. enterocolitica,* and other

Table 17–3. Differentiation of the Three Species (New Classification) of **Salmonella**

	S. choleraesuis	S. enteritidis*	S. typhi
Stern's glycerol fuchsin	−	(+)	−
Simmons' citrate	−	(+)†	−
Ornithine decarboxylase	(+)	(+)	−
Gas from glucose	(+)	(+)	−
Dulcitol	(−)	(+)	(−)
Arabinose	−	+	−
Rhamnose	+	(+)	−
Trehalose	−	+	+

*Includes all salmonellae except *S. choleraesuis* and *S. typhi*.
†( ) most.

closely related species cause infections in humans and animals. The important species are dealt with in some detail further on.

Erwinia **and** Pectobacterium

Organisms of these genera are mainly plant pathogens.

ANTIGENIC NATURE AND SEROLOGY

E. coli. Identification of the serotypes of this species is not carried out routinely in most veterinary diagnostic laboratories because sera are not readily available. Serotyping could be of value in identifying serotypes that are frequently enterotoxin producers. The antigens used to designate serotypes are as follows:

1. Somatic or O antigens: designated by Arabic numerals, e.g., 0133.
2. K (surface or envelope) antigens: thermolabile—L and B antigens; thermostable—A antigen. They are designated by the letters L, B, or A, with an Arabic number, e.g., K4.
3. H or flagellar antigens: designated by H followed by an Arabic number, e.g., H2. If there are no flagella, it is designated NM (nonmotile).

An example of a complete designation is 0111:B4:H2.

Salmonella.

1. Somatic or O antigens: designated by Arabic numerals; group classification is based on several of these antigens.
2. Flagellar antigens: phase 1: Designated by small letters of the alphabet, more or less specific for the salmonella. Isolates must be in this phase before they can be typed. Phase 2: Designated by Arabic numerals; less specific, and duplicated in other bacterial species.
3. K antigens (capsular or envelope): "Vi" antigen, "M" antigen, and so forth. These antigens may interfere with agglutinability of O antisera.

An example of a complete designation is *S. typhimurium*, 1,3,5,12:i:1, 2.

In most veterinary diagnostic laboratories the salmonella isolates are examined serologically in order to determine their group. Group identification is based on the possession of certain somatic or O antigens. Salmonella O antisera are available commercially covering groups A through I. The procedure is a simple slide agglutination test. It is usual to test an isolate first against a polyvalent O serum covering groups

Table 17–4. Important Diseases Caused by Salmonella

Group A:	S. paratyphi	Paratyphoid fever in humans.
Group B:	S. abortivoequina	Abortion in mares.
	S. schottmuelleri	Paratyphoid fever in humans.
	S. typhimurium	Gastroenteritis in humans; most prevalent species causing infections in various animal species.
Group C₁:	S. choleraesuis	Secondary invader in hog cholera; may be associated with necrotic enteritis in swine. Infections in humans.
Group C₂:	S. newport	Infections in humans, various animals, and especially cattle.
Group D:	S. enteritidis	Infections in various animals; gastroenteritis in humans.
	S. gallinarum	Fowl typhoid.
	S. pullorum	A severe infection of chicks and poults known as bacillary white diarrhea or pullorum.
	S. typhi	Typhoid fever in humans.
	S. dublin	Severe infections in calves.
Group E₁:	S. anatum	Keel disease in ducklings; infections in humans and animals.

A to I. If this is positive, then tests are conducted with the individual group sera. Further serologic characterization is carried out in reference laboratories.

RESISTANCE

Like most vegetative forms of bacteria, *Salmonella* are not especially resistant to physical and chemical influences. Sunlight and desiccation kill them readily; freezing does not.

ISOLATION AND CULTIVATION

The organisms grow well on ordinary unenriched culture media. Selective media are available that favor the growth of some genera (see Tables 17–5 and 17–6). Tissues, feces, or intestinal material is usually submitted for culture.

Procedures for isolation and cultivation are outlined in Table 17–7.

The colonies of the various enterobacteria on blood agar look very much the same with few exceptions. However, colonies on selective media show considerable differences among genera (see Table 17–5).

IDENTIFICATION

After observing the kinds and numbers of colonies, several are inoculated in triple sugar iron agar (TSI). This medium is used for fermentation of lactose, sucrose, and dextrose, and production of H_2S and gas. It is inoculated first into the butt, then streaked on the slant and incubated for 18 hours at 37°C. THe following reactions may be obtained:

1. Alkaline slope (red) and acid butt (yellow): dextrose fermentation only.
2. Acid slope (yellow) and acid butt (yellow): lactose or sucrose fermentation or both; dextrose fermentation.
3. Blackening along the stab line: H_2S production.

Table 17–5. Appearance of Important Enterobacteria on Selective Media

Enterobacteria	Brilliant Green Agar	MacConkey Agar
Coliforms: E. coli Enterobacter Klebsiella	Inhibited. If present, are yellowish-green	Grow and are red. Enterobacter and Klebsiella may be larger and mucoid.
Proteus	Grow; don't spread; yellowish-green. Sucrose-negative: strains are colorless.	Grow and spread. Colorless.
Salmonella	Grow. Red due to peptone hydrolysis.	Grow; colorless.

4. Gas bubbles in agar: some fermentative enterobacteria produce gas while many others do not.

The reactions on TSI are observed (Table 17–8). These, along with the so-called IMViC reactions (indole, methyl red. Voges-Proskauer [acetyl-methyl carbinol], citrate [utilization]) and the other reactions listed in Table 17–9, will identify the principal genera. The definitive identification of some species of enterobacteria can be determined from Table 17–10.

All strains of *Proteus* species may spread or swarm over the agar plate; swarming is inhibited if the agar is increased to 4%. The spreading edges of two different strains of *Proteus* on an agar plate are inhibited before union takes place (Dienes' phenomenon). In contrast, the spreading edges of the same strain fuse imperceptibly. This can be of epidemiologic significance in urinary tract infections.

TREATMENT

Tetracyclines, chloramphenicol (especially for *S. typhi*), nitrofurans, ampicillin, neomycin, and sulfonamides have all been employed. There are multiple resistant strains. The plasmids involved are transferred among enteric organisms by conjugation. Included in the plasmid (R factor) is the resistance transfer factor (RTF) and genes for resistance to several drugs. They appear to diminish permeability to the corresponding drugs. There are complex interrelations among the enteric bacteria. Serologic type may be based on a small difference in a single macromolecule. There are great opportunities for genetic recombination. In salmonellosis there may be carriers after treatment.

IMMUNITY

E. coli bacterins are used to immunize cows and sows in order to prevent disease in their young. However, because of antigenic heterogeneity, they are considered of limited value. Mini-cell and pilus vaccines have been developed and appear to be of value. Sows have been vaccinated orally with field cultures of *E. coli*. An attenuated live *S. typhimurium* vaccine is used in cattle in England. Various salmonellae such as *S. choleraesuis* and *S. typhimurium* are incorporated in bacterins, alone or with other bacteria. An *S. dublin* bacterin is used to prevent salmonellosis in calves. Because immunity to salmonellosis is probably predominantly cell-

Table 17–6. Media for the Isolation and Identification of the Enterobacteriaceae

Medium	Key Nutrients	Indicators	Detected	Inhibitors	Bacteria Inhibited	Bacteria Favored
Selenite F broth	Lactose	None	—	Sodium selenite	Coliforms	*Salmonella, Shigella, Proteus,* Paracolons
Tetrathionate broth	None	None	—	Bile salts, iodine	Coliforms, gram-positives	*Salmonella, Shigella,* Paracolons
Triple sugar iron agar (TSI)	Glucose 0.1%, lactose 1.0%, sucrose 1.0%	Phenol red, ferrous ammonium sulfate	Carbohydrate fermentation, H_2S production	None	None	All
MacConkey agar	Lactose	Neutral red	Lactose fermentation	Bile salts, crystal violet	Gram-positives	Enteric bacteria and other gram-negatives
Brilliant green agar	Lactose, sucrose	Phenol red	Lactose or sucrose fermentation	Brilliant green	Coliforms, *Shigella*	*Salmonella, Proteus,* Paracolons
Simmons' citrate agar	Sodium citrate	Bromthymol blue	Growth from citrate as sole source of carbon	None	Bacteria unable to use citrate as sole C source	Citrate-positive organisms
MR-VP broth	Glucose	Add after incubation to two different culture tubes: methyl red	Acid from glucose = +	None	—	—
		VP1 (alpha naphthol) VP2 (KOH)	Acetyl-methyl carbinol from glucose = +	None	—	—
Tryptone broth (for indole)	Tryptophan	Add Kovac's reagent after incubation	Indole production from tryptophan	None	—	—

Table 17–7. *Sequence of Procedures for the Isolation and Identification of Enterobacteria*

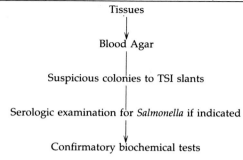

Tissues

Blood Agar

Suspicious colonies to TSI slants

Serologic examination for *Salmonella* if indicated

Confirmatory biochemical tests

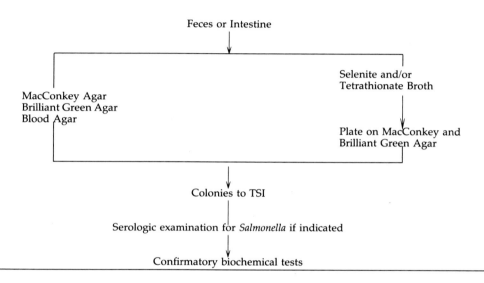

Feces or Intestine

MacConkey Agar
Brilliant Green Agar
Blood Agar

Selenite and/or
Tetrathionate Broth

Plate on MacConkey and
Brilliant Green Agar

Colonies to TSI

Serologic examination for *Salmonella* if indicated

Confirmatory biochemical tests

mediated, there is some question as to the value of bacterins.

PUBLIC HEALTH SIGNIFICANCE

Salmonella

Reservoir and Sources of Infection. The carrier state may be considerable in domestic (including poultry) and wild animals; turtles and other pets may also shed salmonellae. Human patients, both sick and convalescent, and subclinical carriers may shed organisms.

Other sources are feces of humans and animals; whole eggs, especially duck eggs, egg products, meat and meat products, and poultry; and fertilizers and animal feeds prepared from bones, fish meal, and meat.

Transmission. Infections and epidemics are usually traceable to various food products derived from meat, eggs, milk, and poultry. Other means of infection derive from the contamination of food and water with rodent feces, from infected food handlers, and from contaminated equipment and utensils. Sporadic cases occur from direct contact with an infected animal or person.

Yersinia pestis

Synonym. *Pasteurella pestis.* The genus *Yersinia* has been created for *Pasteurella pestis* and *Pasteurella pseudotuberculosis.* These species resemble the Enterobacteriaceae more closely than the classic pasteurella. The remaining species in the genus, *Y. enterocolitica,* causes disease resembling that caused by *Y. pseudotuberculosis.* It has been recovered from many animal species and from humans. All species are facultative intracellular parasites. The genus was isolated and described by Kitasato and Yersin independently in 1894.

Pathogenesis and Pathogenicity. A toxin is produced, but its role in pathogenesis is not clear.

Table 17–8. Reactions of Some Important Enterobacteria on Triple Sugar Iron Agar

Slant	Butt	Gas	H₂S	Sugars* Attached (Acid)	Probable Identification
A	A	−	−	G, L, (S)	*Escherichia coli*
A	A	+	−		
A	A	+	−	G, L, S	*Klebsiella*
K	A	+	−	G	*Salmonella*
K	A	−	+	G	
K	A	+	+	G	
A	A	+	+	G, L (S)	*Proteus*
K	A	−	−	G	
K	A	+	−	G	
K	A	+	+	G	
K	A	+	+	G	*Arizona*
A	A	−	−	G, L, S	*Serratia*
A	A	+	−	G, L, S	
K	A	−	−	G	
A	A	+	−	G, L, (S)	*Citrobacter*
A	A	+	+	G, L, (S)	
K	A	−	−	G	
K	A	+	+	G	
K	A	−	−	G	*Providencia*
K	A	+	−	G	
K	A	−	−	G	*Yersinia*

*K = alkaline; A = acid; L = lactose; S = sucrose; G = glucose; L, (S) = lactose and/or sucrose.

Table 17–9. Differentiation of the Principal Genera and Some Species of the Enterobacteriaceae

Test	*Escherichia*	*Shigella*	*Salmonella*	*Arizona*	*Citrobacter*	*Klebsiella*	*Enterobacter cloacae*	*Enterobacter aerogenes*	*Hafnia*	*Serratia*	*Proteus vulgaris*	*Proteus mirabilis*	*Providencia*
Indole	+	−/+	−	−	−	−/+	−	−	−	−	+	−	+
Methyl red	+	+	+	+	+	−	−	−	+/−	−/+	+	+	+
Voges-Proskauer	−	−	−	−	−	+	+	+	+/−	+	−/+	−/+	−
Simmons' citrate	−	−	d	+	+	+	+	+	+/−	+	d	+	+
H₂S gas (TSI)	−	−	+	+	+/−	−	−	−	−	−	+	+	−
Urease	−	−	−	−	dw	+w	+w	−	−	dw	+	+	−
Motility	+/−	−	+	+	+	−	+	+	+	+	+	+	+
Lysine	d	−	+	+	−	+	−	+	+	+	−	−	−
Ornithine	d	d	+	+	d	−	+	+	+	+	−	+	−
Phenylalanine	−	−	−	−	−	−	−	−	−	−	+	+	+
Gas from glucose	+	−	+	+	+	+	+	+	+	+/−	+/−	+	−
Lactose	+	−	−	d	d	+	+	+	−/+	−/+	−	−	−
Sucrose	d	−	−	−	d	+	+	+	d	+	+	d	d

Key: (+) = 90% of isolates positive; (−) = 90% of isolates negative; (d) = delayed positive (3 to 5 days); (w) = weak reaction; (+/−) = majority positive; but less than 90% positive; (−/+) = majority negative, but less than 90% negative.

(Adapted from Koneman, E.W., Allen, S.D., Dowell, V.R., Jr., and Sommers, H.M.: Diagnostic Microbiology. Philadelphia, J.B. Lippincott Co., 1979.)

Table 17-10. Differentiation of Some Enteric Bacteria by Biochemical Tests*

- = 0–10% of strains positive
(-) = 11–25% of strains positive
d = 26–75% of strains positive
(+) = 76–89% of strains positive
+ = 90–100% of strains positive

	Indole production	Methyl red	Voges-Proskauer	Citrate (Simmons')	Hydrogen sulfide (TSI)	Urease (Christensen's)	Phenylalanine	Lysine decarboxylase	Arginine dihydrolase	Ornithine decarboxylase	KCN (growth in)	Motility	Gelatin liquefaction	Malonate	Glucose (gas)	Lactose	Sucrose	Mannitol	Dulcitol	Salicin	Adonitol	Inositol	Sorbitol	Arabinose	Raffinose	Rhamnose	Esculin hydrolysis	ONPG (β-galactosidase)
Citrobacter amalonaticus	+	+	-	(+)	-	(+)	-	-	(+)	+	+	+	-	(-)	+	d	(-)	+	-	d	-	-	+	+	-	+	-	+
C. Diversus	+	+	-	+	(+)	(+)	-	-	d	+	-	+	-	+	+	d	-	+	d	(-)	+	-	+	+	d	+	-	+
C. freundii	-	+	-	+	+	d	-	-	d	(-)	+	+	-	-	+	d	d	+	d	-	-	-	+	+	-	+	-	+
Edwardsiella tarda	+	+	-	-	+	-	-	+	-	+	-	+	-	-	+	-	-	-	-	-	-	-	-	-	-	-	-	-
E. tarda biogroup 1	+	+	-	-	+	-	-	+	-	+	-	+	-	-	d	-	d	-	-	-	-	-	-	-	-	-	-	-
Enterobacter aerogenes	-	-	+	+	-	-	-	+	-	+	+	+	-	+	+	+	+	+	-	+	+	+	+	+	+	+	+	+
E. cloacae	-	-	+	+	-	d	-	-	+	+	+	+	-	(+)	+	+	+	+	d	+	-	(-)	+	+	+	+	d	+
E. gergoviae	-	d	+	+	-	+	-	+	+	+	+	+	-	+	+	d	+	+	-	+	-	-	-	+	+	+	d	+
Escherichia coli	(+)	+	-	-	-	-	-	(+)	(+)	d	-	d	-	-	+	+	d	+	(-)	d	(-)	(-)	(+)	+	d	(+)	d	+
E. coli (inactive)	(+)	+	-	-	-	-	-	d	(-)	(-)	-	(-)	-	-	(+)	(-)	(-)	+	d	-	-	(-)	(+)	+	(-)	d	-	d
Hafnia alvei	-	d	d	-	-	-	-	+	-	+	+	d	-	d	+	-	-	+	-	(-)	-	-	-	+	-	+	d	+
Klebsiella oxytoca	+	d	d	+	-	+	-	+	-	-	+	-	-	+	+	+	+	+	d	+	+	+	+	+	+	+	+	+
K. pneumoniae ss. *pneumoniae*	-	(-)	+	+	-	+	-	+	-	-	+	-	-	+	+	+	+	+	d	(+)	+	+	+	+	+	+	(+)	+
Morganella morganii	+	+	-	-	-	+	+	-	-	+	+	+	-	-	(+)	-	-	-	-	-	-	-	-	-	-	-	-	-
Proteus mirabilis	-	+	(-)	d	+	+	+	-	-	+	+	+	+	-	+	-	d	-	-	-	-	-	-	-	-	-	-	-
P. vulgaris	+	+	-	(-)	+	+	+	-	-	-	+	+	+	-	+	-	+	-	-	+	-	-	-	-	-	-	(+)	-
Providencia alcalifaciens	+	+	-	+	-	-	+	-	-	-	+	+	-	-	(+)	-	(-)	-	-	(+)	+	-	-	-	-	-	-	-
P. rettgeri	+	+	-	+	-	+	+	-	-	-	+	+	-	-	(+)	-	(-)	+	-	d	+	+	-	-	d	d	d	-
P. stuartii	+	+	-	+	-	d	+	-	-	-	+	(+)	-	-	-	-	d	d	-	-	-	+	-	-	-	-	d	-
Salmonella subgenus 1	-	+	-	+	+	-	-	+	d	+	-	+	-	-	+	-	-	+	+	-	-	d	+	+	-	+	-	-
subgenus 111 ("Arizona")	-	+	-	+	+	-	-	+	(+)	+	-	+	+	+	+	d	-	+	-	+	-	-	+	+	-	+	+	+
Serratia liquefaciens	-	(+)	(+)	+	-	-	-	+	-	+	+	+	+	-	d	-	+	+	-	+	-	d	+	+	d	(+)	(-)	+
S. marcescens	-	(-)	+	+	-	(-)	-	+	-	+	+	+	+	-	d	-	+	+	-	+	d	(+)	+	-	-	d	+	+
S. odorifera	d	(+)	(+)	+	-	-	-	+	d	d	+	+	+	+	d	+	d	+	-	+	d	-	-	+	d	+	d	+

*Reproduced with permission from Carter, M.E.: Enterobacteria. *In* Diagnostic Procedures in Veterinary Bacteriology and Mycology. Edited by G.R. Carter. 4th Ed. Springfield, Ill., Charles C Thomas, 1984.

Plague is fundamentally a disease of rats and wild rodents. Humans are considered accidental hosts.

Bubonic and pneumonic forms of plague in humans can be epidemic. The disease is transmitted by fleas. Fleas become infected from rats in which the disease is bubonic and similar to that seen in humans. Buboes is the term used for infected lymph nodes. The bubonic form can give rise to the pneumonic form, which is highly contagious and usually fatal if not treated.

Sylvatic plague occurs in wild rodents other than rats. At least 38 species of wild rodents, including marmots and squirrels, have been found to be susceptible. Fleas transmit it to humans and other rodents. Sylvatic plague has given rise to outbreaks of bubonic and pneumonic plague.

Between 1910 and 1951, 523 cases of bubonic plague in humans were reported in the United States, and the fatality rate was 65%. Outbreaks have occurred in California, Louisiana, Florida, Texas, and Washington. In addition, sporadic cases have been reported from Arizona, Idaho, New Mexico, Nevada, Oregon, and Utah. Fortunately, many of the foci of sylvatic plague are situated in sparsely populated and isolated rural districts where the fleas of wild rodents do not have the opportunity to bite human populations.

Isolation, Cultivation and Identification. The organism is not fastidious. Identification is made on the basis of the criteria presented in Table 17–11. It is closely related to *Y. pseudotuberculosis*, with which it shares many antigens. It differs from this organism in that it is nonmotile.

Yersinia pseudotuberculosis

Synonym. *Pasteurella pseudotuberculosis.*

Pathogenicity. This organism produces pseudotuberculosis in various rodents, guinea pigs, cats, chinchilla, and turkeys; epididymo-orchitis of rams; and occasional infections in swine. The infection in small animals initially involves the mesenteric nodes, with spread from the caseous abscesses to the liver and spleen particularly.

In humans, infections simulating typhoid and appendicitis (mesenteric adenitis) occur.

Identification. *Y. pseudotuberculosis* is motile at 22°C; *Y. pestis* is not. See Table 17–11 for additional differential characteristics.

Yersinia enterocolitica

Pathogenicity. This organism, which resembles *Y. pseudotuberculosis*, causes gastroenteritis, mesenteric adenitis, and a wide variety of infrequent infections in humans. It seems likely that the reservoir of *Y. enterocolitica* is the intestine of wild and domestic animals. Many of the infections in animals resemble those caused by *Y. pseudotuberculosis*. Ileitis, gastroenteritis, and mesenteric adenitis are probably the most common disease processes.

Isolation has been made from chinchilla, hares, deer, rabbits, dogs, pigs, mink, various avian species, and goats, cattle, and sheep. The organism has been isolated from a considerable percentage (25%) of mesenteric nodes of swine and also from tongues (35%).

Identification. The organism can be cultivated without difficulty by a "cold enrichment" procedure like that used for *Listeria monocytogenes*. Growth is better at room temperature or lower than 37°C. Identification is made on the basis of morphologic, cultural, and biochemical characteristics (see Table 17–11).

Y. enterocolitica shares an antigen with the classic *Brucella* species and thus may give rise to false *Brucella* agglutination reactions. There are more than 30 serotypes, many of which do not appear to be pathogenic. New species *Y. intermedia*, *Y. frederiksenii*, and *Y. kristensenii* have been proposed for strains that differ biochemically from those of human origin.

Treatment. Both *Y. pseudotuberculosis* and *Y. enterocolitica* are susceptible to tetracyclines, trimethoprim-sulfamethoxazole, aminoglycosides, kanamycin, and chloramphenicol.

Because the *Yersinia* are facultative intracel-

Table 17–11.   Differentiation of Yersinia Species

					(Oxidase-negative; Optimum Temperature 25 to 30 C)	Acid			
Species	Motile 25 C	Indole	MR	VP	Urease	Glucose	Lactose	Sucrose	Salicin
Y. pestis	–	–	+	–	–	+	–	–	(+)*
Y. enterocolitica	+	–	+	+	+	+	–	+	–
Y. pseudotuberculosis	+	–	+	–	+	+	–	–	+

*( ) most.

lular parasites and because the infections they cause may be acute, early and adequate treatment is particularly important.

SUGGESTED CLINICAL EXAMPLES

An outbreak of edema disease in pigs.

An outbreak of salmonellosis in pigs.

An outbreak of salmonellosis in calves.

A problem of calf scours (colibacillosis) in a dairy herd.

Arizona infections in turkey poults.

Outbreaks of pullorum disease and fowl typhoid.

Scours and diarrhea in young pigs, lambs, puppies, or foals.

SOURCES FOR FURTHER READING

Edelman, R., and Levine, M.M.: Summary of a workshop on enteropathogenic *Escherichia coli*. J. Infect. Dis., *147*:1108, 1983.

Edwards, P.R., and Hewing, W.H.: Identification of Enterobacteriaceae. 3rd Ed. Minneapolis, Burgess Publishing Co., 1972.

Ewing, W.H.: Differentiation of Enterobacteriaceae by Biochemical Reactions. Atlanta, Centers for Disease Control, 1973.

Ghosh, A.C.: An epidemiological study of the incidence of infection with salmonellae in broilers and broiler breeders in Scotland. Br. Vet. J., *129*:243, 1972.

Giannella, R.A.: Pathogenesis of *Salmonella enteritis* and diarrhea. *In* Microbiology. Edited by D. Schlessinger. Washington, D.C., American Society for Microbiology, 1975.

Gordon, R.F.: Avian salmonellosis. *In* The Veterinary Annual. Edited by C.S.G. Grunsell. Bristol, England, Scientechnica, 1971.

Greenfield, J., Bigland, C.H., and Dukes, T.W.: The genus *Arizona* with special reference to Arizona disease in turkeys. Vet. Bull., *41*:605, 1971.

Jack, E.J.: Salmonella abortion in sheep. *In* The Veterinary Annual. Edited by C.S.G. Grunsell. Bristol, England, Scientechnica, 1971.

Moon, H.W.: Mechanisms in the pathogenesis of diarrhea: A review. J. Am. Vet. Med. Assoc., *172*:443, 1978.

Morse, E.V., et al.: Salmonellosis in *Equidae:* A study of 23 cases. Cornell Vet., *66*:198, 1976.

Robinson, R.A.: Salmonella infection: Diagnosis and control. N. Z. Vet. J., *18*:259, 1970.

Rubin, R.H., and Weinstein, L.: Salmonellosis. New York, Stratton, 1977.

Sojka, W.J.: *Escherichia coli* in Domestic Animals and Poultry. Farnham Royal, England, Commonwealth Agricultural Bureau, 1965.

Sojka, W.J., Slavin, G., Brand, T.F., and Davies, G.: A survey of drug resistance in salmonella isolated from animals in England and Wales. Br. Vet. J., *128*:189, 1972.

18

Pseudomonas

PRINCIPAL CHARACTERISTICS

The pseudomonads are gram-negative, aerobic (sugars split by oxidation), medium-size rods. They are motile, catalase- and oxidase-positive, and some species produce soluble pigments.

Upward of 150 species have been described; they are found widely in nature. Three species are of considerable pathogenic significance in animals:

1. *P. aeruginosa,* which causes miscellaneous infections;
2. *P. pseudomallei,* which causes melioidosis; and
3. *P. mallei,* which causes glanders.

The natural habitat of the first two species is water, soil, and decaying vegetation. *P. aeruginosa* may also be found on the skin, mucous membranes, and in feces. *P. pseudomallei* only occurs naturally in tropical areas.

P. maltophilia, P. stutzeri, and other pseudomonads rarely cause infections in animals.

Pseudomonas aeruginosa

PATHOGENESIS

Some strains of *P. aeruginosa* possess pili, which facilitate adherence to epithelial cells with subsequent colonization. Among the metabolites and other substances that may play a role in the production of disease are two water-soluble pigments (see further on), a hemolysin, a leukocidin, proteinases, a pyocyanase (bacteri-

cidal for some bacteria), endotoxin, and a mucinous slime. A protein exotoxin (exotoxin A) is produced that is lethal for mice; it is considered important in virulence. Many strains pathogenic in humans have been found to produce this toxin.

PATHOGENICITY

This species is a frequent contaminant in disease processes, and isolation alone is not necessarily significant. Its significance in mixed infections, particularly with streptococci and staphylococci, may be questionable. Isolation in pure culture strongly indicates pathogenicity.

Pseudomonas aeruginosa is an opportunist in weakened tissues (burns), wounds, debilitated patients, individuals with malignancies and immunodeficiencies, and young animals. It may replace bacteria that have been eliminated from infectious processes by antimicrobial treatment, and it sometimes causes a fatal septicemia. Infections are rare in healthy, normal individuals.

Some diseases or conditions with which *P. aeruginosa* has been associated are

1. Horse: abortion.
2. Cattle: mastitis, abortion.
3. Dog: prostatitis, cystitis, dermatitis, and outer ear infections.
4. Fowl: septicemia.
5. Mink: hemorrhagic pneumonia.
6. Wound infection and abscesses in all animals; urinary infections.
7. Humans: wound, urinary, and inner ear infections and fatal infections involving

156

lungs, heart valves, meninges, and brain; also nosocomial infections.

SPECIMENS

Specimens: urine and pus.

ISOLATION AND CULTIVATION

All strains grow well on ordinary nutrient media. Colonies are irregular, spreading, translucent, 3 to 5 mm in diameter, and may show a bluish-metallic sheen. Beta-hemolysis is usually observed around colonies growing on blood agar plates. A distinctive aromatic odor is usually apparent, regardless of the medium used.

P. aeruginosa does not grow anaerobically and thus its lack of growth is a reliable test for anaerobiosis.

Medium-sized, gram-negative rods are seen in smears. They cannot be distinguished morphologically from the enteric bacteria.

IDENTIFICATION

Two pigments are commonly produced by these bacteria, both of which are water-soluble: pyocyanin (bluish-green), which is chloroform-soluble, and "blue pus bacillus" fluorescein or pyoverdin (yellowish-green), which is not chloroform-soluble. Both pigments may be found in media, but not always. Occasionally a strain will produce a dark red pigment (pyorubin) or a brown-black pigment (pyomelanin). If pyocyanin is produced, this can be extracted from a slant culture by pouring chloroform over it. All strains are oxidase-positive.

Fluorescein fluoresces under ultraviolet light but *P. fluorescens*, an occasionl contaminant, also produces it; however, this species does not grow well at 37° C.

Other features of *P. aeruginosa* are motility by polar flagella and gelatin liquefaction. It is oxidase-positive, peptonizes litmus milk, utilizes citrate, is indole-negative, and reduces nitrate. The oxidation/fermentation (O/F) test is positive for oxidation. Differential features of the more important pseudomonads are listed in Table 18–1.

ANTIGENIC NATURE

The species is heterogeneous, with 17 serotypes based on differences in O antigens. Strains can be typed by bacteriophages and pyocins (bacteriocins), but serotyping is less cumbersome. Killed vaccines are used in burn patients and to prevent hemorrhagic septicemia in mink.

RESISTANCE

In general these organisms resemble other vegetative bacteria except that they are more resistant to high dilutions of quaternary ammonium compounds and phenolic compounds. Pus is protective. They have been known to survive in quaternary ammonium disinfectants containing hard water or fragments of cork and plastic. With adequate moisture, *P. aeruginosa* can survive for long periods on water faucets, utensils, floors, instruments, baths, humidifiers, and respiratory care equipment.

TREATMENT

Infections due to *P. aeruginosa* do not usually respond well to chemotherapy. Gentamicin and other aminoglycosides such as amikacin, tobramycin, and colistin (polymyxin E) are used, but resistant forms develop during prolonged treatment. Carbenicillin and polymyxin are also employed. In severe infections carbenicillin may be combined with gentamicin. Because of the high concentration of polymyxin in the urine, this drug is especially effective in *Pseudomonas* urinary infections. Neither streptomycin nor the tetracyclines are too active. Sulfonamides, especially sulfadiazine, sulfamerazine, and sulfamethazine, are sometimes of value. Multiple type drug resistance due to R factors is encountered.

Multiple *P. aeruginosa* infections are uncommon in veterinary practice. When encountered, proper isolation procedures, strict sanitary measures, and effective disinfection are necessary for control.

Pseudomonas pseudomallei

This organism is found in tropical soils and water in the Far East and Australia.

MODE OF INFECTION

In both humans and animals, the organisms are thought to gain entry by inhalation, ingestion, or through wounds and abrasions.

PATHOGENICITY

The disease in humans and animals varies from a benign pulmonary form to a systemic form with visceral nodules (little pus unless secondary bacteria) and a terminal septicemia.

Although the disease in animals can be septicemic, often it is chronic and characterized by

Table 18–1. ***Differentiation of Important* Pseudomonas *Species***

	P. aeruginosa	*P. maltophilia*	*P. fluorescens*	*P. pseudomallei*	*P. mallei*
Glucose oxidation	+	+	+	+	+
Maltose oxidation	–	+	V*	+	–
SS agar	+	–	+	–	–
Oxidase	+	–	+	+	–
Motility	+	+	+	+	–
Cetrimide agar	+	–	+	+	–
Growth at 42 C	+	V	–	–	–
Pigment	Pyocyanin: water and chloroform-soluble; Fluorescein: water-soluble; Pyorubin: occasional strains	None, but a yellow to brown water-soluble tyrosine produced	Fluorescein: waer-soluble	None	None

*V–variable reactions.

nodules in the lungs, liver, spleen, lymph nodes, and subcutis. The acute disease occurs more often in young animals. In spite of extensive lesions, animals may appear normal. Among the animals infected are cattle, sheep, pigs, horses, dogs, cats, primates, and rodents.

Criteria for identification are given in Table 18–1.

TREATMENT

Sulfonamides and broad-spectrum antibiotics are effective, but the treatment of choice appears to be trimethoprim-sulfamethoxazole. The response depends largely upon the extent of the lesions.

Pseudomonas mallei

HABITAT AND OCCURRENCE

P. mallei is an obligate pathogen of horses, other solipeds, humans, and carnivores. The disease it causes, which is called glanders (farcy), has been eradicated from North America and Western Europe. However, it still occurs in parts of Asia, Eastern Europe, and Africa.

MODE OF INFECTION

The organisms usually enter via the respiratory tract.

PATHOGENICITY

No exotoxin has been described; endotoxin is probably significant. Glanders is a contagious, usually chronic disease of equines characterized by the formation of tubercles or nodules (granulomas) that frequently break down to form ulcers. Three forms of the disease are seen, depending upon the principal location of the lesions, viz., nasal, pulmonary, or skin.

Humans, and particularly members of the cat family, may be infected. All infections usually terminate fatally if not treated.

SPECIMENS

Specimens: tissue containing early tubercles or pus from ulcers.

ISOLATION AND IDENTIFICATION

P. mallei grows on blood and serum agar and is oxidative rather than fermentative. For identification, see Table 18–1.

TREATMENT, IMMUNITY, AND CONTROL

The most effective drugs are streptomycin and sulfadiazine. No vaccines or bacterins are used.

Control is by mallein testing (analogous to tuberculin testing), with the elimination of reactors. Mallein is injected intrapalpebrally. Immunity is predominantly cell-mediated.

SUGGESTED CLINICAL EXAMPLES

Canine otitis externa yielding *P. aeruginosa*.
Bovine mastitis due to *P. aeruginosa*.
Endometritis in a mare due to *P. aeruginosa*.
Thoracic puncture wound in a calf due to *P. aeruginosa*.
Melioidosis in dogs returning from Southeast Asia.
Melioidosis in primates.
Examination of imported horses for glanders.

SOURCES FOR FURTHER READING

Arenstein, M.S., and Sanford, J.P. (eds.).: Symposium on *Pseudomonas aeruginosa*. J. Infect. Dis., *130*(Suppl.): 1974.
Bergen, T.: Bacteriophage typing and sero-grouping of *Pseudomonas aeruginosa* from animals. Acta Pathol Microbiol. Scand., *80B*:351, 1972.

Cottew, G.S.: Melioidosis in sheep in Queensland. A description of the causal organism. Aust. J. Exp. Biol. Med. Sci., *28*:677, 1950.

Dogget, R.G. (ed.): *Pseudomonas aeruginosa:* Clinical Manifestations of Infection and Current Therapy. New York, Academic Press, Inc., 1979.

Franklin, M., and Franklin, M.A.: A Profile of *Pseudomonas.* New Jersey, Beecham Pharmaceuticals, 1971.

Gilardi, G.L.: *Pseudomonas* species in clinical microbiology. Mt. Sinai J. Med., NY, *43*:710, 1976.

Howe, C., Sampath, A., and Sponitz, M.: The *Pseudomallei* group: A review. J. Infect. Dis., *124*:598, 1971.

Liu, P.V.: Extracellular toxins of *Pseudomonas aeruginosa.* J. Infect. Dis., *130*(Suppl.):94, 1974.

Lusis, P.I., and Soltys, M.A.: *Pseudomonas:* A review. Vet. Bull., *41*:169, 1971.

Palleroni, N.J.: The *Pseudomonas* Group. Durham, England, Meadowfield Press Ltd., 1978.

Redfearn, M.S., Palleroni, N.J., and Stanier, R.Y.: A comparative study of *Pseudomonas pseudomallei* and *Bacillus mallei.* J. Gen. Microbiol., *43*:293, 1966.

Stedham, M.A.: Melioidosis in dogs in Vietnam. J. Clin. Vet. Med. Assoc., *158*:1948, 1971.

Woods, D.E., et al.: Role of pili in adherence of *Pseudomonas aeruginosa* to mammalian buccal epithelial cells. Infect. Immun., *29*:1146, 1980.

19

Pasteurella and Francisella

There is no justification for including *Francisella* with *Pasteurella* other than convenience and tradition. *F. tularensis* was once, with little justification, called *Pasteurella tularensis*.

Pasteurella

PRINCIPAL CHARACTERISTICS

Species of *Pasteurella* are gram-negative small rods or coccobacilli. They are non-motile, non-spore-forming, aerobic, facultatively anaerobic, and fermentative (except for *P. anatipestifer*).

Bergey's Manual of Systematic Bacteriology lists the following official species:
1. *P. multocida:* may occur as commensals in the upper respiratory and digestive tract of a number of animal species.
2. *P. haemolytica:* may occur as commensals in the upper respiratory and digestive tract of a number of animal species.
3. *P. pneumotropica:* may occur as commensals in the upper respiratory and digestive tract of a number of animal species.
4. *P. ureae:* found in the upper respiratory tract of humans.
5. *P. gallinarum:* commensal in upper respiratory tract of chickens; occasionally causes low grade respiratory infections in chickens.
6. *P. aerogenes:* commensal in the intestine of swine; rarely pathogenic.
7. *P. anatipestifer:* a nonfermenter that really does not belong in the genus *Pasteurella*.

DISTRIBUTION AND HABITAT

Pasteurella organisms are distributed worldwide. The above-listed species (except for *P. urease*) occur as commensals in the upper respiratory and digestive passages of animals, e.g., *P. multocida* is found in the mouth of cats and the tonsils and nasal passages of swine; *P. haemolytica* is found in the nasopharynx of some normal cattle and sheep.

Pasteurella multocida

HISTORICAL
The first significant report of an organism of this species was made by Bollinger in 1878.

MODE OF INFECTION

Infection may be acquired by contact, inhalation, or ingestion; rarely it is transmitted by biting arthropods.

PATHOGENESIS

As in other gram-negative infections, endotoxins no doubt play a role in pathogenesis. Various environmental stresses play an important role in predisposition to infection. Passage of the infecting agent from animal to animal results in enhancement of virulence. *P. multocida* is a frequent secondary invader in pneumonic disease; however, it may also be a primary cause of disease, as in fowl cholera and epizootic hemorrhagic septicemia; when it is primary, septicemia frequently occurs.

unstable
to heat

A thermolabile toxin is produced by some strains, particularly those type D cultures recovered from swine. Some investigators think that the latter cultures, along with *Bordetella bronchiseptica*, have a causal role in atrophic rhinitis of swine.

PATHOGENICITY

The diseases with which *P. multocida* is associated are too numerous to discuss fully. It may be a primary agent but more frequently it is a secondary invader when resistance of the animal is reduced by various stresses.

It is a primary or more frequently a secondary invader in pneumonia of cattle, swine, sheep, goats, and other species. As a secondary invader it is frequently involved in the bovine "shipping fever complex" and in enzootic pneumonia of pigs. It is considered the primary cause of fowl cholera and epizootic hemorrhagic septicemia of cattle and water buffaloes. The latter disease occurs in many tropical and subtropical countries but is rare in the United States and South America. It is one of the causes of the pleuropneumonia form of "snuffles" in rabbits, it is a cause of severe mastitis of cattle and sheep, and it is responsible for a variety of sporadic infections in animals, including encephalitis, meningitis, and abortion.

Because dogs and cats harbor these organisms in their mouths as commensals, bites of humans and other animals are frequently infected with them. A wide variety of infections have been reported in humans: sinusitis, bronchiectasis, peritonitis, appendicitis, and septicemia.

DIRECT EXAMINATION

Bipolar organisms can be demonstrated in blood smears in septicemias. This is of minor significance except as an aid in the diagnosis of epizootic hemorrhagic septicemia.

SPECIMENS

Specimens are selected according to the location of the infectious process. The organisms survive well in transport media and refrigerated and frozen tissues.

ISOLATION AND CULTIVATION

Definitive diagnosis is based upon isolation and identification of *P. multocida*. Good primary growth requires media enriched with serum or blood. Colonies appear after incubation for 24 to 48 hours at 37°C. They are usually of moderate size, round, and grayish. Some strains produce large mucoid colonies. Fresh cultures have a characteristic odor.

Smears reveal small, gram-negative rods and coccobacilli. Marked pleomorphism is not uncommon.

IDENTIFICATION

Of special significance are nonmotility, indole production, lack of hemolysis, and production of oxidase (see Table 19–1). In contrast, *P. haemolytica* is beta-hemolytic, indole-negative, and grows on MacConkey agar. Cultures of *P. multocida* are occasionally encountered that are aberrant in one or two biochemical characteristics. Those from dogs and cats vary considerably from those from bovine and swine and may ultimately be recognized as distinct species.

EXPERIMENTAL ANIMALS

Mice and rabbits are susceptible to most strains. Lethal infections develop within one or several days. Mouse inoculation is occasionally used to recover *P. multocida* from heavily contaminated specimens, e.g., nasal swabs from pigs.

ANTIGENIC NATURE

Types have been identified on the basis of differences in capsular substances (polysaccharides): types A, B, D, and E.

1. Type A: causes fowl cholera and many other infections of various animals.
2. Type B: causes hemorrhagic septicemia in Asia, the Middle East, and Southern Europe.
3. Type D: recovered relatively infrequently from various infections in many animals but frequently from pneumonia and atrophic rhinitis in swine.
4. Type E: causes hemorrhagic septicemia in Africa.

Capsular types may be subdivided further into somatic types (16 thus far) on the basis of serologic differences in lipopolysaccharides (somatic or O antigens). A serotype is designated by the capsular type, followed by the number representing the somatic type, e.g., serotype B:2 is a cause of hemorrhagic septicemia.

TREATMENT

The following antibacterial drugs have been widely used: penicillin and streptomycin; tetracyclines; sulfonamides, including sulfamera-

Table 19–1. Differentiation of **Pasteurella** *Species*

	Principal Hosts	Mac-Conkey	Oxidase	Urease	Indole	Fermentation Glucose	Fermentation Lactose	Fermentation Sucrose
P. multocida	Various	−	+	−	+*	A	−*	A
P. haemolytica	Various	+	+	−	−	A	A*	A
P. pneumotropica	Rodents	−	+	+	+	A	A	A
P. ureae	Humans	−	+	+	−	A	−	A
P. gallinarum	Chickens	−	+	−	−	A	−	A
P. anatipestifer	Ducks	−	−	−	−	−	−	−
P. aerogenes	Swine	+	+	+	−	A	−	A

*Some exceptions.

zine and sulfamethazine; and chloramphenicol if strains are resistant to the less toxic drugs. Sulfaquinoxaline is the drug of choice in fowl cholera. For many years antibiotic resistance was uncommon, but currently some clinical isolates have displayed multiple resistance.

IMMUNITY

Immunity is predominantly humoral.

Pasteur's first vaccine was developed to prevent fowl cholera. It was an attenuated strain that was not altogether satisfactory. In recent years vaccines consisting of live attenuated strains, administered in drinking water, have been employed to prevent fowl cholera. A live attentuated vaccine is being employed to prevent pneumonic pasteurellosis in cattle.

Whole–broth killed cultures (bacterins) with a high concentration of organisms, some containing adjuvants, have been used widely to prevent the following P. multocida infections:

1. Fowl cholera: there is a problem of different serotypes resulting in bacterin "breaks," i.e., the causal serotype may not be in the bacterin.
2. Shipping fever: with or without P. haemolytica and the viruses of PI-3 and IBR.
3. Pneumonia in sheep: with P. haemolytica.
4. Epizootic hemorrhagic septicemia: type B or type E strains.

Hyperimmune serum is seldom used because it is expensive and because of the occurrence of different serotypes.

Pasteurella haemolytica

Two different biotypes of P. haemolytica have been identified, viz., biotype A and biotype T. They differ in a number of characteristics, including pathogenicity, antigenic nature, and biochemical activity (Table 19–2).

PATHOGENICITY

Some strains of P. haemolytica elaborate a soluble cytotoxin that kills alveolar macrophages and other leukocytes, thus breaching the lung's primary defense mechanism.

This species has a primary or secondary role in pneumonia of cattle, goats, and sheep and is frequently recovered from the bronchopneumonic lungs of cattle with shipping fever. Other important diseases in which this organism is involved are mastitis of ewes and septicemia of lambs.

Laboratory animals are refractory to experimental infection.

A distinct variety of P. haemolytica can cause infrequent low-grade infections in poultry.

ISOLATION AND CULTIVATION

Direct examination is of limited value.

Media containing serum or blood are required for good growth. Colonies are round, grayish, and usually somewhat smaller than those of P. multocida. They are usually surrounded by a zone of beta-hemolysis. This zone varies considerably and may be no larger than the colony, and thus it is not apparent unless the colony is removed. Bovine blood is more suitable than that of sheep or horses for the demonstration of hemolysis.

IDENTIFICATION

Smears from colonies disclose small gram-negative rods or coccobacilli. Of special significance in identification are the fact that they are beta-hemolytic, indole-negative, nonmotile, and grow on MacConkey agar (see Table 19–1). What appears to be a distinct variety of P. haemolytica can frequently be recovered from the upper respiratory tract of chickens and turkeys. It differs in hemolysis, which is stronger, and biochemically from typical cultures of P. haemolytica.

Table 19–2. Differential Characteristics of the Two Biotypes of Pasteurella haemolytica

	Biotype A	Biotype T
Acid production from L-arabinose, D-xylose,	+	−
trehalose, salicin	−	+
Susceptibility to penicillin	High	Low
Serotypes†	1, 2, 5, 6, 7, 8, 9, 11, 12	3, 4, 10
Principal location in natural host	Nasopharynx	Tonsils
Principal disease association	Pneumonia of cattle and sheep; septicemia of nursing lambs	Septicemia of feeder lambs

*Reproduced with permission from Biberstein, E.L.: Biotyping and serotyping *Pasteurella haemolytica*. *In* Methods in Microbiology. Vol. 19. Edited by T. Bergan and J.R. Norris, London, Academic Press, 1978.
†Based on difference in capsular antigens.

TREATMENT

This is essentially the same as for *P. multocida.* Multiple drug resistance is encountered.

ANTIGENIC NATURE AND IMMUNITY

P. haemolytica is heterogeneous and somewhat resembles *P. multocida* in that it has capsular and somatic varieties. The somatic antigens are so complex that serotypes are designated according to differences in capsular substances, e.g., type 1 is the most common type in bovine pneumonia. There are more than a dozen types.

Immunity is thought to be predominantly humoral.

Bacterins containing both *P. haemolytica* and *P. multocida* are widely used in cattle and sheep, although their value is questionable. Claims of efficacy in the prevention of bovine pneumonic pasteurellosis have been made for a live unattenuated vaccine administered to cattle intradermally.

Pasteurella pneumotropica

This organism can be recovered from the nasopharynx of some guinea pigs, rats, hamsters, mice, dogs, and cats. It is usually a secondary invader in pneumonic disease in mice and rats. It is not a significant pathogen in dogs and cats.

It resembles *P. multocida* culturally but can be distinguished biochemically (see Table 19–1). Some strains may split sugars with the production of gas.

Pasteurella anatipestifer

P. anatipestifer causes infectious serositis, a highly acute disease of ducklings, various water fowl, chickens, turkeys, and pheasants. This disease has often had an adverse effect on the commercial duck industry. A widely distributed serofibrinous exudate is found in the acute form of the disease.

Francisella tularensis

Synonym. *Pasteurella tularensis*

As mentioned previously, this intracellular parasite bears little resemblance to the *Pasteurella* species other than size and morphology.

PATHOGENESIS

The manner in which *F. tularensis* causes disease is not understood. Endotoxin is probably an important factor; exotoxin has not been found. Immunity is primarily cell-mediated, and the lesions are granulomatous.

The human disease may assume several forms, but the most common is the ulceroglandular form, with the development of papule, ulcer, and lymph gland enlargement, in that order. Depending upon the portal of entry the other forms are the oculoglandular, pneumonic, and typhoidal. All forms may give rise to the systemic form, but the latter two are considered the most serious. The characteristic lesions are small, granulomatous abscesses in lymph nodes and viscera following bacteremia.

MODE OF INFECTION

Humans may become infected as a result of contact with infected animals or their discharges; animal bites; ingestion of contaminated water and partially cooked meat; and inhalation of fecal droplets of ticks.

PATHOGENICITY

Tularemia is principally a disease of wild animals; however, humans as well as some domestic animals and fowl are susceptible. In nature, the disease is frequently transmitted from infected to susceptible hosts by insect vectors. These include wood ticks, dog and rabbit ticks, the deer fly, fleas, and lice.

The prevalence of tularemia in wild rabbits in the United States has been estimated to be approximately 1%. In North America, the cottontail rabbit is the reservoir of infection for nearly 70% of the human cases. Other naturally susceptible animals are squirrel, opossum, beaver, woodchuck, muskrat, skunk, coyote, fox, cat, sheep, deer, bullsnake, game birds, and domestic fowl.

Small, necrotic, granulomatous foci in the liver, spleen, and lymph nodes use the characteristic gross lesions observed in wild rabbits.

ISOLATION AND CULTIVATION

Note: The organism is highly infectious for humans.

It grows well on cystine-blood agar; cystine is essential for growth. Colonies are minute and dewdrop-like, yielding small, gram-negative rods and coccobacilli. There is a characteristic greenish discoloration surrounding the colonies.

Guinea pig inoculation is sometimes used to overcome contaminants. The organism can be recovered without difficulty from necropsied, terminally ill guinea pigs.

IDENTIFICATION

Biochemical tests are difficult to perform and are not usually carried out. The fluorescent antibody (FA) procedure is widely used to identify the organisms. Identification of specific agglutinins in the sera of guinea pigs inoculated with infectious material is confirmatory.

TREATMENT

Streptomycin is the drug of choice. Early treatment will usually eliminate organisms from lesions.

IMMUNITY

This is predominantly cell-mediated. A live attenuated vaccine is used in people whose risk of infection is high.

SUGGESTED CLINICAL EXAMPLES

Severe enzootic pneumonia (secondary *P. multocida*) in a piggery.

An outbreak of fowl cholera in range turkeys.

An outbreak of epizootic hemorrhagic septicemia in cattle.

Severe enzootic *Pasteurella* pneumonia in sheep.

Severe shipping fever in feedlot cattle.

Bovine mastitis due to *P. multocida* involving a herd.

Septicemia in neonatal lambs due to *P. haemolytica*.

Suspected tularemia in a wild rabbit.

SOURCES FOR FURTHER READING

Bain, R.V.S., de Alwis, M.C.L., Carter, G.R., and Gupta, B.K.: Hemorrhagic septicemia. FAO Animal Production and Health Paper, No. 323. Rome, Food and Agricultural Organization of the United Nations, 1982.

Biberstein, E.L.: Biotyping and serotyping of *Pasteurella haemolytica*. *In* Methods in Microbiology. Edited by T. Bergan and J.R. Norris. New York, Academic Press, Inc., 1978.

Brennan, P.C., Fritz, T.E., and Flynn, R.J.: *Pasteurella pneumotropica*: Cultural and biochemical characteristics, and its association with disease in laboratory animals. Lab. An. Care, 15:307, 1965.

Carter, G.R.: Pasteurellosis: *Pasteurella multocida* and *Pasteurella haemolytica*. Adv. Vet. Sci., 11:321, 1967.

Collins, F.M.: Mechanisms of acquired resistance to *Pasteurella multocida* infection: A review. Cornell Vet., 67:103, 1977.

Frank, G.H., and Wessman, G.E.: Rapid plate agglutination procedure for serotyping *Pasteurella haemolytica*. J. Clin. Microbiol., 7:142, 1978.

Heddleston, K.L., Gallagher, J.E., and Rebers, P.A.: Fowl cholera: Gel diffusion precipitin test for serotyping *Pasteurella multocida* from avian species. Avian Dis., 16:925, 1972.

Kilian, M., Frederiksen, W., and Biberstein, E.L. (eds.): *Haemophilus, Pasteurella* and *Actinobacillus.*. New York, Academic Press, 1981.

Leibovitz, L.: A survey of the so-called "anatipestifer syndrome." Avian Dis., 16:836, 1972.

Markham, R.J.F., and Wilkie, B.N.: Interaction between *Pasteurella haemolytica* and bovine alveolar macrophages: Cytotoxic effect on macrophages and impaired phagocytosis. Am. J. Vet. Res., 41:18, 1980.

Reilly, J.R.: Tularemia. *In* Infectious Diseases of Wild Mammals. Edited by J.W. Davis. Ames, Iowa State University Press, 1970.

Rutter, J.M., and Luther, P.D.: Cell culture assay for toxigenic *Pasteurella multocida* from atrophic rhinitis of pigs. Vet. Rec., 114:393, 1984.

20

Actinobacillus

PRINCIPAL CHARACTERISTICS OF *Actinobacillus*

Species of the genus *Actinobacillus* are gram-negative, nonmotile, small rods. They are non-spore-forming, aerobic, facultatively anaerobic, and fermentative.

The following species are recognized as official by *Bergey's Manual of Systematic Bacteriology:* (1) *A. lignieresii;* (2) *A. equuli;* (3) *A. suis* (causes septicemia and other infectious processes in young pigs); and (4) *A. capsulatus* (causes arthritis in rabbits).

There are two unofficial species: (1) *A. actinoides,* which produces pneumonia in calves and seminal vesiculitis in bulls; it is probably the same as *Haemophilus sommus;* and (2) *A. seminis,* which causes epididymitis in young rams—a disease resembling that caused by *Brucella ovis*—and purulent polyarthritis and gangrenous mastitis in sheep.

All of these organisms probably occur as commensals, giving rise to exogenous and endogenous infections.

Actinobacillus lignieresii

HISTORICAL

A. lignieresii was described by Lignieres and Spritz in 1902 as one of the causes of bovine actinomycosis.

DISTRIBUTION AND HABITAT

It is worldwide in distribution and occurs as a commensal in the alimentary tract of cattle.

MODE OF INFECTION

The organism usually produces a sporadic, endogenous disease, but on occasion several animals may be infected. It gains entrance to the oral mucosa through injuries to the tissue. *developing or originating w/in the organism*

PATHOGENICITY

Actinobacillosis is seen most commonly in cattle, less commonly in sheep, and rarely in pigs, dogs, and humans. Lesions usually consist of multiple, granulomatous abscesses. In cattle and sheep, these occur most frequently around the head and neck region. The lesion commences as a firm nodule that eventually ulcerates and discharges a viscous, white to faintly green pus that contains small granules. The granules are greyish-white and usually less than 1 mm in diameter. By comparison, the sulfur granules of actinomycosis are several millimeters in diameter.

Unlike actinomycosis, the infection is spread via the lymphatics. Lesions may involve the tongue (wooden tongue), lungs, and less frequently other internal organs. Rarely, granulomatous abscesses occur in the udder of the sow.

Several cases of an acute, suppurative bronchopneumonia have been described in humans.

DIRECT EXAMINATION

Small, gram-negative rods are demonstrable within granules. The granules are examined in the same manner as those from actinomycosis: wash, examine granule under a coverslip in 10% NaOH, then smear and stain. The granules in

165

actinobacillosis are small (< 1 mm), grey, and white.

SPECIMENS

Pus and necrotic material from early, nondischarging lesions are submitted.

ISOLATION AND CULTIVATION

A. lignieresii can be recovered consistently if clinical material is seeded onto serum or blood agar and incubated at 37°C; 10% CO_2 stimulates growth.

Small, translucent, smooth, and glistening colonies resembling those of *P. multocida* are evident in 24 to 48 hours. Stained smears disclose small gram-negative rods or coccobacilli.

IDENTIFICATION

The organism can only be identified precisely by biochemical criteria (see Table 20–1).

IMMUNITY

Little is known about the immune response in this disease. The granulomatous nature of the lesions suggests a strong component of cellular immunity.

TREATMENT

Advanced cases are not usually treated. In others, surgical drainage along with a broad-spectrum antibiotic or a sulfonamide is employed. Potassium iodide given orally is useful. Treatment must be prolonged.

Actinobacillus equuli

Synonym: *Shigella equirulis*

HABITAT

This organism is commonly found in the intestinal tract of normal horses.

MODE OF INFECTION

Mode of infection is probably by ingestion. Infrequently it may be via the umbilicus or across the placenta (prenatal). *Strongylus* larvae may carry the organism into arteries.

PATHOGENICITY

In foals the disease caused by *A. equuli* is called shigellosis or viscosum infection ("sleepy foal disease"). Many foals develop the disease within a few hours or days of birth. Those dying within 24 hours of life have a severe enteritis. Those living for several days develop a purulent nephritis, frequently with concomitant pneumonia and joint infections.

The following manifestations may be seen in older horses: lameness due to purulent arthritis; infected aneurysms leading to systemic involvement; and infrequent abortion in mares.

Septic arthritis, endocarditis, suppurative nephritis, septicemia, and mastitis are occasionally seen in swine.

SPECIMENS

Affected tissues, purulent material, feces, and blood are submitted.

ISOLATION AND CULTIVATION

The organism grows well on blood agar. The colonies of fresh isolates are rough in appearance but mucoid in character, probably due to a mucinous ("sticky") capsule. They may lose their mucoid character on transfer. Some strains are beta-hemolytic.

IDENTIFICATION

The principal differential features are given in Table 20–1.

CONTROL AND TREATMENT

Immunization is not practiced, and little is known about the immunology of the infection.

Table 20–1.   Differentiation of Actinobacillus *Species*

	A. lignieresii	*A. equuli*	*A. suis*	*Past. haemolytica*
Hemolysis	—	V	+	+
MacConkey	+	V	(+)	+
Oxidase	+	+	+	+
Urease	(+)	+	(+)	—
Gelatinase	—	V	—	—
Lactose (acid)	(+)	+	+	(+)
Sucrose (acid)	+	+	(+)	+

Key: V = variable; (+) = most positive.

Strains are antigenically heterogeneous. Good sanitation at parturition, with disinfection of the umbilicus, is important. Prophylactic treatment of all foals shortly after birth with penicillin and streptomycin, or tetracyclines has been effective.

SUGGESTED CLINICAL EXAMPLES

Actinobacillosis in a bull.
Mammary actinobacillosis in a sow.
Multiple cases of actinobacillosis in calves.
Viscosum infection in neonatal foals.
Actinobacillus equuli infection of a verminous aneurysm with subsequent systemic infection.

SOURCES FOR FURTHER READING

Allen, J.G.: Bronchopneumonia in calves in Western Australia associated with *Actinobacillus actinoides*. Aust. Vet. J., *52*:100, 1976.

Baker, J.R.: An outbreak of neonatal deaths in foals due to *Actinobacillus equuli*. Vet. Rec., *90*:630, 1972.

Campbell, S.G., Whitlock, R.H., Timoney, J.F., and Underwood, A.M.: An unusual epizootic of actinobacillosis in dairy heifers. J. Am. Vet. Med. Assoc., *166*:604, 1975.

Kilian, M., Frederiksen, W., and Biberstein, E.L. (eds.): *Haemophilus, Pasteurella, Actinobacillus*. New York, Academic Press, 1981.

Mair, N.S., et al.: *Actinobacillus suis* in pigs. J. Comp. Pathol., *84*:113, 1974.

Phillips, J.E.: Actinobacillosis. *In* The Veterinary Annual. Edited by W.A. Pool. Bristol, John Wright & Sons Ltd., 1965–66.

Phillips, J.E.: Antigenic structure and serological typing of *Actinobacillus lignieresii*. J. Pathol. Bacteriol., *93*:463, 1967.

Phillips, J.E.: *Actinobacillus*. *In* Bergey's Manual of Systematic Bacteriology. Vol. 1. Edited by N.R. Krieg. Baltimore, Williams & Wilkins, 1984.

Till, D.H., and Palmer, E.P.: A review of actinobacillosis with a study of the causal organism. Vet. Rec., *72*:527, 1960.

Watt, D.A., Banford, V., and Nairin, M.E.: *Actinobacillus seminis* as a cause of polyarthritis. Aust. Vet. J., *46*:515, 1971.

Windsor, R.S.: *Actinobacillus equuli* infection in a litter of pigs. Vet. Rec., *92*:178,1983.

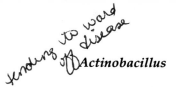

21

Campylobacter and Vibrio

Principal Characteristics of *Campylobacter*

Campylobacter organisms are spirally curved (one or more spirals), gram-negative, pleomorphic rods; they are motile, microaerophilic to anaerobic, and oxidase-positive. They do not attack carbohydrates.

In contrast, *Vibrio* organisms are aerobic, facultatively anaerobic, and fermentative.

More than 10 species of *Campylobacter* and of *Vibrio* are listed in *Bergey's Manual of Systematic Bacteriology*. Only several are considered pathogenic for animals. *Campylobacter* spp. are found on the mucous membrane of reproductive tracts, in the intestinal tract, and in the oral cavity of humans and animals. Some *Vibrio* species are free-living.

Campylobacter fetus

Synonym: *Vibrio fetus* var. *venerealis* and var. *intestinalis*.

Historical

C. fetus was first recognized as a cause of abortion in cows by McFadean and Stockman in 1909.

Distribution and Mode of Infection

C. fetus is widespread. It is transmitted by ingestion or fomites. It is also present in semen and is spread venereally by the bull but not by the ram.

Pathogenicity

There are two subspecies. Subspecies *venerealis* is found in the prepuce of the bull and the genital tract of the cow and heifer. It produces both infections and the carrier state in cattle. It also causes infertility (epizootic bovine infertility) and occasionally abortion in cattle. Subspecies *fetus* is found in the intestine of cattle, sheep, and pigs. It causes abortion in cattle (sporadic) and sheep (multiple).

Effects are considered to be due in part to endotoxins. The uterine mucosa is infected with *Campylobacter* ss. *venerealis*, resulting in a metritis. As a consequence, the embryo may die and be resorbed. The organism may be shed from the uterus for a long period.

Specimens

Special methods are employed for the collection of cervical mucus and preputial secretions for culture. Filtration may be used to aid recovery; *Campylobacter* can pass through a 0.65 μm membrane filter.

Direct Examination

C. fetus can be demonstrated in the fetal stomach contents by relief or negative staining and by phase microscopy. A specific fluorescent antibody reagent can be used to identify *C. fetus*, but it does not distinguish between subspecies.

Isolation and Cultivation

In order to recover and grow the organism, the material submitted must be fresh.

Special media containing antibiotics are available to reduce growth of contaminants. An atmosphere containing 10% CO_2 should be used. Air should be reduced to one third and replaced with nitrogen for ss. *venerealis.*

Fine pin-point colonies are seen after 3 to 6 days of incubation. Smears reveal small, gram-negative rods that assume various forms—short and long, both curved and S-shaped. Long wavy filaments may be seen in some cultures.

IDENTIFICATION

Most nonpathogenic strains of *Campylobacter* are catalase-negative. One of these is *C. sputorum* ss. *bubulus,* which is found in the genital tract of male and female cattle and sheep.

The two subspecies of *C. fetus* are distinguished on the basis of the following:

	ss. *venerealis*	ss. *fetus*
H₂S production in special medium	−	+
Growth in 1% glycine (See also Table 21–1)	−	+

SEROLOGIC DIAGNOSIS

The serum agglutination test may be of value if interpreted carefully. Sera should be taken from several aborting cows three weeks to four months after abortion. The cervical mucus agglutination test is useful.

ANTIGENIC NATURE AND SEROLOGY

There are considerble antigenic differences among subspecies although they are composed of strains that are closely related serologically and immunologically.

RESISTANCE

Campylobacter spp. do not survive outside the host for more than several hours unless protected from drying and sunshine.

TREATMENT

Campylobacter spp. are susceptible to a number of antibiotics, but treatment is not usually feasible. Losses caused by the bovine disease may be reduced with penicillin and streptomycin. Irrigation of the uterus and prepuce with streptomycin is sometimes carried out.

IMMUNITY

Bacterins composed of killed *C. fetus* ss. *venerealis* combined with adjuvants such as oil, alum, or related compounds are of some value in cattle, but immunity is of short duration. Vaccination has been used in an effort to eliminate the carrier state in bulls. Bacterins are also used to prevent the ovine disease. The relative importance of humoral and cell-mediated immunity is not known, but it seems likely that the former is most important in protective immunity.

CONTROL OF EPIZOOTIC BOVINE INFERTILITY

Semen is routinely treated with streptomycin and penicillin. Breeding by artificial insemination will result in eventual elimination of *C. fetus* ss. *venerealis.* Infected bulls should be removed. *C. fetus* ss. *venerealis* can be eliminated from a herd but ss. *fetus* cannot.

Campylobacter sputorum

This species contains three subspecies: ss. *sputorum,* ss. *bubulus,* and ss. *mucosalis.* The first two are not pathogenic; the last, which is discussed here, is thought to be pathogenic. All are catalase-negative.

Campylobacter sputorum ss. mucosalis

There is considerable evidence that this organism is involved in the etiology of swine proliferative enteritis. This is a complex that includes intestinal adenomatosis, necrotic enteritis, regional ileitis, and proliferative hemorrhagic enteropathy. These are diseases of post-weaned and adult pigs characterized by an enteritis varying in severity from chronic to peracute and involving mainly the ileum.

An organism called *C. hyointestinalis* has also been recovered from lesions of swine proliferative enteritis.

Campylobacter jejuni (C. fetus ss. jejuni)

At one time this organism was thought to be the cause of a disease called "winter dysentery" of cattle. Although it can be recovered from animals with the disease, its primary role has not been demonstrated.

C. jejuni occurs frequently as a commensal in the intestinal tract of many species of domestic and wild animals, including birds and poultry. Dogs and cats frequently shed this organism in their feces, and there are claims that it can cause a febrile enteritis with diarrhea in these animals. *C. jejuni* is an important cause of enteritis in human beings. Among the signs are fever, abdominal pain, nausea, vomiting, blood in the stool, and diarrhea. Infections have been traced to animal and human carriers and food and water contaminated by feces.

C. jejuni is the cause of avian infectious hepatitis (vibrionic hepatitis) of chickens. This is a widespread disease characterized by a low mortality, high morbidity, chronic course, and hemorrhagic and necrotic changes in the liver.

Campylobacter coli

This organism was mistakenly thought to be the cause of swine dysentery. It occurs as a commensal in the intestinal tract of poultry, swine, and human beings and is not yet known to be pathogenic.

It is difficult to distinguish from *C.jejuni*.

ISOLATION AND IDENTIFICATION

Those species just discussed are isolated using essentially the same procedures as described for *C. fetus*. Special measures such as filtration, the use of antibiotics, and below surface sampling (*C. sputorum* ss. *mucosalis*) are used to reduce contaminants. Growth is slow and colonies of the various species resemble those of *C. fetus*, except that those of *C. sputorum* ss. *mucosalis* have a dirty yellow appearance.

In avian hepatitis *C. jejuni* can be demonstrated in bile by phase microscopy. This organism grows readily in a candle jar.

Identification is based on growth characteristics and biochemical reactions (see Table 21–1).

TREATMENT

Among the drugs that have been used to treat human, canine, and feline infections caused by

C. jejuni are erythromycin, the aminoglycosides, chloramphenicol, and the tetracyclines.

PRINCIPAL CHARACTERISTICS OF *Vibrio*

Vibrio organisms are spirally curved gram-negative rods of varying shapes. They are motile, aerobic and facultative anaerobes and are oxidase-positive and fermentative.

Vibrio cholerae is the cause of human cholera and *Vibrio parahaemolyticus* is a contaminant in seafoods, and causes food poisoning in humans, with enteritis.

Vibrio metschnikovii

This organism, which resembles *V. cholerae*, has been recovered on several occasions from chickens with enteritis in Europe.

PATHOGENICITY

V. metschnikovii is considered the cause of an acute and frequently fatal gastroenteritis of young chickens, and other fowl. The presence in the intestinal tract of a sanguineous, yellow-grey fluid is considered characteristic.

ISOLATION, CULTIVATION, AND IDENTIFICATION

The organism is aerobic and grows readily at room or incubator temperature on unenriched media or blood agar. The colonies are small, round, yellowish and glistening. Stained smears reveal small, gram-negative curved rods not unlike other *Vibrio*. It is identified on the basis of growth and biochemical characteristics.

Table 21–1. *Differentiation of Important* Campylobacter *Species and Subspecies*

Species and Subspecies	Principal Hosts	Catalase	Nitrate Reduction	H₂S TSI	H₂S Lead Acetate Strips	Growth in 1% Glycine	Growth in 3.5% NaCl	Growth at 25C
C. fetus ss. *venerealis*	Cattle	+	−	−	−	−	−	+
ss. *fetus*	Cattle, sheep, swine	+	−	−	+	+	−	+
C. jejuni	Cattle, sheep, dog, avian	+	−	−	+	+	−	−
C. sputorum ss. *sputorum*	Humans	−	+	+	+	+	−	+
ss. *bubulus*	Cattle, sheep	−	+	+	+	+	+	(+)
ss. *mucosalis*	Swine	−	+	+	+	−	−	
C. fecalis	Cattle, sheep	+	+	+	+	+	(+)*	−
C. coli	Swine, chickens	+	−	+	+	+	−	−
C. hyointestinalis	Swine	+	−	+	+	+	−	+

*( ) = most.

PUBLIC HEALTH SIGNIFICANCE

Veterinarians, farmers, packing house workers, and others associated with cattle and sheep occasionally sustain infections due to *C. fetus.* Diseases attributed to these infections are abortions, enteritis, endocarditis, and fever with bacteremia. Human infections with *C. jejuni* were discussed earlier.

SUGGESTED CLINICAL EXAMPLES

An outbreak of epizootic bovine infertility in a dairy herd.

An outbreak of *Campylobacter* abortion in sheep.

An outbreak of "winter dysentery" in stabled cattle.

Suspected *Campylobcter jejuni* enteritis in a dog.

SOURCES FOR FURTHER READING

Andrews, P.J., and Frank F.W.: Comparison of four diagnostic tests for detection of bovine genital vibriosis. J. Am. Vet. Med. Assoc., *165*:8, 1974.

Blaser, M.J., et al.: Campylobacter enteritis: Clinical and epidemiologic features. Ann. Intern. Med., *91*:179, 1979.

Blaser, M.J., LaForce, F.M., Wilson, N.A., and Wang, W.L.L.: Reservoirs of human campylobacteriosis. J. Infect. Dis., *141*:665, 1980.

Bryner, J.H., Foley, J.W., and Thompson, K.: Comparative efficacy of ten commercial *Campylobacter fetus* vaccines in the pregnant guinea pig: Challenge with *Campylobacter fetus* serotype A. Am. J. Vet. Res., *39*:3, 1978.

Butzler, J.P. (ed.): Campylobacter Infection of Man and Animals. Boca Raton, Florida, CRC Press Inc., 1984.

Fox, J.G., Moore, R., and Ackerman, J.I.: Campylobacter jejuni-associated diarrhea in dogs. J. Am. Vet. Med. Assoc., *183*:1430, 1983.

Gibson, C.D., Dreher, W.H., and Zemjanis, R.: Simplified technique for collection of preputial samples from bulls for isolation of *Vibrio fetus.* J. Am. Vet. Med. Assoc., *157*:6, 1970.

Laing, J.A.: *Vibrio fetus* Infection of Cattle. FAO Agricultural Studies No. 51. Rome, Food and Agricultural Organization of the United Nations, 1960.

Lawson, G.H.K., Rowland, A.C., and Wooding, P.: The characterization of *Campylobacter sputorum* subspecies *mucosalis* isolated from pigs. Res. Vet. Sci., *18*:121, 1975.

Mellick, R.W., Winter, A.J., and McEntee, K.: Diagnosis of vibrios in the bull by fluorescent antibody technique. Cornell Vet., *55*:2, 1965.

Prescott, J.F., and Brein-Mosch, C.W.: Carriage of *Campylobacter jejuni* in healthy and diarrheic animals. Am. J. Vet. Res., *42*:164, 1981.

Smibert, R.M.: The genus *Campylobacter.* Ann. Rev Microbiol., *32*:673, 1978.

Smibert, R.M.: Genus *Campylobacter. In* Bergey's Manual of Systematic Bacteriology. Vol. 1. Edited by N.R. Krieg. Baltimore, Williams & Wilkins, 1984.

Veron, M., and Chatelain, R.: Taxonomic study of the genus *Campylobacter* Sebald and Veron and designation of the neotype strain for the type species, *Campylobacter fetus* (Smith and Taylor) Sebald and Veron. Int. J. Syst. Bacteriol., *23*:122, 1973.

Winter, A.J., Burda, K., and Dunn, H.O.: An evaluation of cultural technics for the detection of *Vibrio fetus.* Cornell Vet., *55*:431, 1965.

22

Haemophilus

Principal Characteristics of *Haemophilus*

Species of the genus *Haemophilus* are small, gram-negative rods and filaments. They are nonmotile, aerobic and facultatively anaerobic and require X or V factor or both.

More than a dozen species are listed in *Bergey's Manual of Systematic Bacteriology.* Most are associated with humans and animals as commensals on mucous membranes of the upper digestive, respiratory, and genital tracts. Some are potential pathogens. They require one or both of the following factors for growth: (1) X factor: requirement for the iron porphyrin, hemin; supplied by blood agar or chocolate agar; (2) V factor: nicotinamide adenine dinucleotide (NAD) or one of its riboside precursors; supplied by fresh yeast extract or staphylococcal growth.

The hosts and X and V factor requirements of some important species are given below.

Mode of Infection

This is most frequently by inhalation. Fomites may be involved. Infections may be endogenous or exogenous. *[handwritten: originating outside the organism]*

Pathogenesis

Virulence is associated with capsule (polysaccharide) formation, and it is likely that endotoxin has an important role. Young or previously unexposed animals are most susceptible. Stresses and crowding may be contributory.

H. influenzae gains entrance to human tissues via the respiratory tract, usually with an initial nasopharyngitis. If this infection is not checked, it may lead to sinusitis, otitis media, and pneumonia. If a bacteremia develops, joint infections and meningitis may follow. An essentially similar pathogenesis is seen with some of the varieties of *Haemophilus* that infect animals, e.g., *H. parasuis*, *H. paragallinarum*, and *H. pleuropneumoniae*. Disease caused by the unofficial species *H. somnus* probably has a somewhat similar development.

Haemophilus somnus

Because this organism does not require either the X or V factor, it cannot be classed as a true *Haemophilus*.

H. somnus infection of cattle is manifested by three principal syndromes: (1) respiratory involvement, with pneumonia and bacteremia; (2) localization in the central nervous system, with thromboembolic meningoencephalitis; and (3) joint infection accompanied by arthritis. More than one syndrome may be seen in the same animal. The neural manifestation of the disease is frequently fatal. Outbreaks are often associated with stress and are frequently seen in feedlot cattle.

Organisms can be demonstrated from brain lesions. Isolation can be made on media supplemented with blood and yeast in 10% CO_2 (mandatory). Definitive identification requires several biochemical tests.

Species	Hosts	Requirement for X	V
H. influenzae	Humans	+	+
H. parainfluenzae	Humans and cats; probably cattle, sheep, fowl	−	+
H. parasuis	Swine	−	+
H. pleuropneumoniae	Swine, sheep, cattle	−	+
H. haemoglobinophilus	Dogs (preputial sac)	+	−
H. paragallinarum	Chickens	−	+
H. aphrophilus	Humans	+	−
H. avium	Poultry	−	+
H. paracuniculus	Rabbit	−	+
*H. agni**	Sheep	−	−
*H. somnus**	Cattle	−	−
*H. equigenitalis**	Horses	−	−
H. influenzaemurium†	Mice	+	−
H. ovis†	Sheep	+	−

*Unofficial; by current standards they do not qualify for inclusion in the genus.
†Not included in the current *Bergey's Manual* (1984).

Haemophilus pleuropneumoniae (H. parahaemolyticus)

This organism has come into prominence in recent years as a frequent cause of an acute, subacute, or chronic pleuropneumonia of swine. The disease called contagious pleuropneumonia is usually seen in pigs up to 5 months of age and is characterized by a serofibrinous pleuritis and a fibrinous pneumonia. Septicemia, meningitis, and arthritis are seen, particularly in nursing pigs.

On culture there is beta-hemolysis, and the CAMP test is positive. Definitive identification requires certain biochemical tests. Seven different capsular types have been identified.

Haemophilus parasuis

H. parasuis is a secondary invader in swine influenza and the primary agent of Glasser's disease, a disease of young pigs characterized by a polyserositis and occasionally meningitis. The signs and lesions resemble those of polyserositis due to *Mycoplasma hyorhinis*.

Haemophilus paragallinarum

H. paragallinarum is the cause of infectious coryza. This disease has both acute and chronic forms and is characterized by nasal discharge, sneezing, and edema of the face. There are high morbidity and low mortality rates sometimes with marked economic losses because of the reduction in growth and egg production.

PATHOGENICITY OF SOME SPECIES OF LESSER IMPORTANCE

H. agni has been recovered from six- to seven-month-old lambs with septicemia in California.

There have been no recent reports of its occurrence. It may be the same as *Histophilus ovis*.

H. haemoglobinophilus (H. canis) has been recovered from the genital tract of dogs.

H. influenzaemurium causes respiratory infections and conjunctivitis in mice.

H. aphrophilus has been shown to cause endocarditis in humans.

H. avium is a nonpathogenic commensal that can be confused with *H. gallinarum*. In contrast to this organism, it is catalase-positive.

H. ovis has been reported twice in sheep, as a commensal and as a cause of bronchopneumonia.

H. paracuniculus has been isolated from rabbits. Its significance is not known.

ISOLATION AND IDENTIFICATION

The most important species of *Haemophilus* in animal disease will grow on blood agar, with a *Staphylococcus* streak (growth) providing the V factor. Blood agar supplies sufficient hemin. If *Haemophilus* is suspected, blood plates with a staphylococcus streak should be incubated in air containing 10% CO_2. *H. somnus* does not grow initially without CO_2.

Plates are incubated for 24 to 48 hours. Small dewdrop colonies appear after 24 hours of incubation. If the V factor is required, the small colonies will appear near the *Staphylococcus* streak (satellite growth).

For practical purposes identification is based on morphologic and colonial characteristics, X or V factor requirement or both and host, lesions, and clinical signs. Species can be identified using a number of biochemical tests; however, because of the fastidious growth requirements of these organisms, such tests are not carried out routinely in the diagnostic laboratory. For precise identification, reference should be made to *Bergey's Manual of Systematic Bacteriology*, Vol. 1, 1984. Some differential characteristics of the more important species are given in Table 22–1.

RESISTANCE

Haemophilus species are fragile. They are sensitive to sunlight and drying and are readily killed by common disinfectants.

IMMUNITY

Immunity to *Haemophilus* species is thought to be predominantly humoral. Most species are antigenically heterogeneous. A number of serotypes of *H. somnus* and *H. paragallinarum* have been identified. Specific capsular antibodies are considered important in protection. Bacterins are used to prevent infectious coryza, contagious pleuropneumonia of swine, and *H. somnus* infection in cattle.

TREATMENT

Haemophilus spp. are susceptible to penicillin, tetracyclines, sulfonamides, chloramphenicol, and erythromycin. Drugs are usually administered in food or water.

Haemophilus equigenitalis

This organism causes contagious equine metritis (CEM), an acute, highly contagious venereal disease of mares and female ponies characterized by a metritis, cervicitis, and copious, purulent vaginal discharge. Abortions may occur within the first 60 days. Stallions are infected and spread the disease during coitus but show no clinical signs. Spread may also be by contaminated equipment and attendants.

The disease has been reported from the United Kingdom, France, Australia, and many other European countries and Japan.

PATHOGENESIS

The infectious process appears to be confined to the mucous membrane of the uterus, cervix, and vagina, with accompanying endometritis, cervicitis, and vaginitis. There has been no evidence of spread to other tissues and organs. No lesions are seen in the stallion.

DIAGNOSIS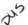

Clinical: The copious mucopurulent discharge occurring after breeding or during the breeding season should be highly suspicious.

Laboratory: The disease can only be diagnosed definitively by the isolation and identification of the causal agent. The following tests have been used: complement fixation, agglutination (plate and tube), and passive hemagglutination. Infected stallions are serologically negative, as are some carrier mares.

LABORATORY SPECIMENS

Swabs from the cervix, urethra, and clitoral fossa, including the clitoral sinuses of the mare and the urethral fossa and penile sheath of the stallion, should be sent to the laboratory, refrigerated, in a transport medium (preferably Amies) as soon after being collected as possible.

ISOLATION AND IDENTIFICATION

The causal agent has been provisionally named *Haemophilus equigenitalis*, although by some criteria it does not belong in the *Haemophilus* genus. The organism can be isolated on chocolate agar that has been incubated for several days in air containing 5 to 10% CO_2. Small colonies similar in appearance to those of other *Haemophilus* spp. appear after 24 hours of incubation. Although fastidious and rather unreactive biochemically, *H. equigenitalis* can be shown to be oxidase, catalase, and phosphatase-positive. Some stimulation of growth is obtained with the X factor but not the V factor. Strains both sensitive and resistant to streptomycin

*Table 22–1. Some Differential Characteristics of Important **Haemophilus** spp.*

Species	Required		Indole	Urease	Hemolysis	CAMP Reaction	Catalase	Oxidase	Acid: Glucose	CO_2 Enhances Growth
	X	V								
H. parasuis	−	+	−	−	−	−	+	−	+	−
H. paragallinarum	−	+	−	−	−	−	+	−	+	+
H. avium	−	+	−	−	−	−	+	−	+	−
H. pleuropneumoniae	−	+	−	+	+	+	−	V	+	−
H. somnus	−	−	+	−	V	−	−	+	+	+
H. equigenitalis	−	−	−	−	−	−	+	−	−	+

have been isolated. Some differential characteristics are listed in Table 22–1.

TREATMENT

Intrauterine irrigation with nitrofurazone, ampicillin, or penicillin daily for 5 to 10 days is effective. Ampicillin or penicillin are given parenterally for the same period. The penis should be cleaned and the prepuce irrigated on at least five occasions with chlorhexidine and nitrofurazone. One week after treatment, mares and stallions must be checked to determine if they are negative for the organism after three successive cultures at weekly intervals.

Conception rates for mares and breeding rates for stallions return to normal the following breeding season.

IMMUNITY

Immunity would seem to be a low order. There is evidence that previously infected mares can be reinfected several weeks after being culturally negative.

CONTROL AND PROPHYLAXIS

If the disease is suspected, state and federal veterinary officials should be notified. The suspected infected stallion should not be used for further breeding until shown to be culturally negative. All suspected or known to be infected animals should be kept under strict isolation until shown to be negative by culture.

The organism is fragile, and evidence indicates that it will not survive in discharge material outside the host for more than several days.

SUGGESTED CLINICAL EXAMPLES

Cases of *Haemophilus somnus* infection in a beef cattle feedlot.

Cases of Glasser's disease in a swine herd.

An outbreak of contagious pleuropneumonia in swine.

An outbreak of contagious equine metritis.

SOURCES FOR FURTHER READING

Biberstein, E.L., and White, D.C.: A proposal for the establishment of two new *Haemophilus* species. J. Med. Microbiol., 2:75, 1969.

Biberstein, E.L.: *Haemophilus. In* Diagnostic Procedures in Veterinary Bacteriology and Mycology. Edited by G.R. Carter. 4th Ed. Springfield, Ill., Charles C Thomas, 1984.

Drerkes, R.E., and Hanna, S.A.: Epizootiology and pathogenesis of *Haemophilus somnus* infection. J. Am. Vet. Med. Assoc., 163:866, 1975.

Kilian, M., Nicolet, J., and Biberstein, E.L.: Biochemical and serological characterization of *Haemophilus pleuropneumoniae* (Matthews and Pattison, 1961). Shope 1964 and proposal of a neotype strain. Int. J. Syst. Bacteriol., 28:20, 1978.

Kilian, M., Frederiksen, W., and Biberstein, E.L. (eds.): *Haemophilus, Pasteurella* and *Actinobacillus*. New York, Academic Press, 1981.

Kreig, N.R. (ed.): Bergey's Manual of Systematic Bacteriology. Vol. 1. Baltimore, Williams & Wilkins, 1984.

Little, T.W.A., and Harding, J.D.J.: The comparative pathogenicity of two porcine *Haemophilus* species. Vet. Rec., 88:540, 1971.

Matsumoto, M., and Yamamoto, R.: Protective quality of an aluminum hydroxide absorbed broth bacterin against infectious coryza. Am. J. Vet. Res., 36:579, 1975.

Panciera, R.J., Dahlgren, R.R., and Rinker, H.B.: Observations on septicemia of cattle caused by a *Haemophilus*-like organism. Pathol. Vet., 5:212, 1968.

Shigidi, M.A., and Hoerlein, A.B.: Characterization of the *Haemophilus*-like organisms of infectious thromboembolic meningoencephalitis of cattle. Am. J. Vet. Res., 31:1017, 1970.

Sutherland, A.K., and Simmons, G.C.: Glasser's disease of swine. Aust. Vet. J., 23:91, 1947.

Taylor C.E.D., et al.: The causative organism of contagious equine metritis. 1977. Proposal for a new species to be known as *Haemophilus equigenitalis*. Equine Vet. J., 10:136, 1978.

23

Bordetella and Moraxella

Principal Characteristics of *Bordetella*

Species of the genus *Bordetella* are small, gram-negative rods and coccobacilli. They are aerobic, oxidase-positive, and do not ferment carbohydrates (metabolism respiratory). There are both motile and nonmotile species.

Only three official species are described:
1. *Bordetella bronchiseptica:* natural hosts are animals; causes respiratory disease.
2. *B. avium:* (unofficial): causes rhinotracheitis of turkey poults.
3. *B. pertussis:* natural host is humans; causes whooping cough.
4. *B. parapertussis:* natural host is humans; causes parapertussis, a mild form of whooping cough.

Bordetella bronchiseptica

Habitat

B. bronchiseptica is a commensal in the upper respiratory tract of dogs, cats, swine, rabbits, horses, guinea pigs, rats, and possibly other animals.

Mode of Infection and Transmission

Infections may be endogenous or exogenous. Inhalation is the principal mode of infection. Spread is by direct and indirect contact and fomites.

Pathogenesis and Pathogenicity

Infections result in respiratory disease that is usually subacute to chronic in nature.

A dermonecrotoxin is produced, but its role in disease is not clear.

In the dog, it is a secondary invader in the pneumonia of canine distemper, and it is sometimes involved in the etiology of "kennel cough." *Study of factors involved in disease, cause of disease.*

It causes pneumonia in swine, usually in the age range of three to eight weeks, which has a tendency to be chronic. It is considered the principal cause of infectious atrophic rhinitis of swine.

In wild and laboratory rodents such as guinea pigs, rabbits (snuffles), and rats, it produces upper respiratory and pneumonic infections.

Respiratory infections have also been reported in the cat, ferret, and horse.

Isolation and Cultivation

The organism is aerobic, can be cultured on blood or serum agar, and may be beta-hemolytic. Small, circular, dewdrop colonies appear in 48 hours. On further incubation, colonies enlarge, becoming flat and glistening. Stained smears disclose small gram-negative rods or coccobacilli.

Special media are available for culturing material from nasal swabs in the testing of swine herds for *B. bronchiseptica* and thus infectious atrophic rhinitis. These media greatly reduce the number of extraneous bacteria.

Identification

B. bronchiseptica is motile, indole-negative, and does not produce H_2S. Urease is produced, and the tests for oxidase and catalase are positive.

176

Litmus Milk: alkaline, turning from blue to black in 5 to 10 days. Because drug resistance has been encountered in *B. bronchiseptica,* it is advisable to carry out susceptibility tests on isolates. Carbohydrates are not fermented. For additional criteria, see Table 23–1.

EXPERIMENTAL ANIMALS

Fatal infections can be produced in guinea pigs by the injection of fresh cultures intraperitoneally.

IMMUNITY

The antigenic nature of *B. bronchiseptica* has not been studied in any detail. It has an antigenic relationship with *Brucella* and is antigenically related to the other members of the *Bordetella* genus.

Immunity appears to be mainly humoral. It is included in mixed and other bacterins to aid in the prevention of respiratory disease and infectious atrophic rhinitis in swine. It is combined with *Pasteurella multocida* in bacterins to prevent snuffles in rabbits. It is sometimes used with other agents to produce antisera to aid in the prevention and treatment of the pneumonia encountered in distemper. Bacterins are used to prevent "kennel cough" in dogs. A live avirulent vaccine has been licensed for use in sows (intramuscular) and piglets (intranasal) to prevent atrophic rhinitis.

TREATMENT AND CONTROL

Sulfonamides are administered to swine in their feed or water for several weeks; the drug is present on nasal mucous membranes. Bacterins are used in young pigs and sows prior to farrowing. Before an animal is considered free of the infection, at least three successive nasal swabs should be negative for *B. bronchiseptica.*

PUBLIC HEALTH SIGNIFICANCE

B. bronchiseptica occasionally causes a whooping cough-like disease in humans.

Bordetella avium

Synonym: *Alcaligenes faecalis.*

This organism is the cause of the economically important disease of turkeys and chickens called rhinotracheitis. There was some doubt as to whether the organism belonged to the *Alcaligenes* or *Bordetella* genus, but a recent comprehensive study that included DNA hybridization has placed it in the latter group.

B. avium resembles *B. bronchiseptica* in its growth and cultural characteristics, but it differs from it in that it does not produce urease. Additional differential characteristics are provided in Table 23–1.

PRINCIPAL CHARACTERISTICS OF *Moraxella*

Moraxella are small, gram-negative aerobic, nonmotile rods. They are catalase- and oxidase-

Table 23–1. *Differential Characteristics of Some Nonfermentative Gram-Negative Bacteria*

TSI and Kligler's: alkaline slant, neutral butt, no gas, and no H₂S production	Principal Host	Beta-Hemolysis	Growth on MacConkey Agar	Growth on Salmonella, Shigella	Oxidase	Motility	Pigment	Gelatinase	Nitrate Reduction	Urease	Citrate	Oxidation Maltose	Oxidation Xylose	Oxidation Glucose
Acinetobacter calcoaceticus var. *anitratus*	Animals and humans	−*	+	(+)	−	−	−	V	−	−*	+	−*	+*	+
var. *lwoffi*	Animals and humans	−*	+	−	−	−	−	−*	−	−*	+*	−	−	−
Alcaligenes faecalis	Humans and animals	−	+	(+)	+	+	−	−	V	−	+	−	−	−
Bordetella avium	Turkeys, chickens	−	+	+	+	−	−	−	−	−	−	−	−	−
Bordetella bronchiseptica	Animals	+*	+	−	+	+	−	−*	+	+	+	−	−	−
Moraxella bovis	Cattle	+	−	−	+	−	+	−	−	−	−	−	−	−
Moraxella species	Animals	−	V	−	+	−	−*	V	V	V	−*	−	−	−*

*some exceptions, V = variables, (+) = most strains positive.

positive, do not utilize carbohydrates, and do not require X and V factors.

Of the six species described in *Bergey's Manual of Systematic Bacteriology* only one, *M. bovis*, is significant in animal disease.

Moraxella bovis

HABITAT

The organism may be found as a commensal on the conjunctiva or in the nasopharynx of cattle.

TRANSMISSION

M. bovis is probably spread most commonly by insects but it can also be spread by contact.

PATHOGENESIS AND PATHOGENICITY

M. bovis is considered the cause of pinkeye, infectious keratoconjunctivitis or infectious ophthalmia of cattle. Both young and adult cattle are susceptible. It is seen more commonly in the beef breeds and is aggravated by grazing in tall grass, by a dry dusty environment, and by insects. Some *M. bovis* strains possess pili that may aid in adherence and colonization.

ISOLATION AND CULTIVATION

Good growth is obtained on standard media; it is enhanced by the addition of blood or serum. Colonies are usually round, translucent, grayish-white, 1 to 2 mm in diameter, and surrounded by a narrow zone of clear hemolysis. After 48 to 72 hours, colonies enlarge and become somewhat flattened, with raised centers.

Stained smears reveal gram-negative or gram-variable coccobacilli, usually occurring in pairs and less frequently in short chains. *M. bovis* is nonmotile, nonsporeforming, and encapsulated.

IDENTIFICATION

No acid is produced in the usual fermentation media. Litmus milk becomes alkaline; *M. bovis* does not reduce nitrates, does not form indole, and liquefies gelatin slowly (see Table 23–1).

IMMUNITY

Immunity to the disease is of short duration and relapses are common. Autogenous and commercial bacterins have been used, but there is some question as to their value.

TREATMENT

Cattle are confined to shady areas, and adequate vitamin A is provided. Chloramphenicol, penicillin, nitrofurazone, and tetracyclines are administered locally (topically) or by subconjunctival injection. Repeated applications are required. Measures should be taken to control insects.

SUGGESTED CLINICAL EXAMPLES

An outbreak of *Bordetella* pneumonia in young pigs.

Attempted eradication of infectious atrophic rhinitis from a swine herd.

An outbreak of *Bordetella* infections in a guinea pig colony.

An outbreak of infectious keratoconjunctivitis in a herd of Herefords.

SOURCES FOR FURTHER READING

Arora, A.K., Killinger, A.H., and Mansfield, M.: Bacteriologic and vaccination studies in a field epizootic of infectious bovine keratoconjunctivitis in calves. Am. J. Vet. Res., 37:803, 1976.

Baptista, P.J.H.P.: Infectious bovine keratoconjunctivitis: A review. Br. Vet. J., 135:255, 1979.

Barner, R.D.: A study of *Moraxella bovis* and its relation to bovine keratitis. Am. J. Vet. Res., 13:132, 1952.

Bemis, D.A., Carmichal, L.E., and Appel, M.F.G.: Naturally occurring respiratory disease in a kennel caused by *Bordetella bronchiseptica*. Cornell Vet., 67:282, 1977.

Fisk, S.K., and Soave, O.A.: *Bordetella bronchiseptica* in laboratory cats from Central California. Lab. An. Sci., 23:33, 1973.

Goodnow, R.A.: Biology of *Bordetella bronchiseptica*. Microbiol. Rev., 44:722, 1980.

Goodnow, R.A., Shade, F.J., and Switzer, W.P.: Efficacy of *Bordetella bronchiseptica* bacterin in controlling enzootic atrophic rhinitis. Am. J. Vet. Res., 40:58, 1979.

Kersters, K., et al.: *Bordetella avium* sp. nov., isolated from the respiratory tracts of turkeys and other birds. Int. J. Syst. Bacteriol., 34:56, 1984.

McCandlish, I.A.P., Thompson, H., Cornwell, H.J.C., and Wright, N.G.: A study of dogs with kennel cough. Vet. Rec., 102:298, 1978.

McCandlish, I.A.P., Thompson, H., and Wright, N.G.: Vaccination against canine bordetellosis: Protection from contact challenge. Vet. Rec., 102:479, 1978.

Pugh, G.W., Jr., Hughes, D.E., and McDonald, T.J.: The isolation and characterization of *Moraxella bovis*. Am. J. Vet. Res., 27:957, 1966.

Pugh, G.W., Jr., et al.: Bovine infectious keratitis: *Moraxella bovis* as the sole etiologic agent in a winter epizootic. J. Am. Vet. Med. Assoc., 161:481, 1972.

Pugh, G.W., Jr., et al.: Experimental infectious bovine keratoconjunctivitis: Effects of feeding colostrum from vaccinated cows in development of pinkeye in calves. Am. J. Vet. Res., 41:1611, 1980.

Smith, I.M., and Baskerville, A.J.: A selective medium facilitating the isolation and recognition of *Bordetella bronchiseptica*. Res. Vet. Sci., 27:187, 1979.

24

Brucella

PRINCIPAL CHARACTERISTICS OF *Brucella*

Brucella are gram-negative, nonmotile, non-spore-forming small rods. They are aerobic and carboyxphilic, catalase- and urease-positive, and produce no acid from carbohydrates in conventional peptone media.

They are not found living apart from animals and all are pathogenic, facultative intracellular parasites with a predilection for the reticuloendothelial system and the reproductive tract and organs. The following species are recognized:

- *B. abortus,*
- *B. melitensis,*
- *B. suis,*
- *B. ovis,*
- *B. canis,*
- *B. neotomae: recovered from sand rats.*

HISTORICAL

Brucella melitensis was identified by Bruce in Malta in 1887. *B. abortus* was first recognized by Bang in 1897, and *B. suis* was discovered by Traum in 1914. In 1918, Alice Evans showed the taxonomic relationship between *B. abortus* and *B. melitensis* and identified the first *Brucella* of human origin in the United States.

MODE OF INFECTION

The common routes of infection in humans and animals are via the mucous membranes of the digestive tract, genital tract (cow or sow from bull and boar), and skin.

PATHOGENESIS OF BRUCELLOSIS

The organism passes from the point of entry via the lymphatics to the regional lymph nodes, and after multiplication to the thoracic duct and then via the bloodstream to the parenchymatous organs and other tissues. The brucellae are principally intracellular in macrophages, and granulomatous foci develop in lymphatic tissues, liver, spleen, bone marrow, and other locations. On occasion these granulomatous foci or nodules may abscess. Hypersensitivity to elements of brucella organisms, including endotoxin, may play a role in pathogenesis.

The predilection that brucellae have for the placenta, fetal fluids, and testes of the bull, ram, and boar is attributed to erythritol. This polyhydric alcohol has been shown to stimulate the growth of *Brucella*. It is not present in the human placenta.

Brucella abortus, B. melitensis, B. suis and *B. canis*

PATHOGENICITY

Cattle. Brucellosis is one of the most important diseases of cattle. It has great public health and economic significance. The disease in cattle is almost always caused by *B. abortus*.

The organism is highly infectious and usually gains entrance to the body as a result of (1) ingestion of food, water, and milk contaminated with uterine discharges, urine, or feces of an infected animal; (2) penetration of the broken or unbroken skin; or (3) service by an infected bull.

The incubation period is usually from 30 to 60 days. In the cow the infection localizes, usually after a bacteremia, in the placenta of the gravid uterus (placentitis). If the animal is not pregnant, there is usually localization in the udder (interstitial mastitis) and adjacent lymph nodes. Organisms are shed in the milk. It may also localize in the liver, lungs, or spleen, where it produces granulomatous foci. Cows may remain infected for years.

In the bull, infection may localize in the testicle, epididymis, or seminal vesicle, and abscessation is a common sequela. Noninfected bulls usually do not become infected as a result of serving an infected cow, but infected bulls infect cows.

The consequences of the bovine disease are loss of calves due to abortion at six months or later (about one third of infected animals usually abort), and sterility or infertility of either the male or female.

CONTROL. Bovine brucellosis has been eliminated from several countries and from many states in the United States. The procedure that has been followed involves blood testing (agglutination test) of all cattle, and the removal of reactors (titer 1:100 or higher). So that cattle will be less susceptible to reinfection, calfhood vaccination is recommended and in some circumstances is mandatory. The attenuated live vaccine (strain 19) is used in female calves four to eight or three to seven months of age. They develop an agglutination reaction, which usually decreases or disappears soon. If the reaction at 1:200 or higher persists past 30 months of age, the animal is considered a reactor. Because strain 19 may cause infertility in some male calves, its use is restricted to females.

The card test, which uses only one serum dilution and stained antigen, is rapid, sensitive, and useful as a field screening test. The agglutination and complement-fixation tests have been adapted to the rapid microtiter system. A number of other tests are performed when the specificity of the reaction is in doubt or in the case of persisting vaccinal reactions.

The brucellosis ring test for agglutinins shed from the udder is performed three times each year on milk from herds whose milk is being sold. If there are reactors to this very sensitive test, or if there is any evidence of brucellosis in a herd, a blood test is carried out. Areas are designated as "Modified-Certified Brucellosis Area" or "Certified Brucellosis-Free Area." The first is so-called when no more than 5% of the herds and not more than 1% of the cattle are found to be infected and the second when no more than 1% of the herds and not more than 0.2% of the cattle are found to be infected over an 18-month period. Regulations and procedures relating to the brucellosis eradication program are involved, and students are referred to publications of the U.S. Department of Agriculture for further details.

Swine. Although low in the United States, the incidence in swine is difficult to estimate, because testing is not compulsory. *B. abortus* and *B. melitensis* rarely infect swine.

Swine of all ages are susceptible. Nursing pigs may become infected as a result of ingesting milk from diseased sows. Older animals usually become infected by ingesting contaminated food, water, or soil. Infected boars transmit the disease by coitus. Swine brucellosis is characterized by abortion, sterility, birth of stillborn or weak pigs, focal abscessation in various organs, spondylitis, and lameness. If given sufficient time, many animals will fully recover and free their tissues of the organism. Abortion may occur at any time during gestation; gilts and sows usually abort only once. Unlike cattle, infected sows may eliminate the infection but be susceptible to reinfection.

Brucellosis is a more generalized infection in hogs than in cattle. Following bacteremia, the organism may localize in lymph nodes, spleen, liver, kidneys, uterus, mammary glands, urinary bladder, seminal vesicles, testicles, accessory sex glands, and bones. Unlike *B. abortus* in the cow, *B. suis* may persist for some time in the sow's uterus, causing metritis and sterility. In some instances, it has been isolated from uterine discharges after 30 months.

CONTROL. Three plans are used to eradicate swine brucellosis. (1) Elimination of the infected herd and restocking with brucellosis-free swine. (2) Infected animals are separated from the noninfected ones and eventually slaughtered. The noninfected gilts, boars, and weanling pigs serve as the nucleus for a clean herd. Testing is carried out frequently and all infected animals are removed. (3) If the incidence of infection is low, reactors are removed and the herd is retested at 30-day intervals. Reactors are removed until the entire herd is negative on retest.

Swine do not react immunologically (humoral)

to the same degree that cattle do, and consequently the agglutination test is less reliable.

Following two consecutive negative herd tests not less than 90 days apart, the herd is eligible for Validated Brucellosis-Free Herd status. Vaccination is not employed.

Dog. *B. abortus* and *B. suis* have been isolated occasionally from sporadic infections in dogs. Canine brucellosis caused by *B. canis* was first recognized as a problem in beagle breeding kennels. The disease is known to be widely distributed throughout the general dog population, although the incidence is low. The mode of infection, transmission, and pathogenesis of the canine disease resembles that of brucellosis in cattle, swine, or goats. Expelled tissues and vaginal discharges of aborted bitches and the urine of infected males are primary sources of the infectious agent. Other means of transmission are copulation and nursing.

The incubation period after oral administration is six to 21 days. The bacteremic phase of the disease may last as long as two years, and other than a lymphadenopathy, dogs show little evidence of infection. Infected bitches usually abort in the last trimester. Those puppies that are not dead when aborted soon die. Following abortion there is a yellow-brown to dark brown discharge that persists for one to six weeks. Another possible result of infection of the bitch is resorption of the fetuses. Infections of bones may give rise to chronic osteomyelitis and spondylitis.

Prostatitis, epididymitis, and testicular atrophy with decreased spermatogenesis are common in the male and may result in irreversible sterility.

DIAGNOSIS. This is accomplished by the agglutination test and by isolation of the organism from blood, urine (male), fetal organs, and vaginal swabs. A positive agglutination reaction of 1:200 or higher with the mercaptoethanol test indicates infection. The slide screening agglutination test is reliable when negative, but positive samples should be retested by the tube test.

CONTROL. Treatment is not practiced. The disease is eliminated by blood testing, followed by elimination of reacting dogs. Only dogs free of brucellosis, i.e., those that are negative to at least two tests, are added to brucellosis-free breeding kennels. A satisfactory vaccine has not yet been developed.

Humans. Infections are caused by the three classic species and *B. canis*. In heavy swine-raising areas, *B. suis* infections are more prevalent; *B. melitensis* infections are seen in goat-raising areas, and *B. abortus* infections in areas with infected cattle. Pasteurization has greatly reduced the incidence of brucellosis in humans.

Organisms are thought to penetrate the unbroken skin and mucous membranes. Sources are laboratory infections, infected cows (obstetric work); and unpasteurized milk and other dairy products. Slaughterhouse workers and veterinarians frequently contract the disease.

The disease can vary from quite mild to very severe. The incubation period ranges from eight to 90 days. Those under 14 years of age are less susceptible. There is usually a bacteremia resulting in a variety of symptoms, including undulating fever, profuse perspiration, and rheumatic and neuralgic pains. The course is variable and relapses are frequent. Most patients totally recover within a year or two, even without treatment. The organism may localize in the liver, lymph nodes, or bones. Symptoms in the chronic form are thought to be caused by hypersensitivity to *Brucella* protein. Infections due to *B. suis* and *B. melitensis* may be more serious than those caused by *B. abortus*. Infections due to strain 19 have been reported.

DIAGNOSIS. The agglutination test may be negative in chronic infections. The Coombs test, which detects incomplete antibody, is usually positive in cases of chronic disease. The skin test utilizes brucellergen or brucellin (delayed type hypersensitivity); a positive test indicates infection or previous exposure.

TREATMENT. Treatment is effective if begun early. Tetracyclines are used alone or with streptomycin for at least a month. Treatment of the chronic disease is not always satisfactory because of inaccessible foci (or focus), often in bone.

Goats. Although accurate data are not available, tests indicate that the incidence of *Brucellosis* in goats in the United States is approximately 1%. The majority of infections in goats are due to *B. melitensis*.

Horse. *B. abortus* and *B. suis* have been recovered, along with other organisms, from cases of fistulous withers and poll evil. Brucellae have also been recovered from osteoarthritic lesions in various locations in the horse.

Sheep. *B. abortus* causes occasional infections, resulting in abortions.

Table 24–1. Differentiation of Brucella Species and their Biotypes†

Species	Urease	Oxidase	Biotype	CO₂ Require-ment	H₂S Production	Growth on Dyes*					Agglutination in Sera		
						Thionin			Basic Fuchsin				
						A	B	C	B	C	A	M	R
B. melitensis	V	+	1	–	–	–	+	+	+	+	–	+	–
			2	–	–	–	+	+	+	+	+	–	–
			3	–	–	–	+	+	+	+	+	+	–
B. abortus	+	+	1	V	+	–	–	–	+	–	+	–	–
			2	+	+	–	–	–	+	+	+	–	–
			3	V	+	+	+	+	+	+	+	–	–
			4	V	+	–	+	–	+	+	–	+	–
			5	–	–	–	+	+	+	+	+	+	–
			6	–	V	–	+	+	+	+	+	+	–
			7	–	V	–	+	+	+	+	+	+	–
			9	V	+	–	+	+	+	+	+	+	–
B. suis	+	+	1	–	+	+	+	+	–	–	+	–	–
			2	–	–	–	+	+	–	–	+	–	–
			3	–	–	+	+	+	+	+	+	–	–
			4	–	–	+	+	+	+	±	+	+	–
B. canis	+	+		+	–	+	+	+	–	+	–	–	+
B. ovis	–	–		+	–	+	+	+	–	+	–	–	+
B. neotomae	+	+		–	+	–	–	+	–	–	+	–	–

*Species differentiation is obtained on tryptose agar with the following graded concentrations of dyes: thionin concentration (A) 1:25,000, (B) 1:50,000, (C) 1:100,000: basic fuchsin concentration (B) 1:50,000, (C) 1:100,000.

†(Modified from Alton, G.G., Jones, L.M., and Pietz, D.E.: Laboratory Techniques in Brucellosis. 2nd Ed., 1975. Courtesy of the World Health Organization, Geneva and from Meyer, M.E.: Brucella. In Diagnostic Procedures in Veterinary Bacteriology and Mycology. Edited by G.R. Carter. 4th Ed. Springfield, Ill., Charles C Thomas, 1984, reprinted with permission.)

DIRECT EXAMINATION

Koster's stain is useful in demonstrating brucellae in smears from the placenta in bovine abortion. Cells of the chorion are packed with organisms.

ISOLATION AND CULTIVATION

Good growth is obtained on tryptose, potato, liver infusion, and blood agar. Colonies are round, entire, smooth, glistening, and translucent. Young colonies are 1 to 2 mm in diameter; they may become 5 to 8 mm on continued incubation. *B. abortus* requires 10% CO_2 for initial isolation. Plates should be incubated for as long as three weeks.

Small rods, single or in pairs or in short chains, are seen in smears from colonies.

IDENTIFICATION

The different species can be identified by the characteristics listed in Table 24–1. With additional tests, a number of biotypes of each of the classic species can be identified.

Monospecific sera to *B. abortus* and *B. melitensis* are used (see Table 24–1). Fluorescent antibody staining is used for generic identification. Organisms from colonies can be presumptively identified as brucellae by a slide agglutination test using *B. abortus* antiserum.

EXPERIMENTAL ANIMALS

Guinea pigs can be readily infected with infectious material. They are useful if material is badly contaminated or the numbers of organisms are very small. Infected guinea pigs will yield pure cultures and develop a significant agglutination titer.

ANTIGENIC NATURE AND SEROLOGY

The three classic strains are closely related and share a number of antigens. Reactions by monospecific sera with other differential properties are of value in identification. *B. canis* and *B. ovis* are antigenically rough and do not possess the A and M antigens.

RESISTANCE

All species are equally susceptible to chemical disinfectants. Organisms are fairly resistant to some environmental conditions, e.g., *B. abortus* will survive for four and a half hours when exposed to direct sunlight; four days in urine; five days on cloth at room temperature; and 75 days in an aborted fetus during cool weather.

IMMUNIZATION

Strain 19 vaccine, a live attenuated strain, was discovered by Buck in 1930. It is not considered transmissible. In vaccinated calves agglutination titers usually fall to negative levels in four to six weeks. As mentioned above, there is the problem of persisting reactors. If an animal is positive (1:200), after 30 months it is considered a reactor. Adjuvant bacterins, e.g., vaccine 45/20, are used in some countries; 45/20 has been used live or dead to reduce losses in adult cattle. Strain 19 has been used similarly. Live, rough (mucoid) cultures have not been effective as vaccines.

Immunity in brucellosis is predominantly cell-mediated.

Brucella ovis

This organism causes a widespread disease of sheep characterized in the ram by orchitis, epididymitis, and impaired fertility, and in some ewes by placentitis and abortion. The ram is more susceptible than the ewe and more rams develop lesions than ewes. Infection of ewes originates almost exclusively from infected rams, and the disease is effectively controlled by the elimination of the rams. Various vaccination procedures have been used successfully to prevent rams from becoming infected.

Control and elimination of the disease are accomplished by complement fixation testing, semen examination (staining and culture), and culling of rams with palpable lesions.

SUGGESTED CLINICAL EXAMPLES

An outbreak of brucellosis in a dairy herd.
An outbreak of brucellosis in a swine herd.
An outbreak of brucellosis in a beagle colony.
Brucella ovis epididymitis in rams.

SOURCES FOR FURTHER READING

Brown, G.M., et al.: Characterization of *Brucella abortus* strain 19. Am. J. Vet. Res., *33*:759, 1972.

Buchanan, T.M., Baber, L.C., and Feldman, R.A.: Brucellosis in the United States, 1960–1972. An abattoir-associated disease. Part. 1. Clinical features and therapy. Medicine, *53*:403, 1974.

Busch, L.A., and Parker, R.L.: Brucellosis in the United States. J. Infect. Dis., *125*:289, 1972.

Carmichael, L.E., and Bruner, D.W.: Characteristics of a newly recognized species of *Brucella* responsible for infectious canine abortion. Cornell Vet., *58*:579, 1968.

Crawford, R.P., Williams, J.D., Huber, J.D., and Childers,

A.B.: Biotypes of *Brucella abortus* and their value in epidemiologic studies of infected cattle herds. J. Am. Vet. Med. Assoc., *175*:1274, 1979.

Elberg, S.S.: Immunity to *Brucella* infection. Medicine, *52*:339, 1973.

Hall, W.A., Ludford, C.G., and Ward, W.H.: Infection and serological responses in cattle given 45/20 vaccine and later challenged with *Brucella abortus*. Aust. Vet. J., *52*:409, 1976.

Harrington, Jr., R., and Brown, G.M.: Laboratory summary of brucella isolations and typing. Am. J. Vet. Res., *37*:1241, 1976.

Hughes, K.L., and Claxton, P.D.: *Brucella ovis* infection. I. An evaluation of microbiological, serological, and clinical methods of diagnosis in the ram. Aust. Vet. J., *44*:41, 1968.

Luchsinger, D.W., and Anderson, R.K.: Longitudinal studies of naturally acquired *Brucella abortus* infection in sheep. Am. J. Vet. Res., *40*:1307, 1979.

Moore, J.A., Gupta, B.M., and Conner, G.H.: Eradication of *Brucella canis* infection from a dog colony. J. Am. Vet. Med. Assoc., *153*:523, 1968.

Nicoletti, P.: Prevalence and persistence of *Brucella abortus* strain 19 infections and prevalence of other biotypes in vaccinated adult dairy cattle. J. Am. Vet. Med. Assoc., *178*:143, 1981.

Smith, H., et al.: Erythritol. A constituent of bovine foetal fluids which stimulates the growth of *B. abortus* in bovine phagocytes. Br. J. Exp. Pathol., *43*:31, 1962.

25

Mycobacteria

PRINCIPAL CHARACTERISTICS OF *Mycobacteria*

Mycobacteria are gram-positive, nonbranching, acid-fast, small rods. They are nonmotile, nonspore-forming, aerobic, and do not have aerial hyphae. They split sugars oxidatively.

Members of this genus may be grouped as follows:
1. The classic species have been recognized for many years as causes of disease in humans and animals:

    M. bovis,

    M. avium,

    M. tuberculosis,

    M. paratuberculosis,

    M. leprae.

2. A number of mycobacteria, called "anonymous" or "atypical," were first placed in categories by Runyon (1969). He established four groups based on rate of growth and pigment production.

    Group I: photochromogenic, producing pigmented colonies only after exposure to light: slow-growing in that it required seven days or more for visible growth.

    Group II: scotochromogenic, i.e., producing pigment in the absence of light; slow-growing.

    Group III: nonphotochromogenic, producing no or slight pigment with exposure to light; slow-growing.

    Group IV.: variable pigmentation; grows rapidly in that there is visible growth in less than seven days.

Many of the organisms within each of these groups have now been speciated on the basis of cultural and biochemical characteristics, and thus the groups introduced by Runyon have been expanded and more precisely defined. The groups and some of the important species are listed in Table 25–1. A number of species have not been listed because they have little or no veterinary significance.

Members of these groups (except for *M. avium*) are not important causes of disease in animals, but they are significant because they can sensitize animals to tuberculin.

TUBERCULOSIS CAUSED BY *M. bovis, M. avium,* AND *M. tuberculosis*

HISTORICAL

M. tuberculosis was probably first seen in tissues by Baumgarten and Koch in 1882. Koch cultivated *M. tuberculosis* and reproduced the disease in the period from 1882 to 1884.

MYCOBACTERIAL CONSTITUENTS

None of the mycobacteria has yet been shown to produce exotoxins. The way in which they produce disease is not known. The chemistry of the tubercle bacilli is quite complex. They have a high concentration of lipids, 20 to 40% dry weight, which is thought to be in part responsible for their resistance to humoral defense mechanisms and to disinfectants, acids, and alkalis.

Table 25–1. Pathogenicity and Source of Some Nonclassic Mycobacteria

Group I	
M. kansasii	Has been isolated from the lymph nodes of cattle, swine, and other animals. Causes pulmonary infections in humans.
M. marinum	Isolation from cold-blooded animals. Causes swimming pool granuloma in humans.
Group II	
M. scrofulaceum	Cervical lymph nodes of animals and children.
M. xenopi	Several reports of isolation from animals.
Group III	
M. avium* (M. avium-intracellu-lare complex)	25 serotypes recognized; 1, 2, and 3 are usually pathogenic for birds. Serotypes 4 to 20 have been isolated from humans and animals but do not produce progressive disease in chickens. A number of serotypes produce tuberculosis in swine mainly involving the lymph nodes. Strains formerly called the Battey bacilli cause serious human infections.
Group IV	
M. fortuitum	Pulmonary infections in humans; skin infections in cats; lymph node infections in cattle.
M. phlei	Soil; nonpathogenic
M. smegmatis	Soil and smegma; nonpathogenic

*Although traditionally one of the classic species, it is listed here because it contains various serotypes that do not produce progressive disease in chickens.

The thick cell wall of mycobacteria is rich in mycolic acid and other complex lipids, making it hydrophobic and impermeable to aqueous stains without heat. Heat is applied in the Ziehl-Neelsen stain.

Some of the specific lipids are the following:

Mycolic Acids. They are β-hydroxy fatty acids that vary in size with species and are responsible for acid-fastness, the property of retaining carbol fuchsin after application of the decolorizer, acid alcohol.

Mycosides. They are responsible for control of cellular permeability (resistance to water-soluble enzymes, antibiotics, and disinfectants). They are associated with cord factor, which is responsible for the characteristic colonial growth of virulent mycobacteria, and wax D, a mycoside that enhances the immune response. Wax D and various proteins induce delayed hypersensitivity.

Glycolipids. They result in toxicity, a granulomatous response, and enhanced survival of phagocytosed mycobacteria.

SOME FACTORS CONTRIBUTING TO TUBERCULOSIS

1. Crowding is important because the dosage of organisms for carriers is higher under crowded conditions, e.g., among stabled cattle as opposed to range cattle.
2. Genetic factors play a role in susceptibility; some races are more susceptible, e.g., American Indian and Eskimo.
3. There is both natural and acquired resistance to tuberculosis, the latter as a result of previous exposure.

PATHOGENESIS

The local manifestations depend upon the route of invasion. In inhalation, the route is via the lungs and tracheobronchial lymph nodes. In ingestion, it is usually through the mesenteric nodes and intestinal wall and to the liver via the portal system. Organisms from nodes may reach the thoracic duct with general dissemination. Animals develop delayed hypersensitivity and

MODE OF INFECTION

M. bovis	M. avium	M. tuberculosis
Organisms leave the host in respiratory discharges, feces, milk, urine, semen, and genital discharges. Infection is by inhalation. Localized lesions of lymph nodes of head and nodes of lungs and parenchyma of lungs are produced. In calves, mode of infection may be by ingestion. Lesions are seen in intestinal wall, mesenteric nodes, liver and spleen, and secondarily in lungs.	Shed in feces; acquired mainly by ingestion of contaminated food, water, and soil. Lesions may be found anywhere but usually involve intestines, liver, spleen, and bone marrow. Lung lesions are infrequent.	Shed in the sputum and respiratory discharges. Direct spread by droplet infection and by fomites. Lesions are found in lungs and lymph nodes principally.

PATHOGENICITY

M. bovis	M. avium (See Table 25–1)	M. tuberculosis
Cattle are a natural host; swine are readily and severely infected. Cases have also been found in dogs, horses, and sheep (rare). Cats are susceptible and may perpetuate the bovine disease. In cattle, there is pulmonary tuberculosis with involvement of associated lymph nodes. Infection of viscera and bones occurs in humans, especially from milk. Chickens are resistant but rabbits and guinea pigs are very susceptible (generalized infections).	Chickens are most susceptible; other birds can be infected. Crowding is an important factor. Water fowl are quite resistant but house birds are susceptible. In swine, disease usually occurs in lymph nodes of the head. Cattle are refractory but sensitized. Mink fed infected chickens will become infected. Infections in humans are of little consequence. Guinea pigs are slightly susceptible.	Occurs in humans, primates, and monkeys, the latter two acquired from humans. Cattle are sensitized by the human organism. In swine, disease usually occurs in lymph nodes of the head and organisms are acquired by eating uncooked garbage. Parrots are susceptible. Chickens are rarely infected. Dogs can be infected. Cats are very resistant. Guinea pigs are susceptible and rabbits are slightly susceptible. In elephants the pulmonary form occurs.

cell-mediated immunity, usually with a lessening of multiplication and dissemination. It is thought that delayed hypersensitivity of an exaggerated level attributable to large amounts of tubercular antigen may have a destructive effect on tissues. Most foci are microscopic and most disappear. Some, however, may persist for years and in some instances may progress to form the characteristic tubercle.

Miliary tuberculosis is an acute form of the disease, with general dissemination and production of large numbers of small tubercles.

DIRECT EXAMINATION

Great care should be exercised in handling suspicious clinical materials.

The organisms can be demonstrated in smears from lesions by employing acid-fast stains. The organisms are small, straight, or slightly curved, and they occur singly or in clumps. They stain red by the Ziehl-Neelsen acid-fast stain.

ISOLATION AND CULTIVATION

Frequently a diagnosis of tuberculosis is made on the basis of the demonstration of typical acid-fast organisms in characteristic lesions.

One procedure for isolation and cultivation in clinical material, e.g., nodules, is as follows:
1. Take mortar: sterile sand and alundum.
2. Add 10 ml of 4% NaOH containing phenol red.
3. After grinding, centrifuge.
4. Neutralize sediment with 2N HCl for a maximum of 30 minutes.
5. Inoculate sediment onto Löwenstein-Jensen slants and egg yolk agar slants and incubate at 37°C for up to eight weeks.
6. The glycerol in the slants has an inhibitory affect on *M. bovis*, which grows better on egg base media without glycerol.

IDENTIFICATION

This is now based principally on cultural, morphologic, growth, and biochemical characteristics. Definitive identification is usually carried out in a reference laboratory. Some of the characteristics used to differentiate important mycobacteria are listed in Table 25–2. The pathogenicity tests shown in Table 25–3 are no longer necessary.

ANTIGENIC NATURE AND SEROLOGY

M. bovis and *M. tuberculosis* are antigenically closely related.

M. avium can be differentiated from the previous two serologically.

M. avium antigenically resembles the so-called Battey bacilli, *M. intracellulare*. Both are sometimes referred to as the *M. avium-M. intracellulare* complex, and both belong in Runyon's group III. The trend now is to refer to the complex as *M. avium* (see Table 25–1).

RESISTANCE

In general mycobacteria are rather resistant to various physical influences and chemical disinfectants. Their considerable resistance is partly due to the presence of lipid in the cell wall. Species causing tuberculosis retain their viability in putrefying carcasses and in moist soil for one to four years and survive for at least 150 days in dry bovine feces. Freezing temperatures have little if any effect. Drying is only effective when the organisms are also exposed to direct sunlight. They are fairly resistant to acids and alkalis; however, phenols (5%), Lysol (3%), cresols, and cresylic acids are fairly effective.

TREATMENT

Treatment may not be feasible or desirable in animals. One of the most useful drugs in the

CULTURAL CHARACTERISTICS

M. bovis	M. avium	M. tuberculosis
Dry, sparse, delicate, nonluxuriant. Growth on solid media incubated at 37°C usually appears within 3–6 weeks.	Moist, slimy, glistening, luxuriant, frequently yellow or gray. Growth on solid media incubated at 40–42°C usually appears within 2–3 weeks.	Dry, crumbly, luxuriant; colonies are usually yellowish with roughened surfaces. Growth on solid media incubated at 37°C usually appears within 2 weeks.

Table 25–2. *In Vitro Tests for Identifying Some Clinically Significant Mycobacteria*

Mycobacterium	43°C	37°C	31°C	Niacin	Nitrate Reduction	Cord Formation	Thiophen-2-carboxylic acid-hydrazide	NaCl Tolerance	Tween Hydrolysis	Chromogenicity	Arylsulfatase at 3 Days	Glycerol Inhibition
M. tuberculosis		M		+	+	+	+	−	−	−	−	+
M. bovis		M		−	−	+	−	−	−	−	−	−
M. avium*	M	M	M	−	−	−	+	−	−	−	−	+
M. kansasii		M	S	−	+	V	+	−	+	+	−	+
M. marinum			S	−	−	−	+	−	+	+	−	+
M. scrofulaceum		M	S	−	−	−	+	−	−	+	−	+
M. xenopi	S	S		−	−	−	+	−	−	+	V	+
M. fortuitum		R	R	−	+	V	+	+	−	−	+	+
M. chelonei		R	R	V	−	−	−	−	−	−	+	+

Key: − = negative—absence or inhibition; + = positive—production or growth; V = variable; R = rapid (1 to 6 days); M = moderate (6 to 14 days); S = slow (more than 14 days).

*Includes strains previously identified as *M. intracellulare*. *M. avium* serotypes 1 and 2 grow best at 43°C; some strains of serotypes 3 through 25 grow best at 22° to 30°C.

(From Thoen, C.O.: Mycobacterium. In Diagnostic Procedures in Veterinary Bacteriology and Mycology. Edited by G.R. Carter. 4th Ed. Springfield, Ill., Charles C Thomas, 1984. Reprinted with permission.)

Table 25–3. *Some Differential Features of Classic Species of* Mycobacterium

(Note: Differentiation of the various mycobacteria requires the examination of a considerable number of characteristics. Only a few are listed below.)

Species	30°C	37°C	44°C	Growth	Stimulated by Glycerol	Susceptibility Guinea Pig	Rabbit	Chicken
M. bovis	−	+	−	Dry, sparse; slow	−	+	+	0
M. avium	+	+	+	Smooth, moist; comparatively rapid	+	+ −	+	+
M. tuberculosis	−	+	−	Dry, crumbly; abundant; slow	+	+	+ −	0

Key: + = definitely susceptible; + − = slightly susceptible; 0 = very resistant

treatment of tuberculosis is isoniazid. It is used with para-aminosalicylic acid or ethambutol and occasionally with streptomycin, constituting "triple therapy." The results are usually excellent and the first three drugs may be given for up to three years, but streptomycin is usually discontinued after several months. Strains may develop resistance to streptomycin, and toxicity to vestibular and auditory nerves may be encountered. Strains are also found that are resistant to isoniazid. Rifampin is also a useful drug that may be used with isoniazid. Isoniazid

has been employed prophylactically to control tuberculosis in zoos and animal parks.

IMMUNITY

Although antibodies are produced in tuberculosis, immunity is primarily cell-mediated. The only agent used to any extent is the BCG vaccine (bacille Calmette Guérin). It is a live bovine strain that was attenuated by growth in potato-glycerin bile medium through several hundred transfers. It is used for the prevention of tuberculosis in children and calves, in whom the disease is prevalent. It has not been used in the United States because it has no place in an eradication program; it sensitizes animals to tuberculin.

Hypersensitivity to tuberculin indicates some resistance to tuberculosis. The tuberculin reaction is sometimes negative (anergy) if the infection is overwhelming or if there is a deficiency in cell-mediated immunity.

FIELD DIAGNOSIS AND CONTROL

In the field, diagnosis is carried out by means of the tuberculin test, which depends upon a reaction of the delayed hypersensitivity type. Several tuberculins are used; all contain mycobacterial proteins, to which infected animals may be hypersensitive. Koch's "Old Tuberculin," which has been used widely in the standardization of tuberculins, is a filtrate of an eight-week-old culture of *M. tuberculosis*. The tuberculin used for the routine testing of cattle in the United States is prepared from strains of *M. bovis*. Avian tuberculin is used in the comparative test (double intradermal) in cattle as well as in swine and poultry. PPD (purified protein derivative) is a relatively pure tuberculin.

The tuberculin tests commonly used are
1. Intradermal: dose 0.1 ml tuberculin; read at 72 hours; firm swelling indicates a positive reaction. This is the most widely used test.
2. Comparative cervical: intradermal inoculation of regular and avian tuberculin at two different sites in the neck. Read at 72 hours by measuring swelling.
3. Ophthalmic: mostly used on primates; 0.1 ml of a 1:10 dilution of regular "bovine" tuberculin is inoculated intradermally into the upper eyelid. Some require three negative tests at 30-day intervals before animals are moved out of quarantine.

The tuberculosis eradication program is based upon the detection and slaughter of infected animals as determined by the tuberculin test. Prior to an organized control program, the infection rate of bovine tuberculosis in the United States was approximately 5%. In 1917, the test and slaughter eradication program was initiated by the Bureau of Animal Industry. By 1940, when the country was accredited, the infection rate had dropped to 0.46%, and by 1957 to 0.156%. At least 85% of the current reactors do not have gross lesions, and it was for this reason that the comparative cervical test was introduced. During this 40-year period over 400 million dollars was spent to control and eradicate the disease.

General Steps in the Control of Bovine Tuberculosis

The system of surveillance followed by the USDA is briefly as follows:
1. When suspected tuberculosis lesions are found in cattle during routine postmortem examination, the veterinary meat inspector submits specimens to the Veterinary Services Diagnostic Laboratory (USDA, Ames, Iowa). If mycobacterial infection is confirmed, the federal veterinarian in charge of the state involved is informed.
2. The regular tuberculin test is then applied to the herd or herds of origin.
3. If the original infection was due to *M. bovis* (based upon pathologic examination or cultivation or both), the procedure of choice is liquidation of the herd. If it is not completely depopulated, the herd is quarantined for 10 months and a series of retests is carried out. Reactors are removed and slaughtered. If infection is extensive, depopulation is always recommended.
4. The comparative test is used mainly after the regular test has revealed questionable responses in routine testing. The action taken on the reactors and those animals classed as suspicious (based upon comparative responses) depends upon their number and the size of the herd. The so-called "scattergram" is used as the guide. Many suspicious and responding animals may have no gross lesions (NGL).

DECONTAMINATION OF INFECTED PREMISES

After depopulation, manure, litter, hay, straw, and other accumulated extraneous material are removed from the stables and barnyard and burned. The stables, building, and barnyard (if structural) are brushed, scraped, and washed down with water under pressure. Within several days, a disinfectant is applied under pressure to saturate the same structures. When depopulation is carried out because of tuberculosis, the premises are not repopulated for at least 30 days. The two disinfectants preferred in tuberculosis eradication are a cresylic compound or sodium orthophenylphenate. Different disinfectants are used for different diseases.

Mycobacterium leprae

M. leprae causes a chronic disease affecting the skin and peripheral nerve trunks. The incubation period may be up to 20 years. It occurs worldwide but is most prevalent in tropical countries and infrequent in countries in temperate regions. It has not been cultivated in vitro, but experimental infections have been produced in the armadillo and in immune-deficient mice and hamsters.

NONCLASSIC MYCOBACTERIA

This includes a large number of species, only a small number of which are pathogenic and clinically significant (see Table 25–1). Some were initially placed in the Runyon groups discussed earlier. They are worldwide in distribution, occurring and living in soil. The species distribution varies with the kind of soil and various climatic and environmental factors. They can sometimes be isolated from animals' feces. Generally severe infections caused by some species of these mycobacteria only occur in humans after impairment of the body's defense mechanisms.

ISOLATION AND IDENTIFICATION

These mycobacteria grow well on Löwenstein-Jensen medium and other culture media used for the growth of mycobacteria. The procedures used for isolation are the same as those referred to earlier for the classic species. Some of the characteristics used for the identification of both classic and nonclassic species are listed in Table 25–2.

SKIN TUBERCULOSIS OF CATTLE

Mycobacteria have been demonstrated from skin lesions consisting of cold, firm, rounded swellings and fluctuant thick-walled abscesses. They occur most commonly in the skin of the lower parts of the leg, and they may soften and ulcerate. Because of the lymphatic distribution of lesions, the term ulcerative lymphangitis has been used. The organisms, which have not been cultivated, may sensitize cattle to tuberculin.

A leprosy of cattle and water buffaloes has been described in the Far East. It is not clear whether or not this condition is distinct from the skin tuberculosis of cattle just described. The distribution of the lesions is similar, and the organisms have not been cultivated in vitro.

FELINE LEPROSY

Cat leprosy is presumed to be an infectious disease caused by an as yet uncultivated *Myco-*
bacterium. The disease is characterized by the formation of single and multiple granulomas or nodules of the skin 1 to 3 cm in diameter. They are painless and move freely. Some may be ulcerous and discharge a slight, serosanguineous exudate. Affected cats are usually in good health and only in rare cases does the disease become generalized.

There is some experimental evidence that the causal agent is identical to *M. lepraemurium*, the cause of rat leprosy, and it has been suggested that cats acquire the infection via rat bites.

Long, slender, acid-fast rods can be demonstrated in smears from the nodules.

Treatment involves the surgical removal of nodules, which do not usually recur. Variable results have been obtained with the antileprosy (human) drug dapsone. Streptomycin and isoniazid are toxic for the cat.

Mycobacterium paratuberculosis

Synonym. Johne's bacillus.

HISTORICAL

This organism was first observed by Johne and Frothingham in 1895. In 1906 Bang demonstrated that the disease was distinct from tuberculosis and caused by a different organism.

DISTRIBUTION

M. paratuberculosis is found worldwide, and cattle, sheep, and goats are the principal ruminants affected. Because there is no national eradication plan for this disease in the United States, it is difficult to determine its precise incidence. It may be sufficiently prevalent in some dairy herds to constitute a real problem.

MODE OF INFECTION

Animals are infected by ingestion of food and water contaminated by feces. The incidence of subclinical cases shedding organisms intermittently may be as high as 15%.

PATHOGENICITY

Little is known regarding the pathogenesis of the disease. Experimental infections can be established orally or intravenously. Dosage of organisms is probably important in establishing infections. Toxic substances have not been demonstrated.

In cattle there is a chronic enteritis, often with

severe diarrhea. The diarrhea in sheep, goats, and other ruminants is usually less severe or absent. The incubation period may be a year or more. Calves are susceptible but do not show signs until adulthood. The disease is usually progressive, leading to emaciation and death. Mortality is caused in large part by the malabsorption of amino acids and the loss of protein into the intestine (protein-losing enteropathy). The ileum and colon are usually involved, and the infection may extend to the rectum in advanced cases. The mucous membrane becomes corrugated and thickened because of epithelioid and giant cells, both of which contain many organisms. Large numbers of organisms may be shed in the feces.

M. paratuberculosis has been isolated from the udder and reproductive tracts of both male and female cattle.

Mice, hamsters, pigs, and horses have been infected experimentally.

DIRECT EXAMINATION

The organisms are often difficult to demonstrate in smears, and failure to demonstrate organisms does not exclude Johne's disease. A number of smears may have to be examined. Thin smears are made from feces, intestinal mucosa (terminal ileum preferred) in the dead animal, and rectal mucosa in the live animal. The rectal smears may only be positive in advanced cases. On the average, the rectal smear will only detect about 25% of infected animals. A small piece of the rectum is pinched out, washed, and then squeezed between two slides. The resulting smear and other smears are stained by the Ziehl-Neelsen method. Johne's bacilli occur singly and in characteristic clumps and stain a pinkish red. Bovine feces frequently yield saprophytic acid-fast organisms that can be mistaken for Johne's bacilli.

A reliable but complicated procedure (laparotomy) is to examine smears of biopsies of mesenteric lymph nodes in the region of the terminal ileum for acid-fast organisms.

ISOLATION AND CULTIVATION

The organism grows very slowly, and cultivation and identification may take months. The feces or tissue is treated for contaminants. A medium containing mycobactin (extract of *M. phlei*) is used. Colonies appear in four to 12 weeks.

IDENTIFICATION

In smears organisms appear as short, thick, small, acid-fast rods similar to the avian tubercle bacillus. Identification is based on cultural (including growth rate and mycobactin dependency), morphologic and staining characteristics and seroagglutination.

ANTIGENIC NATURE AND SEROLOGY

Little is known in this area. The antigenic relationship between this organism and the avian tubercle bacillus is indicated by the fact that animals with Johne's disease often react to avian tuberculin.

RESISTANCE

M. paratuberculosis resembles other mycobacteria in its resistance to physical and chemical influences; it will survive in contaminated stables for months.

CONTROL

The intravenous johnin test will detect about 80% of cases found to be infected by cultural methods. A positive reaction is indicated by a temperature rise of 1.5°F or greater. The complement-fixation test is used as a screening procedure, but it is not as reliable as culture of the feces.

Recent work indicates that an agar gel immunodiffusion test may be as reliable or possibly more reliable than culture for the diagnosis of clinical paratuberculosis.

The following steps are recommended for controlling paratuberculosis:*
1. Animals with persistent diarrhea or chronic weight loss should be isolated or sent to slaughter.
2. Culture the feces from all animals two years old or older every six months and remove and slaughter animals whose cultures are positive and their offspring.
3. Adults from the herd should be sold only for slaughter or to quarantined feedlots. Calves of culturally negative dams may be sold on the open market if they are separated from the dams at birth, raised apart, and have a negative reaction to johnin not more than 30 days before sale.
4. Clean and disinfect the premises after the

---

*Based on Larsen, A.B.: Paratuberculosis: the status of our knowledge. J. Am. Vet. Med. Assoc., *161*:1539, 1972.

removal of infected animals. The cresylic disinfectants and sodium orthophenylphate (when used in the same dilutions that are recommended for disinfecting premises contaminated with *M. bovis)* are suitable for use on premises contaminated with *M. paratuberculosis.*

5. Calf-rearing quarters should have separate cleaning and feeding equipment, which should never be exchanged with the equipment used for the mature animals because calves are easily infected.

6. Continue surveillance (at intervals of not less than five or more than seven months) until there have been four consecutive negative fecal cultures of all animals two years of age or older.

7. Purchase only animals with johnin-negative tests from herds with no history of the disease.

8. If artificial insemination is used, semen should come from culturally negative bulls.

IMMUNITY

Recovery from the disease is rare. Bacterins have been used in sheep and calves with some success, but immunization has not been widely practiced and is not permitted in cattle in some countries. Vaccinated animals may be johnin- and tuberculin-positive.

As in tuberculosis, immunity in Johne's disease is considered to be predominantly cell-mediated.

SUGGESTED CLINICAL EXAMPLES

An outbreak of bovine tuberculosis in an area presumed to be free of tuberculosis.

Avian tuberculosis in a farm laying flock.
A case of feline tuberculosis due to *M. bovis.*
An outbreak of tuberculosis in an animal farm.
A herd of cattle infected with *M. intracellulare.*
A feline skin infection due to *M. fortuitum.*
Johne's disease in a dairy herd.

SOURCES FOR FURTHER READING

Anonymous: Laboratory methods in veterinary mycobacteriology. Ames, Iowa, Veterinary Services Laboratories, APHIS, 1974.
Boughton, E.: Tuberculosis caused by *Mycobacterium avium.* Vet. Bull., *39:*457, 1969.
Dubina, J., Sula, L., Kubin, M., and Varekova, J.: Incidence of *Mycobacterium avium* and *M. intracellulare* in cattle and pigs. J. Hyg. Epidemiol. Microbiol. Immunol., *18:*15, 1974.
Gilmour, N.J.L.: The pathogenesis, diagnosis and control of Johne's disease. Vet. Rec., *99:*433, 1976.
Karlson, A.G., and Thoen, C.O.: *Mycobacterium avium* in tuberculosis adenitis of swine. Am. J. Vet. Res., *32:*1257, 1971.
McLaughlin, A.R., and Moyle, A.I.: An epizootic of bovine tuberculosis. J. Am. Vet. Med. Assoc., *164:*396, 1974.
Merkal, R.S.: Laboratory diagnosis of bovine paratuberculosis. J. Am. Vet. Med. Assoc., *163:*1100, 1973.
Merkal, R.S.: Paratuberculosis: Advances in cultural, serologic, and vaccination methods. J. Am. Vet. Med. Assoc., *184:*939, 1984.
Schaefer, W.B.: Incidence of serotypes of *Mycobacterium avium* and atypical mycobacteria in human and animal disease. Am. Rev. Resp. Dis., *97:*18, 1968.
Sherman, D.M., Markham, J.F., and Bates, F.: Agar gel immunodiffusion test for diagnosis of clinical paratuberculosis in cattle. J. Am. Vet. Med. Assoc., *185:*179, 1984.
Snider, W.R.: Tuberculosis in canine and feline populations. Am. Rev. Resp. Dis., *104:*877, 1971.
Thoen, C.O.: Mycobacterium. *In* Diagnostic Procedures in Veterinary Bacteriology and Mycology. Edited by G.R. Carter. 4th ed. Springfield, Ill., Charles C Thomas, 1984.
Wilkinson, G.T.: A non-tuberculous granuloma of the cat associated with an acid-fast bacillus. Vet. Rec., *76:*777, 1964.
Wilkinson, G.T.: Cat leprosy. *In* The Veterinary Annual. Edited by G.S.G. Grurselh and F.W.G. Hill. Bristol, England, Scientechnica, 1978.

26

Actinomyces, Nocardia, and Dermatophilus

The gram-positive organisms discussed in this chapter are referred to generally as the actinomycetes. Included are the genera, *Actinomyces, Nocardia, Streptomyces,* and *Dermatophilus.* They are sometimes called "higher bacteria" because they have some of the cultural and morphologic characteristics of the fungi. These include extensive filamentation, branching, usually the production of some aerial hyphae with asexual spores or conidia, and rather tenacious colonies. Some produce club-shaped cells and acid-fast elements that bear a resemblance to the corynebacteria and mycobacteria.

Actinomyces

PRINCIPAL CHARACTERISTICS

Actinomyces are gram-positive, nonacid-fast rods that may show branching. They are nonmotile and nonspore-forming; microaerophilic or anaerobic (except for *A. viscosus* and *A. naeslundii);* and catalase-positive (except for *A. viscosus)* and fermentative.

All of the actinomycetes causing disease in animals and humans occur as commensals in the oral cavity.

Significant species are *Actinomyces bovis, A. israelii* (causes actinomycosis in humans), *A. naeslundii* (causes infrequent infections in humans), and *A. viscosus.*

Actinomyces bovis

HISTORICAL

Bollinger described the disease (actinomycosis) and the organism in 1877.

HABITAT

A. bovis is a commensal in the oral cavity of cattle and probably of some other animals.

MODE OF INFECTION

Infections are initiated in wounds of the mucous membrane of the upper digestive tract.

PATHOGENESIS

Exotoxins have not been demonstrated. Organisms grow in the "anaerobic" damaged tissue, causing abscesses. Infectious material may be aspirated into the lungs, producing pulmonary actinomycosis, or swallowed, producing visceral or abdominal actinomycosis.

PATHOGENICITY

A. bovis causes a subacute or chronic progressive disease principally of cattle characterized by the development of indurated, granulomatous, suppurative lesions involving bone and soft tissue. Abscesses discharge through fistulas; tortuous sinuses result from the burrowing process.

Cattle. The disease involves the mandible or

other bony tissue of the head ("lumpy jaw"). Seen less commonly are orchitis, mastitis, and lesions of the liver and other internal organs. Actinomycosis is rare in sheep.

Horses. The organism may be recovered from "fistulous withers" and "poll evil," along with other organisms.

Pigs. In pigs the disease results in abscesses of the liver and other internal organs; in sows it causes chronic granulomatous suppurative mastitis.

Dogs and Cats. Infection is rare in these animals. *A. bovis* and *Actinobacillus lignieresii* are occasionally found together.

Humans. Lesions involve the face, neck, lung, breast, and lymph nodes.

DIRECT EXAMINATION

A small amount of pus is placed in a Petri dish and washed to expose the small 1 to 3 mm sulfur granules associated with the disease. The actinomycotic granules are larger than the greywhite granules seen in actinobacillosis. A granule is transferred to a slide, and a drop of 10% sodium hydroxide is added. A coverslip is placed on the granule, and it is crushed by gentle pressure. In actinomycosis the characteristic "ray fungi" with club-shaped margins can be seen under low power microscopy. The "clubs" are due to a gelatinous sheath and the deposition of calcium phosphate around the terminal filaments. The granule is held together by a polysaccharide-protein complex.

The coverslip is removed and the material spread to make a smear. This is dried, fixed, and stained by the Gram method. If the granules are from an actinomycotic lesion, delicate, intertwined, branching, gram-positive filaments are seen.

ISOLATION AND CULTIVATION

The organism grows well on blood agar, brain heart infusion agar, and thioglycolate broth. An anaerobic atmosphere containing 5 to 10% CO_2 is preferred. Colonies are white, rough, nodular, and difficult to remove. The radiating mycelia can be seen under a dissecting microscope. Small cottony colonies may be seen suspended discretely in thioglycolate broth.

MORPHOLOGY AND STAINING

Gram-stained smears from growth on solid or fluid media reveal masses of gram-positive rods and slightly branched filaments.

IDENTIFICATION

A strongly presumptive identification is usually made on the basis of the gross pathology, characteristic sulfur granules, and demonstration of the gram-positive branching filaments. Cultivation of an organism from characteristic lesions and granules in animals possessing the morphologic characteristics of *A. bovis* is usually considered sufficient for identification.

Definitive differentiation of *A. bovis* from other actinomyces and from anaerobic diphtheroids can be accomplished by various biochemical tests (Table 26–1).

TREATMENT

Establish and maintain drainage of abscesses. In antibiotic therapy penicillin is preferred; tetracyclines, chloramphenicol, and streptomycin have also been used. Potassium iodide or organic iodides may be used, along with penicillin. The visceral form responds least well.

Actinomyces viscosus

This organism differs from other actinomycetes in that it grows aerobically and is catalase-positive. It has been isolated from the human and canine oral cavity, from periodontal disease in humans and hamsters, and most frequently from actinomycosis in dogs. Several isolates have been recovered from other animals.

In the past some of the diagnoses of nocardiosis in the dog may actually have been actinomycosis due to *A. viscosus*. Actinomycosis in the dog is characterized by the presence of actinomycotic granules containing gram-positive, nonacid-fast, filamentous organisms that resemble *A. bovis* morphologically.

Two forms of actinomycosis have been seen in the dog. The more common is the localized granulomatous abscess involving mainly the skin and subcutis. This form responds well to treatment. The other form principally involves the thorax, with or without extension to the abdominal cavity. Pyothorax with granulomatous lesions of thoracic tissues and accumulation of pleural and pericardial fluid containing soft grey-white granules are characteristic of this deep form.

A. viscosus may be cultivated at 37°C on blood and brain heart infusion agar (and broth) but not on Sabouraud agar. Colonies are readily apparent in three to seven days. See Table 26–1 for differential characteristics.

Table 26–1. *Differentiation of* **Actinomyces** *spp. (nonacid-fast; gelatinase and indole-negative)*

Test	A. bovis	A. israelii	A. naeslundii	A. viscosus
Aerotolerance	M or An	M or An	F	F
Catalase	−	−	−	+
Nitrate red	−	+	+	+
Fermentation:				
Mannitol	−	+	−	−
Lactose	−	(−)	−	−
Sucrose	+	+	+	+
Salicin	−	(+)	v	(+)
Glycerol	−	−	−	v
Xylose	−	(+)	−	−
Arabinose	−	(−)	−	−
Raffinose	−	(+)	+	+

Key: M = microaerophilic; An = anaerobic; F = facultative; V = variable; ( ) = most strains.
*Grows better with 10% CO_2.

TREATMENT

Along with surgical debridement and drainage, penicillin, chloramphenicol, tetracyclines, and sulfonamides are effective. Treatment must be prolonged.

Nocardia

PRINCIPAL CHARACTERISTICS

Nocardia are nonmotile, nonspore-forming, gram-positive rods that usually show branching and aerial hyphae. They are aerobic, split sugars by oxidation, and may be partially acid-fast.

Many species, all soil-borne, have been described. Three are considered important pathogens: *N. asteroides* in domestic animals and humans; *N. caviae* in the guinea pig and as a cause of bovine mastitis; and *N. brasiliensis,* one of the causes of nocardiosis in humans.

Nocardia asteroides

HISTORICAL

Nocard (a French veterinarian) was probably the discoverer of this organism or a closely related one *(N. farcinica)* from a disease of cattle—bovine farcy—in 1888.

HABITAT

N. asteroides is found widely distributed in the soil as a saprophyte.

MODE OF INFECTION

Infection is by inhalation or wounds (hands and feet of agricultural laborers). It is not considered contagious and is exogenous.

PATHOGENESIS

The pathogenesis of nocardiosis is somewhat like that of actinomycosis. Infection begins as a nodule or pustule, with subsequent induration. There is usually rupture, with suppuration and regression, followed by exacerbation and spread, with additional abscess formation and production of interlocking sinuses. Toxins have not been demonstrated.

PATHOGENICITY

Nocardiosis is usually a chronic progressive disease characterized by suppurating, granulomatous lesions. Sporadic infections may be seen in many animal species.

Cattle. It occurs as an acute or chronic mastitis with granulomatous lesions and draining fistulous tracts.

Dogs and Cats. There is a localized form of the disease, with subcutaneous lesions (mycetomas) or lymph node involvement or both. In the dog, there is a thoracic form with occasional extension to the abdominal cavity. Like actinomycosis in the dog due to *A. viscosus,* there is a granulomatous pleuritis or peritonitis or both, with the accumulation of pleural, pericardial, and peritoneal fluid. Abscesses may be found in the heart, brain, liver, and kidneys as well. Unlike actinomycosis, granules are not found in infections due to *N. asteroides.* Because the treatments of nocardiosis and actinomycosis are different, it is very important that a correct diagnosis be made.

Humans. The most common forms are pulmonary nocardiosis and a subcutaneous form. The systemic disease with CNS involvement is usually fatal.

DIRECT EXAMINATION

Gram-stained smears of pus reveal gram-positive branching filaments with or without clubs. In most strains the acid-fast stain shows retention of some of the carbolfuchsin.

EXPERIMENTAL ANIMALS

Guinea pigs are susceptible to experimental infection if the organisms are administered in gastric mucin.

ISOLATION AND CULTIVATION

The organism grows on unenriched media and on blood agar and Sabouraud agar, at 25°C or 37°C. Growth is evident in four or five days, and colonies are irregularly folded, raised and smooth, or granular. The color varies from white through yellow to deep orange. Gram-positive partially acid-fast branching mycelial filaments, which break up into bacillary and coccoid forms, are evident under oil immersion. The presence of mycelial elements distinguishes *Nocardia* from saprophytic and atypical mycobacteria. The mycelial forms of *Nocardia* can be readily seen in slide cultures on Sabouraud dextrose agar. The mycelial elements may give regular cultures a powdery appearance.

IDENTIFICATION

A presumptive identification is based on pathology, demonstration of typical organisms in clinical material, and on colonial, cultural, morphologic, and staining chracteristics (partially acid-fast) (Table 26–2).

Streptomyces spp. and *Actinomadura* spp., which also have aerial hyphae, are not usually partially acid-fast and are not pathogenic for mice and guinea pigs. They are occasionally isolated from mycetomas in animals in the tropics.

N. caviae and *N. brasiliensis* are differentiated from *N. asteroides* on the basis of several biochemical reactions (see Table 26–2).

ANTIGENIC NATURE AND SEROLOGY

N. asteroides and *N. brasiliensis* have some antigens in common, and they share antigens with mycobacteria. Little is known regarding the antigenic makeup of *N. asteroides*.

TREATMENT

Treatment consists of surgical debridement and drainage of lesions. Effective drugs are sulfonamides, especially sulfadiazine, novobiocin, and the tetracyclines. Antibiotic administration must be continued for periods as long as 12 weeks. Penicillin is not effective.

There is no effective treatment for nocardial mastitis.

Dermatophilus congolensis

Dermatophilus congolensis is a gram-positive, branching, filamentous rod. It is aerobic, non-spore-forming, and not acid-fast; zoospores are motile.

It is generally agreed that there is only one species. The earlier literature refers to several different species. The disease produced is called streptothricosis or dermatophilosis. It is worldwide in distribution, and although it may affect many animal species, it is seen most frequently in cattle, sheep, goats, and horses.

HISTORICAL

Streptothricosis of cattle was first described by Van Saceghem in 1915 in the Belgian Congo.

HABITAT

As far as is known, *Dermatophilus congolensis* is an obligate parasite living only on animals.

MODE OF INFECTION

Infection is spread by contact, fomites, and biting insects. Moist conditions probably promote its dissemination.

PATHOGENICITY

Streptothricosis or dermatophilosis has been encountered in horses, cattle, sheep, goats,

Table 26–2. *Differentiation of* **Nocardia** *(partially acid-fast, aerial hyphae; catalase-positive, nitrate reduced)*

Species	Decomposition of			
	Casein	Tyrosine	Xanthine	Urea
N. asteroides	−	−	−	+
N. brasiliensis	+	+	−	+
N. caviae	−	−	+	+

dogs, deer, squirrels, and humans. Recent studies indicate that the disease is widely prevalent, especially in cattle. It is an infection involving the superficial layers of the skin and is characterized by the formation of crusts or scabs varying in size from quite small to the size of a 50-cent piece. In advanced cases, large areas of the skin may be involved as a result of coalescence of smaller lesions. Removal of the scab leaves a moist depressed area.

A severe form of the disease has been responsible on occasions for deaths of calves, sheep, and goats.

In sheep, the disease is referred to as mycotic dermatitis and is seen in three forms: (1) dermatitis of the wool-covered areas or lumpy wool; (2) dermatitis of the face and scrotum; and (3) dermatitis of the lower leg and foot, which may result in a severe ulcerative dermatitis referred to as "strawberry foot rot."

Several cases have been described in humans. Infections can be produced experimentally in the rabbit.

DIRECT EXAMINATION

Smears are made from scabs softened with distilled water and then stained by the Giemsa or Gram method. Segmenting filaments and coccoid spores stain deep purple. The spores are seen in packets.

ISOLATION AND CULTIVATION

The organism grows well on blood agar, tryptose agar, and other media. Small, rough, greyish-white colonies appear in 24 to 48 hours; they have fimbriated lace-like borders, enlarge to 4 mm in diameter on further incubation, and become yellowish to yellow-orange. The organism can usually be recovered in the conventional manner on blood agar.

The following procedure has been recommended to overcome the problem of skin contaminants: (1) place scabs in sterile distilled water for 3.5 hours at room temperature, (2) place in candle jar for 15 minutes, and (3) remove loopfuls from surface of water and inoculate onto blood agar or other media; incubate at 37°C.

MORPHOLOGY AND STAINING

Motile zoospores approximately 1 μm in diameter are formed as a result of the septation of hyphal elements; they possess polar flagella. Gram-positive, branching hyphal elements in various stages of segmentation are seen. The hyphal elements are larger and more irregular in shape than the filaments of *Streptomyces* and *Nocardia*.

IDENTIFICATION

This is usually based upon the finding of the characteristic morphologic elements in the Giemsa-stained crusts and scabs and growth of organisms with the cultural features of *D. congolensis*. Definitive identification is made on the basis of certain biochemical properties.

IMMUNITY

Animals can remain infected for long periods; however, when they are cleared of infection, reinfection does not occur. Vaccines have not proved effective in field trials.

TREATMENT

The disease has been effectively treated in some animals by a single large dose of combined penicillin and streptomycin. It is important that both drugs be used. Removal of scabs with a brush and mild soap is recommended before topical application of iodine compounds, copper sulfate, or other solutions.

SUGGESTED CLINICAL EXAMPLES

A case of actinomycosis in a bull.
Actinomycotic mastitis is a sow.
A case of actinomycosis involving the thorax of a dog.
Superficial actinomycosis in a hunting dog.
A case of nocardiosis in a dog.
A case of nocardiosis in a cat.
Bovine mastitis caused by *Nocardia asteroides*.
An outbreak of mycotic dermatitis in sheep.
A case of streptothricosis in a horse.
A severe case of streptothricosis in a calf.

SOURCES FOR FURTHER READING

Albrecht, R., et al.: *Dermatophilus congolensis* chronic nodular disease in man. Pediatrics, 53:907, 1974.
Austwick, P.K.G.: Cutaneous streptothricosis, mycotic dermatitis and strawberry foot rot and the genus *Dermatophilus* Van Saceghem. Vet. Rev. Annot., 4:33, 1958.
Berd, D.: Laboratory identification of clinically important aerobic actinomycetes. Appl. Microbiol., 25:665, 1973.
Davenport, A.A., Carter, G.R., and Schermer, R.G.: Canine actinomycosis due to *Actinomyces viscosus*: Report of six cases. Vet. Med. Sm. An. Clin., 69:1442, 1974.
Davenport, A.A., Carter, G.R., and Beneke, E.S.: *Actinomyces viscosus* in relation to other actinomycetes and actinomycosis. Vet. Bull., 45:313, 1975.

Kurup, P.V., et al.: Nocardiosis: A review. Mycopathology, *40*:194, 1970.

Lloyd, D.H., and Sellers, K.C.: Dermatophilus Infection in Animals and Man. New York, Academic Press, 1976.

Mostafa, I.E.: Bovine nocardiosis (cattle farcy): A review. Vet. Bull., *36*:189, 1966.

Peabody, J.W., and Seabury, J.H.: Actinomycosis and nocardiosis: A review of basic differences in therapy. Am. J. Med., *28*:99, 1960.

Pier, A.C., Richard, J.L., and Farrell, E.F.: Fluorescent antibody and cultural technics in cutaneous streptothricosis. Am. J. Vet. Res., *235*:1014, 1964.

Prescott, J.F.: Campylobacter. *In* Diagnostic Procedures in Veterinary Bacteriology and Mycology. Edited by G.R. Carter. 4th Ed. Springfield, Ill., Charles C Thomas, 1984.

Rhoades, H.E., Reynolds, H.A., Jr., Rahn, D.P., and Small, E.: Nocardiosis in a dog with multiple lesions of the central nervous system. J. Am. Vet. Med. Assoc., *142*:278, 1963.

Roberts, D.S.: Dermatophilus infection. Vet. Bull., *37*:513, 1967.

Stewart, G.H.: Dermatophilus: A skin disease of animals and man. Part I. Vet. Rec., *91*:537, 1972.

Stewart, G.H.: Dermatophilus: A skin disease of animals and man. Part II. Vet. Rec., *91*:555, 1972.

Swerczek, T.W., Schiefer, B., and Nielsen, S.W.: Canine actinomycosis. Zbt. Vet. Med. Bull., *15*:955, 1968.

Watts, T.C., Olsen, S.M., and Rhoades, C.S.: Treatment of bovine actinomycosis with isoniazid. Can. Vet. J., *14*:223, 1973.

27

Spirochetes

There are five genera in the family Spirochaetaceae. However, only the genera *Borrelia*, *Treponema*, and *Leptospira* have species that cause disease in animals and humans. Differentiation of the genera is based mainly on morphology. Spirochetes of the three significant genera are slender, spiral, actively motile, flexible organisms that divide by transverse fission. They are 3 to 500 μm long and 0.2 to 0.75 μm wide.

In nature these organisms are found in water, soil, decaying organic materials, and in or upon the bodies of plants, animals, and humans. The majority are saprophytes, a few are commensals, and some are pathogenic, causing diseases in both animals and humans.

Morphologically spirochetes are relatively slender, helically coiled, round on cross-section, and have a varying number of spirals. The three basic cellular elements are the outer sheath, which encompasses the cell, the axial filament or fibril, and the protoplasmic cylinder, which includes the cell wall and cell membrane. The outer sheath, whose function is not known, appears to act as a unit membrane. That of *Leptospira interrogans canicola* has been shown to be immunogenic.

All these spirochetes have axial filaments that resemble flagella. The axial filaments wind around the protoplasmic cylinder under the outer sheath. It is thought that they may be responsible for motility. Insertion of the axial filament is by a proximal hook and insertion discs. The hook is an extension of the axial filament shaft and bends toward the protoplasmic cylinder. The insertion discs are plate-like and are inserted into a depression at the end of the cell. The number of insertion discs varies with the genus. *Borrelia* have two; *Treponema* has one; and *Leptospira* have three to five.

Motility involves rapid rotation around the long axis, flexation of cells, and locomotion along a helical path. Spirochetes may be anaerobic, aerobic, or facultatively aerobic.

All spirochetes are relatively inactive biochemically, and differentiation by this means is not possible. Identification is usually based on morphologic and antigenic properties.

Although spirochetes are gram-negative when stained by the Gram procedure, they stain poorly. Darkfield microscopy is used because some are too small to be seen with the light microscope. They may be demonstrated by the following special procedures: (1) Giemsa or Wright stain (the larger ones); (2) India ink or nigrosin (negative stain); (3) silver impregnation (coating increases their size); and (4) darkfield microscopy.

Some distinguishing characteristics of the three genera are summarized in Table 27–1.

Borrelia anserina

This is the only species of *Borrelia* that causes significant disease in domestic animals. For the most part speciation of *Borrelia* is based on the arthropod vector.

*Table 27–1. Distinguishing Features of **Borrelia**, **Treponema**, and **Leptospira***

Characteristic	Borrelia	Treponema	Leptospira
Length	8 to 16 μm	5 to 18 μm	6 to 20 μm
Width	0.25 to 0.3 μm	0.25 to 0.3 μm	0.1 to 0.2 μm
Ends	Taper terminally to fine filaments	Pointed, may have terminal filaments	One or both ends have a semicircular hook
Spirals:			
number	4 to 8, loose	6 to 14, regular, angular	Many, fine, tight
amplitude	3 μm	1 μm	0.4 to 0.5 μm
Motility	Lashing, corkscrew-like	Rotating, undulating, stiffly flexible	Spinning, undulating
Cultivation	Readily, anaerobic	Some difficult; aerobic and facultatively anaerobic	Readily, aerobic
Staining:			
Gram	Yes	No	Faint
Giemsa	Yes	Poor	Poor
silver impregnation	Not necessary	Yes	Yes

PATHOGENICITY

B. anserina is the cause of fowl spirochetosis (avian borreliosis), a disease of chickens, ducks, turkeys, and geese. Although an uncommon disease in the United States, it is of considerable economic importance in many countries. The disease is characterized by an acute septicemia with accompanying fever, diarrhea, drowsiness, and emaciation. It is transmitted by the bites of ticks; *Argas persicus* is the principal vector. The organism may be passed in eggs to the next generation of ticks.

The spleen may be enlarged, and anemia is usually present.

DIRECT EXAMINATION

Diagnosis is easily made by demonstration of the organism in carbol fuchsin or Giemsa-stained blood films. It can also be readily observed by darkfield illumination.

ISOLATION AND IDENTIFICATION

B. anserina can be readily cultivated in the chicken embryo and in enriched media containing rabbit tissue. Diagnosis is based upon demonstration of typical *Borrelia* from poultry with characteristic lesions and clinical signs.

TREATMENT, PREVENTION, AND CONTROL

Penicillin and tetracyclines are effective in treatment.

A bacterin made from chicken embryo cultures is used for prevention. Attempts should be made to eliminate ticks.

RELAPSING FEVER

This disease, caused by several *Borrelia* species including *B. recurrentis*, occurs sporadically in the United States. It is characterized by recurrent febrile attacks, during which the organism can be recovered from the blood. It is transmitted from human to human by lice; from animal to animal, especially rodents, by ticks; and from animal to human by ticks. The developmental cycle takes place in ticks. Rodents are probably a natural reservoir.

Borrelia vincenti

This spirochete appears to be a part of the normal flora of the human mouth and, together with other microorganisms, it increases in number in ulcerative conditions of the oral mucous membranes. Oral spirochetes are probably not pathogenic in the sense of being specific etiologic agents of disease. However, an association of these spirochetes, fusiform bacilli, and perhaps some vibrios and cocci, may serve to aggravate if not initiate suppurative infections of the mouth. Herpes virus is a predisposing factor in children. The diseases are trenchmouth (ulcerative disease involving the gums and oral cavity) and Vincent's angina (ulcerative tonsillitis and pharyngitis).

What appear to be similar diseases occur in the mouths of dogs and other animals. Their etiology has not been thoroughly studied.

Treponema hyodysenteriae

This gram-negative, oxygen-tolerant, anaerobic spirochete produces a dysentery in SPF pigs (not germ-free pigs) that is indistinguishable from what in the past has been called vibrionic or swine dysentery. There is evidence that *Bacteroides fragilis* and *Fusobacterium necrophorum* are important secondary agents in the etiology of swine dysentery. Asymptomatic carriers of *T. hyodysenteriae* are encountered.

Pigs of any age may be affected. The disease is manifested by a bloody diarrhea that may terminate in death or a chronic form characterized by a diphtheritic inflammatory process involving the mucosa of the cecum, large intestine, and rectum.

DIRECT EXAMINATION

The demonstration of this organism in material taken from lesions provides a strong presumptive diagnosis of swine dysentery.

The methods used for the demonstration of *T. hyodysenteriae* in mucosa and feces involve the examination of wet mounts with the phase microscope and of Giemsa or Victoria blue stained smears with the light microscope. It is a large flexible spirochete that moves rapidly in a snake-like or eel-like fashion. Considerable experience is necessary in order to distinguish *T. hyodysenteriae* from other spirochetes and from *Campylobacter*.

ISOLATION AND IDENTIFICATION

Isolation is not usually practiced. Diagnosis is usually made on the basis of clinical signs and a positive direct examination.

T. hyodysenteriae can be isolated from filtered feces or ground colonic mucosa on serum-enriched blood agar containing spectinomycin to prevent the growth of bacteria that pass the filters. Plates are incubated anaerobically. The small, white translucent colonies have a zone of clear hemolysis. In contrast, *T. innocens* is weakly beta-hemolytic. Stained smears of *T. hyodysenteriae* disclose a loosely coiled organism.

It is oxidase- and catalase-negative.

A fluorescent antibody procedure has been used effectively for identification.

TREATMENT

Among the compounds used to treat swine dysentery are organic arsenicals, nitroimidazoles, lincomycin, and the macrolides, tylosin, erythromycin, and spiramycin. Some of these drugs and others are administered in feed or water for prophylaxis as well as treatment.

In vitro susceptibility tests may be indicated because antimicrobial resistance to some of these drugs has been encountered.

IMMUNITY

Immunity is predominantly humoral in that hyperimmune serum is protective.

CONTROL

This is particularly difficult because of asymptomatic carriers. Serologic tests such as the ELISA may be useful in detecting these carriers.

Treponema paraluiscuniculi

This organism is the cause of a widespread disease, rabbit syphilis or vent disease. It is a true venereal disease in which lesions consisting of vesicles and scabs are seen mainly involving the prepuce, vagina, and perineal region. Thick scaly crusts persist in the female for months. Penicillin is an effective treatment.

Diagnosis is by the demonstration of organisms from lesions using stains or darkfield microscopy. *T. paraluiscuniculi* has not been cultivated in vitro.

Treponema pallidum

This organism is the cause of syphilis, an important venereal disease of humans.

Leptospira

Leptospirosis is primarily a disease of animals. It is transmitted from animals to humans infrequently.

The basic taxon of the genus *Leptospira* is the serovar (formerly serotype). There are more than 150 parasitic serovars and 16 serogroups. Two species, *L. interrogans* and *L. biflexa*, have been proposed for the "pathogenic or parasitic" and the "saprophytic" leptospires, respectively. As mentioned, the pathogenic leptospires are included in the species *L. interrogans*. In the new classification the former species name, now serovar, is added to *L. interrogans*, e.g., *L. canicola* becomes *L. interrogans canicola* and *L. hardjo* becomes *L. interrogans hardjo*. We will use the older more widely employed names, each of which represents a serovar. The microscopic agglutination test, which is widely used to detect antibodies, is highly serovar-specific. There are both group- and serovar-specific antigens. Serologic procedures are used in the identification of serovars after isolation and cultivation.

Because of insufficient taxonomic data, the various *Leptospira* species are not listed and described in Bergey's Manual of Systematic Bacteriology. There are free-living species as well as species that are parasitic and pathogenic for humans and domestic animals. Each serovar appears to have certain animal species as natural hosts. Some important serovars, their natural hosts (principally in the United States), and their occurrence in domestic animals are given in Table 27–2. Humans and animals may be infected with a wide variety of serovars, although most infections in domestic animals are caused by only a few species of *Leptospira*.

Mode of Infection and Transmission

The source of the organism is urine from infected or carrier animals. Water, litter, and food may serve as fomites. The organisms can live in alkaline water for days. Direct or indirect infection may be via nasal, oral, or conjunctival mucous membranes and abraded skin. *Leptospira* are destroyed in the stomach.

Pathogenesis

After epithelial penetration, there is hematogenous dissemination with localization and proliferation in parenchymatous organs, particularly the liver, for up to 16 days. This causes fever, anemia, subserous and submucosal hemorrhages, conjunctivitis, icterus, and often meningitis and agalactia. The kidney is also infected, frequently resulting in nephrosis and uremia, with shedding of organisms in the urine possibly for months. The lesions, signs, and severity vary with different serovars. Death may occur during the febrile stage or later caused by toxemia resulting from liver and kidney damage. Although the pathogenic mechanisms are not known, there is considerable damage to vascular endothelium.

Canine Leptospirosis

This disease is primarily caused by *L. canicola* and less frequently by *L. icterohemorrhagiae*. Although the exact incidence is unknown, surveys have shown that up to 38% of dogs in various parts of the United States show serologic evidence of exposure or disease.

Infected dogs and rats sporadically shed *Leptospira* in their urine and serve as sources of *L. canicola* and *L. icterohemorrhagiae* infections. Dogs may shed *Leptospira* in their urine for two to six

Table 27–2.   *Important* Leptospira *Species or Serovars and Their Hosts*

Serovars or Species	Known Host (Natural)	Occurrence in			
		Humans	Dogs	Cattle	Swine
icterohemorrhagiae	Rat, mouse	Common	Occasional	Reported	Reported
canicola	Dog, cattle, swine, skunk, jackal	Common	Common	Rare	Occasional
pomona	Cattle, swine, skunk, raccoon, wildcat, opossum	Occasional	Rare	Common	Common
autumnalis	Opossum, raccoon, mouse	Rare	?†	?	?
ballum	Mice, grey fox, rat, opossum, raccoon, wildcat, skunk, rabbit, grey squirrel	?	?	?	?
grippotyphosa	Raccoon, mouse, fox, squirrel, rabbit, bobcat	Rare	Reported	Occasional	Occasional
bataviae	?	Rare	?	?	?
hardjo	Cattle	Rare	?	Common	?
sejroe	Opossum, raccoon, mouse	?	?	Sporadic	?
hebdomadis	Opossum, raccoon	?	?	?	?
australis	Opossum, raccoon, fox	?	?	?	?

*Data principally applicable to the United States.
†Not known.

months; rats usually shed for longer periods of time. Organisms may survive in nature for approximately three weeks if environmental conditions are favorable. The viablity of organisms is influenced by the pH of the urine of dogs and rats, and alkaline pH favors viability.

Clinical. Infections may be latent to severe. A chronic progressive nephritis may follow acute *L. canicola* infection, with death occurring long after the initial infection; however, some dogs recover and renal function is regained. These animals may shed organisms in the urine for long periods. Three principal forms are recognized: (1) the hemorrhagic form, (2) the icteric form, and (3) the uremic form.

Diagnosis. There are six methods of diagnosis:

1. Examination of urine by darkfield microscopy. Experience is required to recognize *Leptospira*. They autolyse rapidly and formalin should be added to preserve them.
2. Serologic tests:
   a. paired sera; look for a fourfold rise in titer;
   b. plate screening test: if positive, do plate dilution test;
   c. plate dilution test: if + 1:64 or 1:128 classed as suspicious, then do the microscopic agglutination test (agglutinatin lysis); this is the preferred serologic procedure. If the titer is 1:300 or higher, it is considered of diagnostic significance. It is preferable to have a fourfold increase in paired sera. However, not all cases of leptospirosis produce significant serologic titers.
3. Isolation, cultivation, and identification: isolation from urine or blood is not usually feasible. Filtration or the addition of 5-fluorouracil may be used to reduce contaminants. *Leptospira* are aerobic and may be cultivated in special media at 30°C.
4. Guinea pig or hamster inoculation: blood, urine, or tissue is used; when bacteremic the experimental animal's blood is used for isolation and cultivation.
5. Histopathology: organisms may be demonstrated in kidney sections with special stains.
6. A fluorescent antibody technique can be used to identify *Leptospira* in tissues and urine sediment.

BOVINE LEPTOSPIROSIS

This disease is principally caused by *L. pomona*. *L. hardjo* causes fewer abortions but results in infertility. Occasionally *L. grippotyphosa*, *L. canicola*, or *L. icterohemorrhagiae* is involved. Three to 11% of cattle show serologic evidence of infection; 2 to 4% are estimated to be actively infected.

Sources. Sources of the organisms are cattle and swine with leptospiruria and wild animals. Cattle may shed for three months, but not in large numbers and irregularly. Outbreaks of leptospirosis are often associated with heavy rainfall. Leptospirosis is infrequent under dry conditions.

Clinical. The infection may be latent in a herd and may be precipitated by stress. Infections are characterized by a variety of clinical signs including fever, diarrhea, anemia, icterus, and hemoglobinuria. Acute infections sometimes result in abortion.

Diagnosis. Diagnosis of bovine leptospirosis is similar in principle to that of the canine disease; serologic tests are used almost exclusively. *Leptospira* are not demonstrable in the fetus.

PORCINE LEPTOSPIROSIS

L. pomona is the principal cause of leptospirosis in pigs. Other serovars are occasionally involved.

Serologic evidence indicates a 3 to 22% level of infection; probably 2 to 4% are actively infected.

Sources. The organisms may be found in swine or cattle, wild animals, and skunks, racoons, opossums, wildcats, or deer. Organisms may be shed for three months; shedding is irregular and not in large numbers.

Clinical. Infections are mostly subclinical or latent. Unthriftiness, abortion, fever, icterus, and anemia are among the signs observed.

Diagnosis. Diagnosis follows that of canine infections; serologic tests are used almost exclusively. *Leptospira* can be recovered from and demonstrated in aborted fetuses.

EQUINE LEPTOSPIROSIS

Leptospirosis appears to be an infrequent disease of horses. Most infections are due to *L. pomona*. There is usually a transient febrile illness, with icterus and occasionally abortions. Recurrent iridocyclitis (moon blindness or periodic ophthalmia) may be a sequela.

IMMUNITY

Immunity appears to be mainly humoral in that the organisms are not intracellular and bacterins (killed organisms) elicit considerable protection, although of short duration (less than a year). The levels of antibody resulting from vaccination are low and do not affect serologic testing. There is little cross-immunity between serovars.

Dogs. Bacterin is composed of *L. canicola* and *L. icterohemorrhagiae.*

Cattle. Bacterin utilizes *L. pomona:* some bacterins contain *L. hardjo* and *L. grippotyphosa* as well. Bacterins are also available that contain as many as five serovars. *Leptospira* may be combined with other antigens, including viruses.

Swine. Bacterin contains *L. pomona.*

TREATMENT AND CONTROL

Combined penicillin and streptomycin are recommended for treatment; early administration is important. Treatment may be of no avail if renal damage is extensive. Heavy doses of streptomycin may eliminate the carrier state. The tetracycline and macrolide antibiotics are also effective.

If leptospirosis is a recurring problem, preventive measures such as effective rat control, fencing off of potentially contaminated ponds and streams, and the careful screening of replacement stock should be implemented. Although *Leptospira* will survive for days in alkaline water, they will only live for about 12 hours in sewage, and they are very susceptible to drying and heat.

PUBLIC HEALTH SIGNIFICANCE

Human beings acquire leptospirosis from infected domestic animals, rodents, and contaminated water. The disease is referred to by several names, including Weil's disease, Fort Bragg fever, and swineherd's disease. Various serovars of *Leptospira*, including *L. canicola*, *L. icterohemorrhagiae*, and *L. pomona*, can infect humans. Veterinarians, slaughterhouse workers, and farmers are at particular risk. The acute form of the human disease is similar to that seen in some animals and is characterized by febrile jaundice and nephritis.

The laboratory diagnosis of the human disease is essentially the same as that described earlier for the dog.

It is thought that treatment will only affect the course of the disease if it is initiated within four days of onset. The same antibiotics are used as recommended for animals.

SUGGESTED CLINICAL EXAMPLES

An outbreak of fowl spirochetosis.

Cases of canine leptospirosis displaying the different forms: hemorrhagic, icteric, and uremic.

An outbreak of bovine leptospirosis in calves or mature cattle or both.

An outbreak of porcine leptospirosis.

SOURCES FOR FURTHER READING

Ellinghausen, H.C., Jr.: Virulence, nutrition and antigenicity of *Leptospira interrogans* serotype *pomona* in supplemented and nutrient deleted bovine albumin medium. Ann. Microbiol. (Inst. Pasteur), *124*:477, 1973.

Ellinghausen, H.C., Jr.: Variable factors influencing the isolation of leptospires involving culture ingredients and testing. Proc. 79th Meeting U.S. Animal Health Assoc., 1975.

Ellis, W.A.: Bovine leptospirosis: Infection by the Hebdomadis serogroup. *In* The Veterinary Animal. Edited by C.S.G. Grunsell and F.G. Hill. Bristol, England, Wright, Scientechnica, 1978.

Ellis, W.A., et al.: Bovine leptospirosis: Microbiological and serological findings in aborted fetuses. Vet. Rec., *110*:147, 1982.

Felsenfeld, O.: *Borrelia.* St. Louis, Missouri, Warren H. Green, Inc., 1971.

Hansen, L.E.: Pathogenesis of leptospirosis. *In* Biology of Parasitic Spirochetes. Edited by R.C. Johnson. New York, Academic Press, Inc., 1976.

Hansen, L.E.: Immunology of bacterial diseases with special reference to leptospirosis. J. Am. Vet. Med. Assoc., *170*:991, 1977.

Johnson, R.C. (ed.): Biology of Parasitic Spirochetes. New York, Academic Press, Inc., 1976.

Solorzano, R.F.: A comparison of the rapid macroscopic slide agglutination test for leptospirosis. Cornell Vet., *57*:239, 1967.

Stringfellow, D.A., et al.: Can antibody responses in cattle vaccinated with a multivalent leptospiral bacterin interfere wtih serologic diagnosis of disease? J. Am. Vet. Med. Assoc., *182*:165, 1983.

Sullivan, N.D.: Leptospirosis in man and animals. Aust. Vet. J., *50*:216, 1974.

Twigg, G.I., Hughes, D.M., and McDiarmid, A.: Occurrence of leptospirosis in horses. Eq. Vet.J., *3*:52, 1971.

Windsor, R.S.: Swine dysentery. *In* The Veterinary Annual. Edited by G.S.G. Grunsell and F.W.G. Hill. Bristol, England. Wright, Scientechnica, 1979.

28

Miscellaneous Potential Pathogens and Nonpathogens

There are a number of bacteria associated with animals, some as commensals and some as transients from the environment, which either do not cause disease or do so only infrequently. Because these organisms may be reported by the clinical microbiology laboratory as occurring in clinical materials, the practicing veterinarian should at least be acquainted with their names and probable origin. Culture purity, condition of the specimen, number of colonies, and repeated isolation must be considered in estimating the significance of these and other ordinarily nonpathogenic organisms. Some of these organisms, such as the *Acinetobacter* species, may replace other organisms in infectious processes that are more susceptible to antimicrobial drugs.

The genera *Streptobacillus* and *Neisseria* and the organism *Bacillus piliformis* are dealt with in this chapter, and information on other potential pathogens and nonpathogens is summarized in Table 28–1.

Neisseria

Neisseria are gram-negative, catalase-positive, oxidase-positive, aerobic cocci. They split sugars by oxidation or not at all.

In smears from cultures, these cocci occur singly or in clumps. Cells taken from body fluids appear as diplococci with adjacent sides flattened.

Six official species are described, and an even larger number of unofficial species is referred to in the literature. Most occur as commensals on the mucous membranes of the upper digestive, respiratory, and genital tracts. Potentially pathogenic species grow best on media enriched with blood or serum.

Members of this genus have only infrequently been reported as causing disease in animals.

1. *N. ovis:** recovered from sheep with keratoconjunctivitis; a commensal on the conjunctiva of sheep and cattle.
2. *N. catarrhalis (Branhamella catarrhalis***): recovered from pneumonic lungs of calves.
3. *N. denitrificans:* isolated from the nasopharynx of guinea pigs.
4. *N. canis:* isolated from the nasopharynx of cats and dogs.
5. *N. meningitidis:* causes meningococcal meningitis of humans.
6. *N. gonorrhoeae:* causative agent of gonorrhea.

The following bacteria somewhat resemble *Neisseria* morphologically:

1. *Acinetobacter calcoaceticus:* see Table 23–1.

---

*Unofficial species.
**New name.

Table 28–1. Miscellaneous Bacteria Recovered from Infrequent Infections and Clinical Specimens

Genus/Species	Gram Stain	Morphology	Oxidation/ Fermentation	MacConkey Agar	Oxidase	Motility	Other	Occurrence and Significance
Aeromonas (*A. hydrophila*)	–	Rod	F	+	+	(+)	–	Fresh and polluted water; fatal infections in animals rare.
Flavobacterium	–	Rod	0	–	+	–	Yellow pigment	Soil and water. Recovered occasionally from clinical materials.
Chromobacterium (*C. violaceum*)	–	Rod	some : 0 some : F		(+)	+	Blue, violet, or black pigment	Soil and water. *C. violaceum*: suppurative pneumonia in cattle, swine, and humans.
Acinetobacter calcoaceticus (Several phenotypic groups)	–	Diplococci, rod	0 or negative	+	–	–	See Table 23–1.	Free-living; genital tract. Animals: fetus, milk, various tissues. Blood cultures: dogs.
Alcaligenes *A. fecalis*	–	Rod	–	+	+	+	See Table 23–1. Urease-negative; nonfermenter	Uncommon in animals. Intestinal tract; not pathogenic.
Achromobacter spp.	–	Rod	0	+	+	+	Acid from glucose	Occasionally from intestinal tract of animals; free-living; not pathogenic; occasionally in clinical specimens.

(+) = most positive.

2. *Moraxella* species: see Chapter 23.
3. *Veillonella* species: anaerobic cocci.

Bacillus piliformis

This interesting gram-negative organism, which is not a member of the *Bacillus* genus, is the cause of Tyzzer's disease.

PATHOGENICITY

The organism probably occurs infrequently in the intestine of rodents. Under circumstances of stress such as experimentation, cortisone treatment, or thymectomy, it causes enteritis and hepatitis. The latter is evidenced by livers with diffusely distributed pale grey necrotic foci. The disease may occur sporadically or as a serious epizootic in mice, rats, gerbils, rabbits, and monkeys. Sporadic infections have been reported in the cat, dog, and foal.

DIRECT EXAMINATION

Smears are made from the necrotic foci in the liver and stained with Giemsa. Long, slender organisms are seen in the cytoplasm of hepatic cells. Very long, thin, tortuous filaments are sometimes seen as well as short bacillary forms and occasionally filaments with moniliform swellings. Tapering and beading of the filaments are characteristic features.

ISOLATION AND CULTIVATION

The organism has not been cultivated on artificial media. It can be cultivated in the yolk sac of embryonated chicken eggs.

TREATMENT AND CONTROL

Broad-spectrum antibiotics in the drinking water are effective against *Bacillus piliformis*. While cleaning and disinfecting, it should be kept in mind that the spores of *B. piliformis* are somewhat resistant. A temperature of 80°C will kill them in 30 minutes. Tyzzer's disease can be prevented by establishing colonies free of *Bacillus piliformis*.

Streptobacillus moniliformis

S. moniliformis is an aerobic, gram-negative, highly pleomorphic rod that forms filaments with moniliform swellings and L forms under certain conditions. Pioneering studies on L forms were carried out with this species. *S. moniliformis* is a normal inhabitant of the upper res-piratory tract of wild and laboratory rats and some other rodents.

PATHOGENICITY

The organism is a secondary invader in chronic murine pneumonia of rats and a primary cause of a disease of mice characterized by septicemia, septic arthritis, hepatitis, and lymphadenitis. Serious infections in turkeys have been attributed to rat bites.

Infections in humans initiated by rat bites (rat-bite fever) are characterized by septicemia and polyarthritis. *Spirillum minus* or *S. minor* (most likely belongs in the genus *Aquaspirillum*) is another cause of rat-bite fever in humans. The organism is carried by rats and mice, and the disease it causes is clinically similar to that caused by *S. moniliformis*.

ISOLATION, CULTIVATION, AND IDENTIFICATION

The organism can be grown in blood or serum-enriched media incubated for at least eight days. Isolation from humans is most readily accomplished with blood cultures. Identification is usually based upon the characteristic cultural and morphologic features of the organism. Confirmation is obtained by a number of biochemical tests.

S. minor has not been cultivated in vitro. It is demonstrable in wet mounts and stained smears.

Legionella pneumophila

This recently named fastidious, gram-negative, small rod is the cause of Legionnaires' disease. The first cases involved members of the American Legion attending a convention in Philadelphia in 1976. The organism was first propagated in guinea pigs and embryonated eggs, but specially formulated media are now available for its cultivation. Since the discovery of *L. pneumophila*, other closely related potentially pathogenic bacteria have been identified, and all have been placed in the family Legionellaceae. They are free-living organisms that are widely distributed in many water-associated environments. No natural infections have been reported in animals.

Diseases caused by this group of organisms may take several forms, of which a multisystem illness with pneumonia is the best known. Only a small number of persons exposed develop clinical disease, and symptoms may be all gradations from asymptomatic or mild to acute. The direct fluorescent antibody procedure can be used for the rapid identification of the organism. Special culture and serologic procedures are available.

Prototheca

Members of this genus are microscopic, colorless achlorophyllic algae of the family Chlorellaceae. They are ubiquitous in nature and are occasionally recovered from clinical specimens, in which they are not usually significant. However, there have been several reports of human and animal infections. The agents are infrequent opportunists that would appear to produce disease only if the host's resistance is impaired. *Prototheca* have been reported to cause bovine mastitis, localized infection in a cat, and disseminated protothecosis in the dog.

Treatment with amphotericin B and ketoconazole has shown promise in human infections.

Small colonies that resemble those of *Cryptococcus* spp. appear on Sabouraud agar (25°C) and blood agar (37°C) in 24 hours. They are hyaline and globose in form, without a capsule. They are larger than bacteria with width and length as great as 13 to 16 μm. Eight or more characteristic endospores are produced by internal segmentation. Five species have been identified using the fluorescent antibody technique.

SUGGESTED CLINICAL EXAMPLES

A case of Tyzzer's disease in the horse.

An outbreak of Tyzzer's disease in a mouse colony.

An outbreak of *Streptobacillus moniliformis* infection in turkeys.

A case of suppurative pneumonia in a pig due to *Chromobacterium violaceum*.

A case of canine protothecosis.

SOURCES FOR FURTHER READING

Carter, G.R., Whitenack, D.L., and Julius, L.A.: Natural Tyzzer's disease in Mongolian gerbils *(Meriones unguiculatus)*. Lab. Ann. Care, *19*:648, 1969.

Carter, G.R., Isoun, T.T., and Keahey, K.K.: Occurrence of *Mima* and *Herellea* species in clinical specimens from various animals. J. Am. Vet. Med. Assoc., *156*:1313, 1970.

Craigie, J.: *Bacillus piliformis* (Tyzzer) and Tyzzer's disease of the laboratory mouse. 1. Propagation of the organism in the embryonated eggs. Proc. R. Soc. Lond. (Biol.), *165*:35, 1966.

Harrington, D.D.: *Bacillus piliformis* infection (Tyzzer's disease) in two foals. J. Am. Vet. Med. Assoc., *168*:58, 1976.

Joseph, P.G., Sivendar, R., Anwar, M., and Fong, S.F.: *Chromobacterium violaceum* infection in animals. Kajian Vet. (Malaysia-Singapore), *3*:55, 1971.

Lyons, R.W.: *Acinetobacter calcoaceticus*. Clin. Microbiol. Newsletter, *5*:87, 1981.

Migaki, G., et al.: Canine protothecosis: Review of the literature and report of an additional case. J. Am. Vet. Med. Assoc., *181*:794, 1982.

Qureshi, S.R., Carlton, W., and Olander, H.J.: Tyzzer's disease in a dog. J. Am. Vet. Med. Assoc., *168*:602, 1976.

Rakich, P.M., and Latimer, K.S.: Altered immune function in a dog with disseminated protothecosis. J. Am. Vet. Med. Assoc., *185*:681, 1984.

Sippel, W.L., Medina, G., and Atwood, M.B.: Outbreaks of disease in animals associated with *Chromobacterium violaceum*. 1. The disease in swine. J. Am. Vet. Med. Assoc., *124*:467, 1954.

29

Rickettsia and Chlamydia

The rickettsiae and chlamydiae are obligate intracellular organisms that are now classed as bacteria. At present they are classified in the orders Rickettsiales and Chlamydiales. They contain the families listed below.

ORDER RICKETTSIALES

Family Rickettsiaceae. These are usually parasites of the gut cells of arthropods; transmission is from arthropod to animal. Capillary endothelium is attacked, producing thrombi that result in hemorrhagic skin rashes. This family is subdivided into tribe I, Rickettsiae, tribe II, Ehrlichieae, and tribe III, Wolbachieae (invertebrates).

Family Bartonellaceae. These bacteria parasitize mammalian erythrocytes; there is an intermediate arthropod host. They are rod-shaped and multiply by division inside or outside the host cell.

Family Anaplasmataceae. These organisms also parasitize mammalian erythrocytes; there is an intermediate arthropod host. They are spherical, multiply intracellularly, and have sac-like appendages. No organelles are seen, as in protozoa.

ORDER CHLAMYDIALES

Family Chlamydiaceae. Transmission is by inhalation and ingestion; there is no arthropodal involvement. Epithelial cells of the lung and mucosal membranes as well as vascular endothelium and mobile phagocytes are parasitized.

SOME FEATURES OF RICKETTSIAE AND CHLAMYDIAE

Only rickettsiae and chlamydiae of the families Rickettsiaceae and Chlamydiaceae are discussed here. There is a lack of basic information on members of the families Bartonellaceae and Anaplasmataceae.

There are fundamental differences between the chlamydiae and the rickettsiae. The latter have cytochromes and their metabolic reactions are aerobic, whereas the former have not been shown to have cytochromes, and their metabolic reactions are essentially anaerobic. The chlamydiae also have a singular developmental cycle, while the rickettsiae multiply by simple binary fission.

Both are now classed as bacteria. They can be seen with the light microscope. All contain DNA and RNA and are susceptible to various antibiotics. They have cell walls that resemble those of gram-negative bacteria. They stain reasonably well with Giemsa, Castaneda, and Macchiavello stains but poorly with Gram's stain. They are small, pleomorphic coccobacillary forms existing as obligate intracellular parasites. They possess many of the metabolic functions of bacteria but require exogenous cofactors from animal cells.

Most rickettsiae and chlamydiae grow readily in the yolk sac of embryonated eggs and in cell cultures. Several species have been grown on artificial media.

RICKETTSIAE

(Excluding Haemobartonellaceae and Anaplasmataceae)

Morphology

Rickettsiae are minute coccobacilli, visible with the light microscope. They are usually about 0.3 μm in width and about 0.5 μm in length.

Toxin Production

Noninfectious (ultraviolet irradiated) rickettsiae are toxic for mice and rats when administered intravenously. Death is caused by damage to endothelial cells, producing loss of plasma, decrease in blood volume, and shock. The toxins have not been isolated and identified. Hemolysins are produced by some typhus rickettsiae.

Mode of Infection

1. In mammals by direct penetration of the skin as a result of the feeding of an infected arthropod (tick, louse, flea, or mite).
2. In arthropods as the result of ingestion of blood of infected animals.
3. From arthropod to progeny by infected ova.
4. By inhalation and ingestion, as in Q fever.
5. By ingestion of infected flukes, as in salmon poisoning.

Pathogenesis

Infections begin in the vascular system; organisms proliferate in endothelial cells and are disseminated via the bloodstream. There is obstruction of small blood vessels because of hyperplasia of infected endothelial cells and resulting small thrombi. Fever, hemorrhagic rash, stupor, shock, and patchy gangrene of subcutis and skin are among the signs and lesions noted.

Pathogenicity

In addition to the diseases listed in Table 29–1, tick-borne fever and bovine petechial fever are thought to be caused by rickettsiae.

Tick-borne fever is a noncontagious, febrile disease of sheep and occasionally cattle kept on tick-infested pastures. The disease has only been reported from Great Britain and Europe.

Bovine petechial fever is a contagious, febrile disease of cattle characterized by edema of the conjunctiva and petechiae of the mucous membranes. Although the course is usually mild, severe cases terminating in death are encountered. The disease has only been reported in Africa.

Diagnosis

The rickettsiae can be cultivated in the yolk sac of embryonated eggs and in cell cultures. Serologic procedures consist of agglutination and complement fixation tests that are available for some of the diseases (Q fever, typhus, and "spotted' fevers).

Heartwater. Giemsa-stained smears from brain tissue; inoculation of susceptible cattle.

Tropical Canine Pancytopenia. Giemsa-stained blood smears; characteristic inclusions in monocytes and neutrophils. Serologic: indirect fluorescent antibody test.

Equine Ehrlichiosis. Essentially the same as for canine ehrlichiosis.

Q Fever. Inoculation of chicken embryos, guinea pigs, and hamsters; detection of organisms in stained smears. Agglutination or complement fixation tests.

Immunity

Immunity is both cellular and humoral. Vaccines consisting of killed organisms are used to prevent epidemic typhus and Rocky Mountain spotted fever. Vaccines are not available for the prevention of the rickettsial diseases of animals.

Treatment

Tetracyclines in combination with a normal immune response are curative.

FAMILY HAEMOBARTONELLACEAE

FELINE INFECTIOUS ANEMIA

Haemobartonella felis causes the widespread disease of cats, feline infectious anemia. It is characterized by acute and chronic forms, both of which lead to anemia. In the acute disease clinical signs include variable fever (103 to 105°C), anorexia, jaundice, and splenomegaly. In the chronic form the clinical signs are less severe and temperatures may be normal or subnormal.

The mode of transmission is not known for certain, but arthropod vectors are thought to be involved. The disease occurs in a latent form in

Table 29–1. Family Rickettsiaceae

Tribe I Rickettsieae { *Rickettsia* / *Coxiella*		Tribe II Ehrlichieae { *Ehrlichia* / *Cowdria* / *Neorickettsia*	
	Disease	Host (Disease)	Transmission
R. rickettsii	Rocky Mountain spotted fever: mild to serious acute, febrile disease. Infections in animals usually mild.	Humans (mainly South Atlantic states)	Endemic in wood, rabbit, and dog ticks. In all tissues of ticks and feces.
Cowdria ruminantium	Africa, Caribbean. Acute septicemia: "heartwater." High mortality.	Cattle, sheep, goats	Ticks.
E. canis (Ehrlichieae occur in cattle and sheep without clinical disease)	Tropical canine pancytopenia or canine ehrlichiosis. Parasites of monocytic cells. Long course; recurrent fever.	Dog	Brown dog tick.
E. equi	Sporadic disease; fever, ataxia, leg edema, thrombocytopenia, anemia. Low mortality.	Horse	Vector not known.
E. potomacensis (proposed)	Potomac horse fever: fever, anorexia, leukopenia, usually diarrhea; mortality as high as 30%	Horse	Vector not known
Neorickettsia helminthoeca / Elokomin fluke fever agent	Salmon poisoning; 90% fatal. Acute, febrile, conjunctivitis, diarrhea. / Similar agent occurring with *N. helminthoeca* or separately.	Dog, bear, raccoon, ferrets.	Fish contain the infected helminth fluke, which encysts in muscles. Dogs eat infested salmon. Flukes mature and release invasive rickettsiae; ova passed → snail → salmon.
Coxiella burnetii	Q fever: febrile pneumonitis. Rarely fatal. / Endemic: some dairy cattle, rats, and many other domestic and wild animals, which serve as reservoir. Occasional abortions.	Humans	Ticks: infected for long periods. Agent in cow's milk, various discharges. Inhalation of contaminated dust; fomites. Differs from other rickettsiae in being relatively resistant to drying and heat.

many cats and becomes clinical as a result of stress or concurrent disease.

Diagnosis

H. felis is a small, coccoid, rod-like or ring-shaped organism. Diagnosis is based upon the demonstration of numbers of characteristic organisms on the surfaces of erythrocytes of peripheral blood or bone marrow in Giemsa-stained smears. A number of smears may have to be examined because *H. felis* may only appear in the blood periodically.

Treatment

Blood transfusions should be given if indicated. Tetracyclines are administered for two to three weeks.

Control and Prevention

External parasites should be controlled and blood donor cats should be screened to prevent the spread of the disease.

FAMILY ANAPLASMATACEAE

ANAPLASMOSIS

The principal rickettsia in this family is *Anaplasma marginale*. It causes anaplasmosis, an arthropod-borne (numerous species of ticks) disease of cattle and other ruminants, which is manifested in acute, subacute, and chronic forms, with fever and varying degrees of anemia and icterus. If untreated the acute disease is frequently fatal.

Anaplasmosis occurs widely in tropical and

subtropical countries, principally in cattle and water buffaloes. Calves under six months are relatively resistant to the clinical disease but may become carriers.

A. ovis is a relatively avirulent rickettsia that sometimes occurs with *A. marginale* in Central Africa. Under some circumstances it can cause clinical anaplasmosis in sheep and goats.

Diagnosis

Anaplasmosis is diagnosed by the demonstration of the organisms as marginal bodies in erythrocytes of Giemsa-stained smears. Severe, prolonged infections with much red cell destruction may show few anaplasmas.

Indirect immunofluorescence assay and the card agglutination, capillary agglutination, and complement fixation tests are used to detect animals that have been exposed or are infected.

Treatment

Tetracyclines are effective if given early. They are also effective in eliminating the carrier state when administered for prolonged periods.

Control and Prevention

Vectors should be reduced. Eradication can be accomplished by the removal of infected animals, although this is not usually feasible.

Premunition of young animals, i.e., deliberate infection with virulent or attenuated *A. marginale*, is widely practiced in tropical and subtropical countries. In adult animals premunition should include concomitant tetracycline administration.

A vaccine consisting of killed organisms is available.

FAMILY CHLAMYDIACEAE

PSITTACOSIS–LYMPHOGRANULOMA VENEREUM GROUP (PLV)

The group antigen is a lipoprotein-carbohydrate complex and there are specific antigens.

Taxonomists now recognize two species of *Chlamydia*, viz., *C. trachomatis* (*Chlamydia* subgroup A) and *C. psittaci* (*Chlamydia* subgroup B). Strains of *C. trachomatis* are now considered to cause trachoma, lymphogranuloma venereum, and inclusion conjunctivitis in humans. Various strains of *C. psittaci* that may only differ serologically are considered to be the cause of the chlamydioses of animals.

CHLAMYDIAE

Morphology and Multiplication

The highly infectious elementary bodies released from cells are spherical in shape, with a diameter of approximately 0.25 μm.

They reproduce as follows. The mature parasites are spherical and from 0.2 μm to 1.0 μm in size. Elementary bodies (0.2 to 0.3 μm) invade host cells, thereby yielding intracytoplasmic inclusions (up to 12 μm) filled with amorphous forms (0.1 μm diameter) that develop after various sequential changes. There is then division and reduction in size with the production of highly infectious elementary bodies in approximately 30 hours.

Toxin Production

Toxins have not been demonstrated from *Chlamydia*.

Mode of Infection

Animals and humans are infected by the inhalation of infectious dust and droplets. In some chlamydioses, e.g., enzootic abortion of ewes, infection may take place by ingestion.

Pathogenesis

The chlamydiae have a predilection for epithelial cells of the mucous membranes, although other tissues in a variety of locations are regularly infected. Pneumonia may develop from the inhalation of infectious dust and droplets. In enzootic pneumonia of ewes the mode of infection is ingestion, and organisms localize in cells of the placenta. Latency is a common feature of chlamydial infections. Latent infections are often activated by various stresses.

Pathogenicity (Table 29–2)

Psittacosis or Avian Chlamydiosis. *C. psittaci* causes psittacosis, a disease of humans and psittacene birds (parakeets, parrots). It is commonly carried in the spleen and kidney of normal-appearing birds. As a result of certain influences or "stresses," the organisms multiply and are shed in the feces in large numbers. The feces dry, producing a dust that is infectious by inhalation to susceptible avian or mammalian hosts.

The disease resulting from the inhalation of fecal dust is initially a pneumonitis. The organisms may spread via the blood, producing very

Table 29–2. Principal Chlamydioses of Animals Caused by **Chlamydia psittaci**

Disease	Characteristics
Feline pneumonitis	A frequent infection of cats; a problem in "cat colonies." Infection is by inhalation, beginning as an upper respiratory infection with conjunctivitis and nasal discharge; consolidation of lung may follow.
Enzootic abortion of ewes (EAE); ovine pneumonitis. EAE is an important widespread disease of sheep and goats.	The organisms causing these two diseases are probably identical or very closely related.
Sporadic bovine encephalomyelitis; Buss disease	Probably widespread but rarely diagnosed; occurs in young calves and less commonly in older cattle. Dyspnea, diarrhea, and lameness are followed by paralysis. This is serofibrinous peritonitis and encephalomyelitis. Mortality as high as 25%.
Polyarthritis of lambs, calves, and swine	Probably worldwide. Among the signs seen in young animals are depression, lameness, swollen joints and tendons, reluctance to move, fever, diarrhea, conjunctivitis, and nasal catarrh.

serious systemic disease. Mortality may be as high as 20% in untreated individuals.

Ornithosis is the name that was given to the chlamydiosis seen in nonpsittacene birds, e.g., pigeons, sparrows, and domestic poultry. Like psittacosis, this disease is also transmissible to humans. Some texts use the term psittacosis and ornithosis synonymously. In turkeys the disease may be economically important.

Psittacosis or ornithosis is controlled by the isolation of imported psittacene birds and administration of chloromycetin or tetracycline in the feed or water for 45 days.

Laboratory Diagnosis

1. Demonstration of organisms in stained smears and sections of lesions, e.g., smears of conjunctival scrapings in feline pneumonitis. Gimenez's stain is preferred for smears. Fluorescein labeled antibody may be used for the specific staining of smears.
2. Isolation and cultivation of organisms are usually done in the yolk sac of the chicken embryo, in mice, and also in irradiated cell cultures. Organisms are detected by staining with fluorescein-labeled antibody. Species identification requires serologic procedures to detect specific antigens.
3. Paired serum samples (for rising titers); complement fixation (group antigen); and immunofluorescence (inhibition test).

Immunity

Immunity is both cell-mediated and humoral. The type-specific antigen stimulates production of protective antibody. Vaccines consisting of suspensions of killed organisms are available for the prevention of feline pneumonitis and enzootic abortion of ewes.

Treatment

Sulfonamides are effective for *C. trachomatis* subgroup A because these organisms synthesize their own folic acid. Subgroup B organisms *C. psittaci* (animal pathogens), require preformed folic acid and thus are not inhibited by sulfonamides. Penicillin results in the production of intracellular spheroplasts and is therefore not recommended. Tetracyclines and chloramphenicol are useful.

SUGGESTED CLINICAL EXAMPLES

A case of canine ehrlichiosis (tropical canine pancytopenia).

A case of salmon poisoning in a dog.

A case of Q fever in a farm family traced to raw cow's milk.

An outbreak of psittacosis among parrots or parakeets.

Examination of a parrot suspected of transmitting psittacosis to its owner.

An outbreak of ornithosis in turkeys.

An outbreak of feline pneumonitis in a cat colony.

An outbreak of enzootic abortion in ewes.

SOURCES FOR FURTHER READING

Davidson, D.E., Jr., et al.: Prophylactic and therapeutic use of tetracycline during an epizootic of ehrlichiosis among military dogs. J. Am. Vet. Med. Assoc., *172*:697, 1978.

Doughri, A.M., Young, S., and Stortz, J.: Pathologic changes in intestinal chlamydial infection of newborn calves. Am. J. Vet. Res., *35*:939, 1974.

Ewing, S.A.: Canine ehrlichiosis. Adv. Vet. Sci., *13*:331, 1969.

Foggie, A.: Chlamydial infections in mammals. Vet. Rec., *100*:315, 1977.

Grayston, J.T., and Wang, S.P.: New knowledge of chlamydiae and the diseases they cause. J. Infect. Dis., *132*:87, 1975.

Haig, D.A.: Tickborne rickettsioses in South Africa. Adv. Vet. Sci., 2:307, 1955.

Keefe, T.J., Holland, C.J., Salyer, P.E., and Ristic, M.: Distribution of *Ehrlichia canis* among military working dogs in the world and selected civilian dogs in the United States. J. Am. Vet. Med. Assoc., *181*:236, 1982.

Kitao, T., Farrell, R.K., and Fukuda, T.: Differentiation of salmon poisoning disease and Elokomin fluke fever: Fluorescent antibody studies with *Rickettsia sennetsu*. Am. J. Vet. Res., *34*:927, 1973.

McCauley, E.H., and Ticken, E.L.: Psittacosis-lymphogranuloma venereum agent isolated during an abortion epizootic in goats. J. Am. Vet. Med. Assoc., *152*:1758, 1968.

Mohan, R.: Epidemiologic and laboratory observations of *Chlamydia psittaci* infection in pet birds. J. Am. Vet. Med. Assoc., *184*:1372, 1984.

Page, L.A., and Grimes, J.E.: Avian chlamydiosis (ornithosis). *In* Diseases of Poultry. Edited by M.S. Hofstad. 8th Ed. Ames, Iowa State University Press, 1984.

Plommet, M., Caponi, M., Gestin, J., and Renoux, G.: Fièvre Q experimentale des bovins. Ann. Rech. Vet., 4:325, 1973.

Seamer, J., and Snape, T.: *Ehrlichia canis* and tropical canine pancytopaenia. Res. Vet. Sci., *13*:307, 1972.

Stortz, J.: *Chlamydia* and *Chlamydia*-Induced Infections. Springfield, Ill., Charles C Thomas, 1971.

Woldhalm, D.G., Stoenner, H.G., Simmons, R.E., and Thomas, L.A.: Abortion associated with *Coxiella burnettii* infection in dairy goats. J. Am. Vet. Med. Assoc., *173*:1580, 1978.

30

Mycoplasmas

HISTORICAL

The first mycoplasmal species, the cause of contagious bovine pleuropneumonia, was discovered by Nocard (French veterinarian) and Roux in 1898. The species discovered later were called pleuropneumonia-like organisms (PPLO).

GENERAL

The mycoplasmas are the smallest and simplest procaryotic cells capable of self-replication. They are classified in families and genera, as shown in Table 30–1. The mycoplasmas that are parasitic and pathogenic for animals are in the families Mycoplasmatacea and Acholeplasmataceae. The ureaplasmas are distinctive in that they hydrolyze urea. The genus *Acholeplasma* is separated from the genera *Mycoplasma* and *Ureaplasma* by the requirement of the latter two for cholesterol.

These procaryotic organisms have no rigid cell wall and consequently are plastic and highly pleomorphic. They are bound by a limiting lipoprotein plasma membrane. Some divide by binary fission, while others have a reproductive cycle, unlike bacteria. In the latter case elongated forms break up into round forms that may pass through a 0.15 μm filter. Most species of *Mycoplasma* utilize either glucose or arginine as their major source of energy.

MORPHOLOGY

Mycoplasmas in smears are seen as coccobacilli; coccal forms, ring forms, spirals, and filaments. They stain poorly (gram-negative), although Giemsa is useful. They are difficult to demonstrate in and from tissues. They range in size from 50–60 to 100–250 nm.

CULTIVATION AND CULTURAL FEATURES

Mycoplasmas are grown on media consisting of beef infusion, peptone, NaCl, 20% horse serum and 10% yeast extract; agar is added to make a solid medium. Inhibitors of bacterial growth, which may be included, are penicillin (gram-positives) and thallium acetate (gram-negatives). Some additives may be required for the growth of some species.

Parasitic mycoplasmas contain 10 to 20% lipid and possess a relatively low content of nucleic acids as compared with bacteria. Some require nitrogen with 5 to 10% CO_2; they may be grown in chicken embryos and cell cultures.

T-mycoplasmas or ureaplasmas produce smaller colonies (T = tiny) than the conventional mycoplasmas. Unlike the other mycoplasmas, they can split urea. Special procedures are required for the cultivation and maintenance of these organisms.

COLONY MORPHOLOGY

After two to six days of aerobic incubation at 37°C, colonies on solid media are 10 to 600 μm in diameter. Under low power magnification colonies appear transparent, flat, and often resemble a fried egg. Colonies grow into the medium and are difficult to remove from the agar surface. Stained colony preparations can be made from

Table 30–1. Families, Genera, and Habitats of Mycoplasmas

Families and Genera	Approximate Number of Species	Cholesterol Requirement	Habitat
Mycoplasmataceae:			
Mycoplasma	>60	+	Animals
Ureaplasma	2	+	Animals
Acholeplasmataceae:			
Acholeplasma	8	–	Animals
A. laidlawii		–	Soil, sewage, etc.
Spiroplasmataceae:			
Spiroplasma	4	+	Plants and insects
Unclassified genera:			
Anaeroplasma	2	Variable	Rumen of cattle and sheep
Thermoplasma	1	–	Burning coal and refuse piles

(Adapted from Joklik, W.K., Willet, H.P., and Amos, D.B. (eds.): Zinsser Microbiology. 18th Ed. Norwalk, Conn., Appleton-Century-Crofts, 1984.)

culture plates using Dienes' stain. It distinguishes mycoplasmas from dwarf bacterial colonies but not from L forms of bacteria.

SPECIAL PROCEDURES

Agar cultures are transferred by pushing a block of agar, colony side down, over another plate with a glass rod. Blocks with colonies are dropped into broth. Care must be taken to obtain pure cultures.

PATHOGENESIS

Many of the mycoplasmas are commensals in the upper digestive, respiratory, and genital tracts. It is known that some species attach to cells by receptors. Some have a predilection for infecting mesenchymal cells lining serous cavities and joints; others parasitize tissues of the respiratory tract, including the lungs. Species show considerable host specificity. They are extracellular parasites and some produce toxins. The fibrinous exudate frequently present in infections protects them from antibody and antimicrobial drugs and contributes to chronicity. Bacterial secondary invaders are not uncommon.

Infections are frequently chronic and low grade. Various stresses predispose to these infections. Experimental disease is often difficult to produce.

MODE OF INFECTION

This is most frequently by inhalation. Infection may be endogenous or exogenous.

IMMUNE RESPONSE

The immune response is predominantly humoral. As in bacterial infections, the first antibodies to appear are IgM and IgA, followed by IgG. The CF antibodies—being mostly IgM—are found early. Autoimmune phenomena have been reported in some *Mycoplasma* infections.

Various procedures are used to detect and measure antibodies, e.g., agglutination, agar gel precipitation, complement fixation, ELISA, and counter-immunoelectrophoresis.

PATHOGENICITY AND PROPERTIES OF AVIAN STRAINS

M. iners. Pathogenicity for fowl has not been demonstrated.

PROPERTIES. It is nonhemolytic. Common substrates are not fermented. It does not agglutinate chicken red cells. It differs antigenically from other avian species.

M. gallisepticum (MG). This is the primary cause of chronic respiratory disease and airsac disease of chickens, turkeys, and other fowl; infectious sinusitis of turkeys; and synovitis. Egg transmission is of major importance.

PROPERTIES. It is beta-hemolytic, ferments a number of carbohydrates, and agglutinates chicken red cells.

M. synoviae (MS). This species is considered the cause of infectious synovitis of chickens and turkeys. Although all synovial membranes may be affected, the lesions involving the hock and wing joints are most apparent. *M. synoviae* has been isolated from the respiratory tracts of chickens and turkeys. Transmission is by eggs.

PROPERTIES. It is pathogenic for chicken embryos and ferments dextrose and maltose but not lactose, sucrose, or mannitol.

M. gallinarum. A nonpathogenic organism found in the respiratory tract of fowl.

PROPERTIES. It is beta-hemolytic, does not ferment common substrates, and does not agglutinate avian erythrocytes.

M. meleagridis (MM). MM causes airsacculitis of turkeys. Transmission is by eggs. It is isolated from semen, vagina, bursa of Fabricius, air sacs, lungs, trachea, and sinuses.

PROPERTIES. It is nonhemolytic and does not ferment glucose.

PATHOGENICITY OF PORCINE STRAINS

M. hyorhinis causes polyserositis and arthritis in young pigs and is a secondary invader in rhinitis and pneumonia. It is frequently found in the upper respiratory tract.

M. hyosynoviae causes arthritis in young and feeder pigs; it is frequently found in the upper respiratory tract.

M. hyopneumoniae (M. suipneumoniae) is the primary cause of enzootic pneumonia of swine, the most widespread pneumonic disease of swine. Ordinarily it is a mild chronic disease whose effects are mainly reflected in delayed weight gains. As a result of various stresses the pneumonia, usually complicated by *Pasteurella multocida,* can become severe.

MYCOPLASMAS OF CATTLE

M. mycoides ss. *mycoides* causes contagious bovine pleuropneumonia (CBPP), a major plague of cattle that is enzootic in parts of Africa and Asia. CBPP is a highly contagious disease characterized by septicemia, frequently followed by localization in the thorax with extensive suppurative lesions involving the lungs, pleura, and pericardium.

Like many other mycoplasmas *M. bovis* can be found as a commensal in the respiratory and genital tracts. It is a frequent cause of mastitis, arthritis, and less frequently of genital infections.

Ureaplasmas have frequently been isolated from the genital tract, pneumonic lungs, semen, and milk of cows. They are not uncommon commensals and have a probable pathogenic potential. Recent reports suggest an etiologic role in bovine granular vaginitis and infertility.

The other mycoplasmas recovered from cattle are listed in Table 30–3.

MYCOPLASMA INFECTIONS OF SHEEP AND GOATS

Several *Mycoplasma* species cause important diseases of sheep and goats. These infections are referred to briefly.

Contagious caprine pleuropneumonia is an acute serofibrinous pleurisy and pneumonia that may involve an entire lobe. It is characterized by red and grey hepatization with characteristic hemorrhagic infarction. A severe arthritis may be a sequela of the bacteremia. This disease has been attributed to *Mycoplasma mycoides* subspecies *capri, M. capripneumoniae,* and *M. mycoides* ss. *mycoides* (large colony). It occurs in Europe, Asia, and Africa, and there is recent evidence that it exists in the United States.

The "small colony" form of *M. mycoides* ss. *mycoides* is the causative agent of contagious bovine pleuropneumonia.

Contagious agalactia is an acute, subacute, or chronic disease of sheep and goats caused by *M. agalactiae* (other mycoplasmas, viz., *M. mycoides* ss. *mycoides*—large colony—and *M. capricolum* are claimed to cause similar syndromes). It is characterized by bacteremia (after ingestion), with localization and inflammatory activity in the udder, uterus, joints (arthritis), and eyes (conjunctivitis). There is interstitial mastitis, which without treatment may lead to extensive fibrosis. Contagious agalactia occurs in

Table 30–2. *A Comparison of Characteristics of Mycoplasmas and L Forms*

Mycoplasma	L-Phase Variants (L Forms) of Bacteria*
Elements of colonies smaller	Elements of colonies larger
Contain less DNA	Contain more DNA
GC ratio lower	GC ratio higher
Do not revert to bacteria	May revert
No antigenic relation to bacteria	Antigenic relations to parent bacterium
Require sterols (except *Acholeplasma* and *Thermoplasma)*	Do not require sterols
Usually pathogenic or parasitic	Not known to be pathogenic
Many pathogenic strains require serum	Serum requirements less absolute
DNA antibody does not relate to bacteria	DNA antibody shows kinship to bacteria

*L-phase variants occur spontaneously or as a result of the action on bacteria of antisera, antibiotics, salts of heavy metals, phage, and so forth.

Mediterranean countries and some regions of Europe, Africa, and Asia.

Polyarthritis in sheep and goats is probably the most common and geographically widespread mycoplasmosis in these species. It is most often caused by *M. capricolum*.

Keratoconjunctivitis in sheep and goats is a worldwide disease caused by *M. conjunctivae*.

M. mycoides ss. *mycoides* (large colony) has been reported to cause epizootics in kids characterized by septicemia, polyarthritis, and pneumonia, with high morbidity and mortality rates. The organism is usually acquired from the milk of shedding females.

Other disease manifestations with which mycoplasmas have been associated are enzootic pneumonia, arthritis, conjunctivitis, vulvovaginitis, infertility, and central nervous system disorders.

MYCOPLASMA INFECTIONS OF DOGS AND CATS

The mycoplasmas that have been recovered from dogs and cats and the diseases attributed to two of them are covered below.

Mycoplasmas of Dogs

Mycoplasma cynos is considered a cause of a rapidly spreading respiratory infection involving the lungs. By itself it may have little significance, but in combination with other bacteria and viruses it may cause a severe pneumonia.

Other species that have been recovered from the dog and whose significance is uncertain are *M. spumans*, *M. maculosum*, *M. edwardii*, *M. molare*, *M. canis*, and *M. opalescens*.

Mycoplasmas of Cats

M. felis causes a unilateral or bilateral conjunctivitis, which begins with papillary hypertrophy of the conjunctival surface, resulting in a deep red, velvety appearance. If untreated within a week, there is a mucoid exudate and occasionally pseudomembrane formation.

M. gateae is also recovered from cats, but its significance is uncertain.

MYCOPLASMAS OF OTHER SPECIES

Most of the mycoplasmas that have been recovered from domestic animals are listed according to animal species in Table 30–3.

SPECIMENS

The particular fragility of these organisms must be considered in the submission of speci-

mens. They should be refrigerated and delivered to the laboratory within 48 hours. Mycoplasmas in tissues can be preserved for longer periods by freezing, preferably on dry ice.

IDENTIFICATION OF MYCOPLASMAS

Th association of a culture with a lesion is suggestive of a particular organism, e.g., a *Mycoplasma* recovered from polyserositis in a young pig would probably be *M. hyorhinis*. Precise identification is sometimes difficult and may require the help of a reference laboratory. Various procedures are used for different species.

1. An agglutination procedure is used to identify avian mycoplasmas. It is sometimes used for the identification of other species.
2. Direct and indirect fluorescent antibody staining is used to identify organisms in smears and colonies on plates.
3. Growth inhibition tests: specific antisera inhibit growth of homologous immunotypes on agar. This is a particularly useful procedure, but antisera are not always available.
4. Other criteria: fermentation of sugars, colony characteristics, pathogenicity, hemagglutination, tetrazolium reduction, hemolysis, and others.

RESISTANCE

Mycoplasma are more fragile than bacteria because of the absence of a cell wall. They are readily killed by drying, sunshine, and the usual means of chemical disinfection.

TREATMENT

Mycoplasma are resistant to sulfonamides and penicillin. Tetracyclines, gentamicin, kanamycin, tylosin, and erythromycin are effective in some infections.

CONTROL

Flocks have been established that are free of avian *Mycoplasma*. Chickens supplying eggs in such flocks must be negative to cultural and serologic procedures. Chicks and eggs are screened so that the flocks are maintained free of *Mycoplasma*.

Herds of pigs free of swine Mycoplasmas and

Table 30–3. Mycoplasmas and Acholeplasmas Associated with Diseases of Animals*

Animal Species Affected	Disease	Organisms
Cattle	Pneumonia	*Mycoplasma mycoides* var. *mycoides*
		M. bovis
		M. dispar
		Ureaplasmas
	Arthritis	*M. bovis*
		M. bovigenitalium
	Mastitis	*M. bovis*
		M. californicum
	Abortion	*M. bovis*
	Vaginitis	Ureaplasmas
		M. bovigenitalium
	Seminal vesiculitis	*M. bovis*
		M. bovigenitalium
	Uncertain	*M. bovirhinis*
		M. alkalescens
		M. arginini
		Acholeplasma modicum
		A. laidlawii
		M. bovoculi
		M. verecundum
		M. canadense
		M. alvi
Swine	Pneumonia	*M. hyopneumoniae*
	Arthritis	*M. hyorhinis*
		M. hyosynoviae
	Uncertain	*M. flocculare*
		M. sualvi
		A. axanthum
		A. granularum
Sheep and Goats	Pneumonia	*M. ovipneumoniae*
	Pneumonia,	*M. mycoides* ss. *capri*
	Arthritis,	*M. mycoides* ss. *mycoides*
	Mastitis	*M. agalactiae*
		M. putrefaciens
	Conjunctivitis	*M. conjunctivae*
	Arthritis	*M. capricolum*
	Uncertain	*M. arginini*
		M. oculi
Horses	Uncertain	*M. equigenitalium*
		M. equirhinis
		M. subdolum
		M. felis
		M. arginini
		M. salivarium
		A. equifetale
		A. hippikon
		A. laidlawii
Rats and Mice	Pneumonia	*M. pulmonis*
	Arthritis	*M. arthritidis*
	Rolling disease	*M. neurolyticum*
Guinea pigs	Uncertain	*M. caviae*
Dogs	Pneumonia	*M. cynos*
	Uncertain	*M. spumans*
		M. maculosum
		M. edwardii
		M. molare
		M. canis
		M. opalescens
Cats	Possibly conjunctivitis	*M. felis*
	Uncertain	*M. gateae*

*(Adapted from Stalheim, O.H.V.: Mycoplasmas of animals. *In* Diagnostic Procedures in Veterinary Bacteriology and Mycology. Edited by G.R. Carter. 4th Ed. Springfield, Ill., Charles C Thomas, 1984.)

other important viral and bacterial pathogens (specific pathogen-free or SPF pigs) have been established from caesarian-delivered pigs raised in isolation.

IMMUNIZATION

Cattle are vaccinated with a live attenuated *M. mycoides* ss. *mycoides* strain to prevent contagious bovine pleuropneumonia.

SUGGESTED CLINICAL EXAMPLES

An outbreak of chronic respiratory disease in broiler chickens.

An outbreak of infectious synovitis in turkeys.

Mycoplasma polyserositis involving pre-weaned pigs.

Mycoplasma arthritis in feeder pigs in the 75 to 175 lb range.

Cases of fulminating enzootic pneumonia in a swine herd.

A herd outbreak of *Mycoplasma* mastitis.

Mycoplasma pneumonia in lambs.

Granular vaginitis and infertility in a dairy herd.

SOURCES FOR FURTHER READING

Afshar, A.: Diseases of bovine reproduction associated with *Mycoplasma* infections. Vet. Bull., *45*:211, 1975.

Allam, N.M., Powell, D.G., Andrews, B.E., and Lemcke, R.M.: Isolation of *Mycoplasma* species from horses. Vet. Rec., *93*:402, 1973.

Doig, P.A., Ruknke, H.L., and Palmer, N.C.: Experimental bovine ureaplasmosis. 1. Granular vulvitis following vulvar inoculation. Can. J. Comp. Med., *44*:252, 1974.

East, N.E., et al.: Milkborne outbreak of *Mycoplasma mycoides* subspecies *mycoides* infection in a commercial goat dairy. J. Am. Vet. Med. Assoc., *182*:1138, 1983.

Jasper, D.E.: *Mycoplasma* and mycoplasma mastitis. J. Am. Vet. Med. Assoc., *170*:1167, 1977.

Jones, G.E.: Mycoplasmas of sheep and goats: A synopsis. Vet. Rec., *113*:619, 1983.

Rosendal, S.: Canine mycoplasmas II. Biochemical characteristics and serological differentiation. Acta Pathol. Microbiol. Scand., *82B*:25, 1974.

Stalheim, O.H.V., and Page, L.A.: Naturally occurring and experimentally-induced mycoplasmal arthritis of cattle. J. Clin. Microbiol., *2*:165, 1975.

Stalheim, O.H.V.: Mycoplasmal respiratory disease of ruminants: A review and update. J. Am. Vet. Med. Assoc., *182*:403, 1983.

Stalheim, O.H.V.: Mycoplasmas of animals. *In* Diagnostic Procedures in Veterinary Bacteriology and Mycology. Edited by G.R. Carter. 4th Ed. Springfield, Ill., Charles C Thomas, 1984.

Tully, J.G., and Whitcomb, R.G. (eds.): The Mycoplasmas. Vol. 2. Human and Animal Mycoplasmas. New York, Academic Press, Inc., 1979.

Whittlestone, P.: Mycoplasmas in diseases of domestic animals. *In* The Veterinary Annual. Edited by C.S.G. Grunsell and F.W.G. Hill. Bristol, England, John Wright, 1973.

Whittlestone, P.: Enzootic pneumonia of pigs (EPP). Adv. Vet. Sci. Comp. Med., *17*:1, 1973.

Wilkinson, G.T.: Mycoplasmas of the cat. *In* The Veterinary Annual. Edited by C.S.G. Grunsell and F.W.G. Hill. Bristol, England, Scientechnica, 1980.

Yoder, H.W., Jr.: Avian mycoplasmas. *In* Diagnostic Procedures in Veterinary Bacteriology and Mycology. Edited by G.R. Carter. 4th Ed. Springfield, Ill., Charles C Thomas, 1984.

Part III

FUNGI

31

Introduction to the Fungi and Fungous Infections

What follows is a very brief introduction to the fungi and the diseases they cause. If time permits, this information should be supplemented by references cited under "Sources for Further Reading."

GENERAL CHARACTERISTICS OF THE FUNGI

For the most part the fungi are nonmotile and possess cell walls that somewhat resemble those of plants in chemical composition and structure. Fungi grow as single cells—the yeasts—or as multicellular filamentous colonies—the molds and mushrooms. The fungi are not photosynthetic, and consequently they are restricted to a saprophytic or parasitic existence. They are abundant and widespread in the soil, on vegetation, and in water, where they subsist on decaying vegetation and wood.

The two principal kinds of fungi are the molds and the yeasts. The main element of the vegetative or growing form of the mold is the hypha, a branching tubular structure 2 to 10 μm in diameter. As growth begins, hyphae become intertwined to form a mycelium. The vegetative mycelium consists of the surface hyphae, while the hyphae that arise above the surface are referred to as the aerial mycelium. Under certain conditions the hyphae of the aerial mycelium produce reproductive cells or spores. These are collectively referred to as fruiting bodies. The hyphae of many fungi are divided by cross-walls called septa.

The yeasts are oval or spherical cells ranging in diameter from 3 to 5 μm. Some varieties of yeasts or yeast-like fungi produce chains of irregular yeast cells that are referred to as pseudohyphae. Some fungi that exist in the mycelial form in nature at room temperature will convert to a yeast form at 37°C or in the tissues of animals. These fungi are called dimorphic. Many of the properties of the fungi that distinguish them from bacteria are summarized in Table 1–1.

The great majority of the fungi that are pathogenic for animals and humans lack sexuality. For this reason only asexual reproduction will be considered. The three mechanisms of asexual reproduction are (1) sporulation followed by germination of the spores (Aspergillus and Penicillium); (2) fragmentation of hyphae (Coccidioides immitis, Geotrichum candidum); and (3) budding of yeast cells (Candida, Cryptococcus).

The various reproductive structures are defined below and referred to later under specific disease-producing fungi.

The sexual stage of a number of the dermatophytic (ringworm) fungi has been observed, e.g., the sexual or perfect stage of Microsporum nanum is called Nannizzia obtusa (ascomycetes). Only the asexual stage is found in infected skin. The sexual stage of Cryptococcus neoformans is called Filobasidiella neoformans.

COMMONLY USED MYCOLOGIC TERMS

Arthrospore: An asexual spore formed by the disarticulation of the mycelium, as can be seen in *Geotrichum candidum*.

Ascospore: A sexual spore characteristic of the true yeasts or ascomycetes. It is produced in a sac-like structure called an ascus. This ascospore results from the fusion of two nuclei and is seen in *Saccharomyces* spp.

Ascus: The specialized sac-like structure characteristic of the true yeasts in which ascospores are produced. This is found in *Saccharomyces* spp.

Blastospore: A spore produced as a result of a budding process along the mycelium or from a single spore, as in *Saccharomyces* spp.

Chlamydospores: Thick-walled, resistant spores formed by the direct differentiation of hyphae, as seen in *Candida albicans* and *Histoplasma capsulatum*.

Clavate: Club-shaped such as the microconidia of *Microsporum nanum*.

Columnella: The persisting dome-shaped upper portion of the sporangiophore, which can be seen in *Mucor* spp.

Conidium: An asexual spore formed from hyphae by abstriction, budding, or septal division, as in *Penicillium* spp.

Conidiophore: A stalk-like branch of the mycelium on which conidia develop either singly or in numbers as found in *Penicillium* spp.

Dematiaceous: A term used to denote the dark brown or black fungi such as *Phialophora* spp., and *Hormodendrum* spp.

Dimorphic: Having two forms or phases, referred to as the yeast form and mycelial form. *Blastomyces dermatitidis* is dimorphic.

Echinulate: Spiny, for example the macroconidia of *Microsporum*.

Endogenous: Originating or produced from within. *Candida albicans* infections are usually considered endogenous.

Exogenous: Originating from without, such as *Histoplasma capsulatum* infection.

Ectothrix: Occurring outside the hair shaft, as does *Microsporum* spp.

Geophilic: Denotes fungi whose natural habitat is the soil, such as *Coccidioides immitis*.

Germ Tube: Tube-like structures produced by germinating spores. They develop into hyphae, as in *Candida albicans*.

Glabrous: The smooth form, for example, the glabrous form of *Geotrichum candidum*.

Hyphae: The filaments that compose the body or thallus of a fungus.

Macroconidia: Large, multicelled conidia; they may be fusiform (spindle-shaped) or clavate (club-shaped). If divided by transverse and longitudinal septations, they are termed muriform (having walls). *Microsporum canis* produces them.

Microconidia: Small, single-celled conidia borne laterally on hyphae. They may be spherical, elliptical, oval, pyriform (pear-shaped) or clavate. *Microsporum canis* produces them.

Mycelium: A mat made up of intertwining, thread-like hyphae.

Nodes: The points on the stolons from which the rhizoids arise, as in *Rhizopus* spp.

Pseudohyphae: Filaments composed of elongated budding cells that have failed to detach, as seen in *Candida albicans*.

Rhizoid: Root-like, branched hyphae extending into the medium, as in *Absidia* spp.

Septate: Has cross-walls or septa in the hyphae, as found in the hyphae of *Aspergillus*.

Sporangiophore: A specialized hypha bearing a sporangium, for example in *Rhizopus* spp.

Sporangium: A closed, often spherical structure in which asexual spores are prouced by cleavage (*Rhizopus*).

Sterigmata: Specialized structures, short or elongated, borne on a vesicle and producing conidia, as seen in *Aspergillus*.

Stolon: A horizontal hypha or runner that sprouts where it touches the substrate. It forms rhizoids in the substrate, as observed in *Absidia* spp.

Vesicle: The terminal swollen portion of a conidiophore, which is seen in *Aspergillus*.

Yeasts: An ill-defined group of unicellular fungi lacking mycelium and reproducing asexually by blastospores and occasionally by sexually produced ascospores. The latter are the true yeasts (*Saccharomyces* spp.).

Zygospore: A thick-walled, sexual spore of the true fungi that results from the fusion of two similar gametangia, as in *Phycomycetes*.

FUNGOUS INFECTIONS: GENERAL CONSIDERATIONS

The fungi causing disease in animals and humans are broadly classified as follows:

1. *Frankly pathogenic fungi:* those that cause

ringworm and the more common mycoses such as blastomycosis and histoplasmosis.

2. *Opportunistic fungi:* those that seldom cause disease. They are widespread in nature, constituting species of a number of genera, e.g., *Penicillium, Aspergillus, Mucor, Absidia,* and *Rhizopus.*

A number of circumstances may give rise to systemic fungous infections:

1. Prolonged administration of antibiotics. Mode of action:
   a. Lowered resistance; mechanisms not known for certain; effect may be on phagocytosis or antibody production.
   b. Interfere with synthesis of vitamins by effect on normal flora, e.g., vitamin K, vitamin B complex components.
   c. Upsets the floral balance, depressing bacteria and favoring fungi, as in intestinal candidiasis.
2. Radiation, steroid therapy, urethane, mustard gas, and folic acid antagonists may activate latent fungous and bacterial infections. Steroids inhibit inflammatory as well as antibody response.
3. Cancer; fungous infections occur in patients with leukemia or lymphoma, particularly if they are being treated with antibiotics. Fungous infections are not uncommon in debilitated patients with terminal malignancies.
4. Immunosuppressive therapy, for example with azathioprine; patients are more susceptible to aspergillosis, cryptococcosis, and various opportunistic fungi.
5. Cytotoxic drugs: ablation of the bone marrow in the treatment of leukemia.
6. Immune deficiencies: T-cell deficiency, thymic hypoplasia, and anergy.

SOME GENERAL FEATURES OF FUNGOUS INFECTIONS

1. Most fungi capable of causing disease in animals and humans are classified among the Fungi Imperfecti (see Chapter 1).
2. Diseases caused by fungi do not usually assume epidemiologic or epizootiologic proportions. Some exceptions are the dermatomycoses and infrequently aspergillosis, histoplasmosis, and cryptococcosis.
3. Conclusive proof that fungi produce classic exotoxins or endotoxins is as yet lacking.

4. Some features of most fungous diseases are
   a. Low invasiveness and low virulence of the organism.
   b. Certain predisposing factors contributing to the establishment of infection.
      i. Production of a necrotic focus by trauma, infection, or ischemia.
      ii. Lowered general resistance.
      iii. Moist environment, e.g., *Candida* infections in humans.
      iv. Exposure to a large number of organisms, e.g., brooder pneumonia.
   c. Chronicity of infection leads to a granulomatous process that resembles the reaction to a foreign body.
   d. Immunity is considered to be more cell-mediated than antibody-mediated.
5. Infected and exposed animals may develop a sensitivity to the fungus in question. The role of this hypersensitivity in connection with pathogenesis and immunity is not clear. It is thought that hypersensitivity may contribute to dissemination of the infection.
6. Fungi are identified principally by the study of cultural characteristics and the microscopic morphology of the so-called "fruiting bodies" or reproductive elements.

IMMUNITY TO FUNGOUS INFECTIONS

IMMUNE RESPONSE

Most of the fungi produce diseases that are characterized by granulomatous lesions not unlike those produced by mycobacteria and other bacterial facultative intracellular parasites. Most fungal infections are asymptomatic, limited, and readily eliminated by the animal. Such exposed animals will usually manifest a positive delayed-type hypersensitivity skin reaction.

Antibodies to the various fungi are found in all the mycotic diseases except the dermatomycoses. In these superficial infections the antibody-producing cells are not stimulated. Antibody titers may be negative or low in asymptomatic or mild infections. It would appear that immunity to fungous infections is more cell-mediated than humoral. Serum antibodies from infected animals do not protect normal animals from experimental infections.

Most animals exposed to or infected by fungi

develop a hypersensitivity of the delayed type that is detectable by inoculation of fungi or their products into the skin. Hypersensitivity to products of fungi spread hematogenously is responsible for the skin eruptions accompanying the dermatomycoses ("id" eruption), candidiasis, and coccidioidomycosis. Hypersensitivity and resistance are closely related in the animal's response to infection. There is a correlation between recovery and the development and persistence of delayed hypersensitivity. When a state of anergy (absence of delayed hypersensitivity reaction) develops in a serious systemic infection, the prognosis is usually poor.

Skin tests analogous to the tuberculin test are used in blastomycosis, histoplasmosis, coccidioidomycosis, and sporotrichosis. Various elements of the fungus are inoculated intradermally. A reaction of the delayed hypersensitivity type constitutes a positive test. A positive test indicates either past or current infection, and the result is considered along with other information in arriving at a diagnosis. The test result may be negative if the animal is anergic.

SEROLOGY OF MYCOTIC INFECTIONS

The serologic diagnosis of mycotic infections of animals has received little attention. Some of the serologic procedures that are employed in important mycoses of humans are mentioned under specific diseases. Not all veterinary diagnostic microbiology laboratories are prepared to carry out these procedures. Assistance is sometimes available through the courtesy of some hospital and public health laboratories.

It should be kept in mind that the skin tests and serologic procedures referred to under specific diseases were developed for use in human beings and that animals may respond somewhat differently.

TREATMENT OF MYCOTIC INFECTION: GENERAL

The polyene antibiotics produced by various *Streptomyces* spp. have revolutionized the treatment of mycotic diseases. The principal drugs in the polyene group are amphotericin B, nystatin, hamycin, and pimaricin. They probably combine with sterols in the cytoplasmic membrane of fungi and adversely affect its function. Sterols are not present in bacteria. They are present in red blood cells, however, and hemolytic anemia can be a side-effect. Renal toxicity is the most serious side-effect seen with amphotericin B.

The drug 5-fluorocytosine, which is useful in the treatment of several mycotic diseases, is thought to interfere with the metabolic pathways of some fungi and as a result is fungistatic. It is relatively nontoxic when given orally. Resistance of *Candida albicans* has been encountered.

The synthetic benzimidazole derivatives, collectively called imidazoles, are recently developed drugs with antifungal activity. They affect the fungal cell wall and cell membrane, resulting in interference with nutrient utilization. Miconazole and ketoconazole appear to be the most useful. Although side-effects are seen, they are not as serious as those that can accompany amphotericin B therapy. Because these drugs are generally less effective than amphotericin B, they are best used in selected cases and occasionally to supplement or replace amphotericin B.

GROUPING OF FUNGOUS DISEASES

The fungous diseases are grouped in subsequent chapters as follows:
1. Dermatophytosis
2. Mycoses Caused by Yeasts and Yeast-like Fungi:
    a. Candidiasis
    b. Cryptococcosis
    c. Geotrichosis
3. Subcutaneous Mycoses:
    a. Sporotrichosis
    b. Chromomycosis
    c. Maduromycosis
    d. Epizootic Lymphangitis
    e. Rhinosporidiosis
4. Systemic Mycoses:
    a. Zygomycosis
    b. Aspergillosis
    c. Blastomycosis
    d. Histoplasmosis
    e. Coccidioidomycosis
    f. Adiaspiromycosis

This is an arbitrary grouping, and occasionally the subcutaneous mycoses may produce systemic disease; conversely, some of the agents causing systemic disease may be confined to the subcutis.

LABORATORY PROCEDURES

The fungi grow well on simple media at room temperature (22 to 25°C). The most commonly used media are variations of Sabouraud dextrose agar. The latter contains peptone, dextrose, and agar and has a pH of 5.6. The low pH inhibits the growth of bacteria. All fungi grow aerobically.

A number of fungi will grow in the yeast phase at 37°C. The media most commonly used at this temperature are blood agar and brain heart infusion agar.

Inocula should be large, and incubation periods as long as a month may be required.

Cycloheximide (Actidione) may be added to Sabouraud agar to inhibit the growth of many saprophytic fungi. It should be remembered that it also inhibits some important fungi: *Pseudoallescheria boydii, Aspergillus fumigatus,* and *Cryptococcus neoformans.* Chloromycetin is added to Sabouraud agar to inhibit bacteria.

A variety of media are used in mycology laboratories for special purposes, such as demonstration of chlamydospores, growth of some dermatophytes, and the presumptive identification of certain yeasts.

SOURCES FOR FURTHER READING

GENERAL

Ainsworth, G.C., and Austwick, K.C.: Fungal Diseases of Animals. 2nd Ed. Farnham Royal, England, Commonwealth Agricultural Bureaux, 1973.

Beneke, E.S., and Rogers, A.L.: Medical Mycology Manual. 4th Ed. Minneapolis, Burgess Publishing Co., 1980.

Campbell, M.C., and Stewart, J.L.: The Medical Mycology Handbook. New York, John Wiley & Sons, 1980.

Conant, N.F., Smith, D.T., Baker, R.D., and Calloway, J.L.: Manual of Clinical Mycology. 3rd Ed. Philadelphia, W.B. Saunders Co., 1971.

Emmons, C.W., Binford, C.H., Utz, J.P., and Kwong-Chung, K.J.: Medical Mycology. 3rd Ed. Philadelphia, Lea & Febiger, 1977.

Haley, L.D., Trandel, J., and Coyle, M.B.: Practical Methods for the Cultures and Identification of Fungi in the Clinical Microbiology Laboratory. Washington, D.C., Cumitech 77, A. Society Microbiology, 1980.

Jungerman, P.F., and Schwartzman, R.M.: Veterinary Medical Mycology. Philadelphia, Lea & Febiger, 1972.

Rippon, J.W.: Medical Mycology. 2nd Ed. Philadelphia, W.B. Saunders Company, 1982.

IMMUNITY AND SEROLOGY

Balows, A., Ausherman, R.J., and Hopper, J.M.: Practical diagnosis and therapy of canine histoplasmosis and blastomycosis. J. Am. Vet. Med. Assoc., *148*:678, 1966.

Coleman, R.M., and Kaufman, L.: Use of the immunodiffusion test in the serodiagnosis of aspergillosis. Appl. Microbiol., *23*:301, 1972.

Kaufman, L.: Serodiagnosis of fungal diseases. *In* Manual of Clinical Microbiology. Edited by E.H. Lennette et al. 3rd Ed. Washington, D.C., American Society of Microbiology, 1980.

Kaufman, L., et al.: Specific immunodiffusion test for systemic candidiasis. J. Infect. Dis., *17*:180, 1973.

Lane, J.G., and Warnock, D.W.: The diagnosis of *Aspergillus fumigatus* infection of the nasal chambers of the dog with particular reference to the value of the double diffusion test. J. Sm. Anim. Pract., *18*:169, 1977.

Palmer, D.F., Kaufman, L., Kaplan, W., and Cavallaro, J.J.: Serodiagnosis of Mycotic Diseases. Springfield, Ill., Charles C Thomas, 1977.

Walter, J.E., and Jones, R.D.: Serologic tests in the diagnosis of aspergillosis. Dis. Chest., *53*:729, 1968.

Ytturraspe, D.J.: Clinical evaluation of a latex particle agglutination test and a gel diffusion precipitin test in the diagnosis of canine coccidioidomycosis. J. Am. Vet. Med. Assoc., *158*:1249, 1971.

THERAPY

Balows, A., Ausherman, R.J., and Hopper, J.M.: Practical diagnosis and therapy of canine histoplasmosis and blastomycosis. J. Am. Vet. Med. Assoc., *148*:678, 1966.

Crounse, R.J.: Effective use of griseofulvin. Arch. Dermatol., *83*:176, 1961.

Kirk, R.W. (ed.): Current Veterinary Therapy VIII, Philadelphia, W.B. Saunders, 1983.

McMullan, W.C., Joyce, J.R., Hanselka, D.V., and Heitman, J.M.: Amphotericin B for the treatment of localized subcutaneous phycomycosis in the horse. J. Am. Vet. Med. Assoc., *170*:1293, 1977.

Medoff, G., and Kobayashi, G.S.: Strategies in the treatment of systemic fungal infections. N. Engl. J. Med., *302*:145, 1980.

Pratt, W.B.: Chemotherapy of Infection. New York, Oxford University Press, 1977.

Pyle, R.L.: Clinical pharmacology of amphotericin B. J. Am. Vet. Med. Assoc., *179*:83, 1981.

Weir, E.C., Schwartz, A., and Buergelt, C.D.: Short-term combination chemotherapy for treatment of feline cryptococcosis. J. Am. Vet. Med. Assoc., *174*:507, 1979.

32

Dermatophytosis (Dermatomycosis)

GENERAL CONSIDERATIONS

The dermatophytes belong in the Fungi Imperfecti. The "perfect state," i.e., the sexual phase, has been demonstrated for several of the dermatophytes, thus transferring them to the class Ascomycetes.

They are highly adapted parasites although several, e.g., *Microsporum gypseum* and *M. nanum,* can survive for long periods in soil (geophilic). On the basis of host preference, fungi associated with the lower animals and humans are termed, respectively, zoophilic and anthropophilic. Some have a broad host range, while others infect only a few animal species (Table 32–1).

Infection by a dermatophyte may result in a state of hypersensitivity to an extract of the dermatophyte. Both the lesions and the immunity are related to this sensitivity. Vesicular lesions may appear on various parts of the body as part of a general allergic reaction. They result from the hematogenous spread of the fungi or its products. These lesions do not contain the organism. They are called dermatophytids or "id" lesions or reactions. They occasionally occur in dogs.

Secondary bacterial invaders such as *Staphylococcus aureus* are not uncommon. Pustules may be formed in hair follicles.

Dermatophytes can hydrolyze keratin. The epidermis and hair are the principal structures attacked in lower animals. The dermatomycoses are almost always superficial.

Characteristically, dermatophytosis is more frequently observed in stabled farm animals than in pastured animals. The incidence is usually higher during winter months, and the disease may clear up spontaneously during spring and summer.

In domestic animals there are no apparent differences in the clinical appearances of infections produced by the different dermatophytes. The lesions in domestic animals are usually characterized by circular, scaly areas of alopecia with or without crust formation. In dogs and cats, lesions occur most frequently on the head and extremities. The head and tail are the most frequent locations in horses and cattle.

Dermatophytosis may be transmitted from animal to animal, or to humans, by direct or indirect contact.

Frequently cases of dermatomycosis believed to be reinfections are only remissions of previously treated clinical infections.

The term "ringworm" denotes a clinical entity rather than an infection caused by a specific dermatophyte. In the lower animals two genera of dermatophytes are encountered, *Microsporum* and *Trichophyton.*

DIFFERENCES BETWEEN IMPORTANT GENERA OF DERMATOPHYTES

Microsporum	*Trichophyton*
Some species fluoresce: *M. canis* regularly, *M. gypseum* poorly or not at all	Most do not fluoresce
Macroconidia occur frequently	Macroconidia are seen less commonly
Some macroconidia are spiny	Macroconidia are thin-walled and not spiny
Location of spores: ectothrix	Location of spores: ectothrix and endothrix

228

Table 32–1. Summary of Principal Characteristics of Important Veterinary Dermatophytes*

Species	Principal Hosts	Fluorescence	Arthrospores	Cultural Features	Macroconidia	Microconidia	Other
M. canis	Dog (70%), cat (98%), humans, monkey, horse	+	Ectothrix, small, mosaic	White to buff; reverse: yellow to orange; rapid grower	Spindle-shaped, frequent	Few, sessile	Accessory structures similar to those of *T. gallinae*
M. gypseum	Dog (20%), horse, cat (10%)	–	Ectothrix, large, chains	Buff; reverse: orange brown to yellow; moderately rapid	Ellipsoidal, septa 2–6, frequent	Sessile or on short sterigmata; clavate	Persists in soil; accessory structures similar to those of *T. gallinae*
M. nanum	Swine	–	Ectothrix, large, chains	White to buff; reverse: red; moderately rapid	Obovoid to ellipsoidal ovate; frequent	Clavate	Persists in soil
T. mentagrophytes var. granular Humans: downy form	Many animal species, including all domestic animals	–	Ectothrix, large, chains	Granular, light buff to tan; reverse: variable red, yellow, etc., fairly rapid	Occurrence variable; spindle or clavate; 5–6 septa	Abundant, pyriform or clavate, sessile	*T. equinum* resembles *T. mentagrophytes*; requires nicotinic acid. Causes ringworm in the horse.
T. verrucosum	Cattle, sheep	–	Ectothrix, large, chains	Deeply folded, white to brilliant yellow; slow	Requires thiamine; long and thin-walled. Rare	Abundant with thiamine; singly ovoid; pyriform or clavate	Chlamydospores; grows better at 37° than at 25°C
T. gallinae	Fowl favus or white comb	–	Ectothrix, large, chains	Radial folds, white to pale rose; reverse: red; moderately rapid	Infrequent; club-shaped and clavate	Singly on hyphae, pyriform to clavate	Chlamydospores, nodular bodies, pectinate bodies, racquet hyphae

*Other dermatophytes are encountered less frequently in the domestic animals. Among these are *T. rubrum*, reported from the dog; *M. audouinii*, reported from the dog and monkey; and *T. schoenleinii*, reported from horses and cats in Europe.

Procedure for the Laboratory Diagnosis of Dermatophytosis

1. If feasible, examine patient in the dark with a Wood's lamp to determine if fluorescence is present. If present, remove some fluorescing hairs with forceps for microscopic examination. Also remove hairs at edge of lesions for examination.

2. Hairs and skin scrapings are examined in 10% or 20% NaOH under a coverslip for the presence of arthrospores. The preparation should be gently warmed for about 10 minutes before examining.

3. Regardless of whether arthrospores are found, material is inoculated onto Sabouraud agar containing cyclohexamide and chloramphenicol. Do not discard plates until they have been incubated at room temperature (25 to 30°C) for at least a month. *T. verrucosum* (cattle) requires a medium supplemented with inositol and thiamine; *T. equinum* requires nicotinic acid. Yeast extract is a satisfactory source of these growth supplements.

4. If fungi grow, examine colonies grossly for morphology, texture, and pigment, as seen from under the colonies. Then examine the mycelium or other material microscopically in a lactophenol cotton blue wet mount. The tape mount is a convenient procedure. The principal morphologic and cultural characteristics of the important dermatophytes of animals are summarized in Table 32–1. The morphology of the macroconidia of the major animal dermatophytes is shown in Figure 32–1. Their demonstration in cultures is significant in identification.

A medium called Dermatophyte Test Medium is available commercially under a number of trade names. When dermatophytes grow on this modified Sabouraud agar (which contains phenol red), they change the yellow medium to red (alkaline), usually within two weeks. This is a useful screening medium. It is advisable to submit positive cultures to a microbiology laboratory for confirmatory examination.

Treatment of Dermatophytosis

The animal or animals should be isolated if possible. Precautions should be taken to prevent human infections.

The following are employed: Whitfield's ointment (salicylic and benzoic acid), which is keratolytic in its action. Tincture of iodine may be painted on the lesions.

Fatty acids such as zinc and sodium salts of

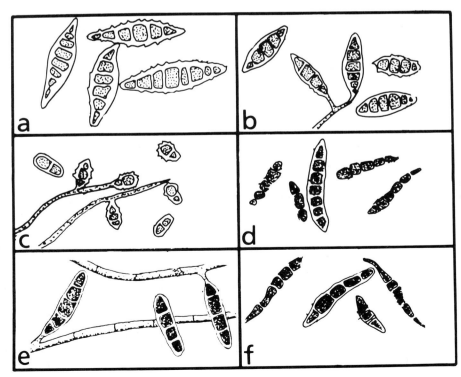

Figure 32–1. Macroconidia of important dermatophytes: a, *Microsporum canis*; b, *M. gypseum*; c, *M. nanum*; d, *Trichophyton mentagrophytes*, e, *T. equinum*; and f, *T. verrucosum*.

propionic, undecylenic, and caprylic acids are useful topically, as are tolnaftate, natamycin (pimaricin), and the imidazole derivatives—miconazole and clotrimazole. Natamycin is a polyene or tetraene antibiotic like nystatin and amphotericin B.

Griseofulvin (from *Penicillium griseofulvum*) is effective when given orally but is too expensive as a rule for large animal use. The drug accumulates in keratinous structures (cornified layer of the epidermis, hair, and nails) and renders them resistant to infection. Prolonged treatment is usually required.

Cattle ringworm usually clears up in the spring after the animals leave the stable. Clorox and other antifungal preparations, including natamycin, are applied as sprays.

SUGGESTED CLINICAL EXAMPLES

Dermatomycosis in the dog, cat, and horse.
Dermatomycosis in stabled cattle.
Dermatomycosis in a swine herd.

SOURCES FOR FURTHER READING

(Note: See also sources for Chapter 31.)
Carrol, H.F.: Evaluation of dermatophyte test medium for diagnosis of dermatophytosis. J. Am. Vet. Med. Assoc., *165*:192, 1974.

Carter, G.R. (ed).: Diagnostic Procedures in Veterinary Bacteriology and Mycology. Springfield, Ill., Charles C Thomas, 1984.

Crounse, R.J.: Effective use of griseofulvin. Arch. Dermatol., *83*:176, 1961.

Dawson, C.O.: Ringworm in animals. Rev. Med. Vet. Mycol., *6*:223, 1968.

Dvorak, J., and Otcenasek, M.: Mycological Diagnosis of Animal Dermatophytoses. The Hague, Dr. W. Junk, N.V., Publishers, 1969.

Gentles, J.C., Dawson, C.O., and Connole, M.D.: Keratophilic fungi on cats and dogs. Sabouraudia, *4*:171, 1965.

Georg, L.K., Kaplan, W., and Camp, L.B.: Equine ringworm with special reference to *Trichophyton equinum*. Am. J. Vet. Res., *18*:798, 1957.

Ginther, O.J.: Clinical aspects of *Microsporum nanum* infection in swine. J. Am. Vet. Med. Assoc., *146*:945, 1965.

Grappel, S.F., Bishop, C.T., and Blank, F.: Immunology of dermatophytes and dermatophytosis. Bacteriol. Rev., *38*:222, 1974.

Kane, J., Padhye, A.A., and Ajello, L.: *Microsporum equinum* in North America. J. Clin. Microbiol., *16*:943, 1982.

Oldenkamp, E.P., and Spanoghe, L.: Natamycin treatment of ringworm in cattle. Netherlands J. Vet. Sci., *102*:124, 1977.

Oldenkamp, E.P.: Treatment of ringworm of the horse with natamycin. Vet. Rec., *11*:36, 1979.

Pratt, W.B.: Chemotherapy of Infection. New York, Oxford University Press, 1977.

Rebell, G., and Taplin, D.: Dermatophytes, Their Recognition and Identification. Revised Ed. Coral Gables, Fla. University of Miami Press, 1970.

Vanbreuseghem, R.: Guide Pratique Mycologie Medicale et Veterinaire. Paris, Masson et Cie, 1966.

33

Mycoses Caused by Yeasts or Yeast-like Fungi

CANDIDIASIS (MONILIASIS, THRUSH)

A number of species of *Candida* can be differentiated by biochemical tests. All *Candida* occur saprophytically. The important species from the standpoint of disease is *C. albicans*. It is a normal inhabitant of the digestive tract, oral cavity, and vagina. Infections are usually endogenous.

The following *Candida* species have been implicated as causes of bovine mastitis: *C. albicans, C. krusei, C. pseudotropicalis, C. rugosa,* and *C. tropicalis.*

PATHOGENICITY

Infections occur most frequently on mucous membranes of the digestive and genital tracts. The young are especially susceptible. Candidiasis involving the gastrointestinal tract may result from prolonged antibiotic therapy. Natural infections in animals appear to be uncommon, and there are few reports in the literature.

Puppies, Kittens, Calves, and Foals. Infection of the oral and intestinal mucous membrane is uncommon. Mycotic stomatitis and enteritis result, and white to gray patches representing pseudomembranous inflammation of the mucous membrane are seen.

Swine. Infections of the lower esophagus and esophageal region of the stomach occur. *C. candidum* may be found in stomach ulcers.

Chickens, Turkeys, and Other Birds. Infec-tions of the mouth, esophagus, and crop occur, with pseudomembranous whitish areas, usually in young animals. Crop mycosis (thrush) may affect a considerable number of young chickens and turkeys.

Humans. The clinical picture varies, depending on the site of infection. The mucous membranes of the mouth, tongue, and genital tract are more commonly involved than the nails and skin. The oral form (thrush), characterized by white patches, occurs not uncommonly in infants. Respiratory tract infections usually involve the lungs. Occasionally endocarditis and bone infections are encountered.

Cows. Mastitis caused by *Candida* is common in cows.

Mares and Cows. *Candida albicans* causes metritis and vaginitis in mares and cows.

Stallions and Bulls. Genital candidiasis is seen in stallions and bulls.

ISOLATION AND CULTIVATION

Organisms can frequently be seen in wet mounts and in smears stained with Gram's stain (gram-positive), where they appear as oval, thin-walled, budding cells and hyphal fragments (pseudohyphae).

They are readily cultivated on blood agar and Sabouraud agar at 22°C and at 37°C. Soft, creamy colonies resembling those of staphylococci are seen in 24 to 48 hours.

IDENTIFICATION

This is accomplished by the demonstration of the large chlamydospores (see Fig. 35–1) or germ tubes characteristic of *C. albicans.* Plates of corn meal or chlamydospore agar are inoculated by cutting into the agar at an angle to the bottom of the plate. If present, the chlamydospores can be seen below the surface in 24 to 48 hours by focusing directly on the line of inoculation.

In order to demonstrate germ tubes, a small amount of serum is inoculated with a light inoculum of growth. After incubation for two hours at 37°C, a drop from the serum sediment is examined microscopically. A germ tube is a filamentous outgrowth from the yeast cell. Unlike in pseudohyphae, there is no restriction at the point of origin.

Species of *Candida* other than *C. albicans* are identified by carbohydrate fermentation and assimilation tests.

ANIMAL INOCULATION

Rabbits are susceptible to intravenous inoculation. Abscesses develop in the kidneys.

TREATMENT

Nystatin (mycostatin) is used in ointments for skin infections and locally for oral and genital infections. It is administered in the feed to treat candidiasis in chickens and turkeys, and intestinal and oral candidiasis in swine, dogs, and cats. Very little of the drug is absorbed orally. It has been administered in the mammary gland to treat mastitis caused by *Candida* species.

Amphotericin B is the most effective drug for the treatment of systemic candidiasis. Flucytosine (5-fluorocytosine) has been used with some success.

Ketoconazole and clotrimazole have been effective in the treatment of mucocutaneous candidiasis in human beings.

CRYPTOCOCCOSIS (TORULOSIS)

There are several species in the genus *Cryptococcus.* Only *Cryptococcus neoformans* is considered potentially pathogenic. It occurs in nature and reaches high concentrations in pigeon droppings and nests. The pigeon is not infected; the organisms colonize feces after they have been passed. Infections are exogenous and are usually acquired by inhalation. Primary foci are most often in the respiratory system, including the paranasal sinuses, with subsequent spread.

PATHOGENICITY

In cattle, only sporadic cases of mastitis have been reported. It is uncommon in sheep and goats.

In the dog and cat, the organisms show a predilection for the central nervous system. Infections of the pharynx and paranasal sinuses are seen, with dissemination to the CNS. A form with subcutaneous granulomas is also seen.

In horses, it is most frequently seen as a paranasal infection, which may or may not spread to other tissues, including the brain.

In humans, infections involving the lungs and central nervous system (cryptococcal meningitis) are most common.

DIRECT EXAMINATION

Yeast-like cells can be seen in wet mounts of cerebrospinal fluid and pus. The large capsule can be seen if clinical material is mixed with India ink or nigrosin (see Fig. 35–1). The yeast-like cells are gram-positive and can be seen in stained smears.

ISOLATION AND CULTIVATION

The organism grows at 37°C and 25°C on blood agar and Sabouraud agar; it is inhibited by cycloheximide. Wrinkled, whitish granular colonies usually appear within a week. They become slimy, mucoid, and cream to brownish in color on further incubation. Budding yeast-like cells with large capsules can be seen in wet mounts.

Most saprophytic strains of *Cryptococcus* species do not grow at 37°C.

IDENTIFICATION

Identification is based in part on cultural and morphologic characteristics, especially the presence of the large capsule (see Fig. 35–1). Members of the genus *Cryptococcus* produce urease on Christensen's urea agar, while *Candida* species do not. Several species of *Cryptococcus* possess capsules, but only *C. neoformans* produces brown colonies on bird seed agar. The latter medium, which contains *Guizotia abyssinica* seeds, can also be used as a selective medium for *C. neoformans.* The various species are identified by carbohydrate assimilation tests. Strains of the true yeast *Saccharomyces* can be distinguished from the cryptococci by the presence of ascospores in the former. The ascospores stain well with methylene blue.

Geotrichum and *Trichosporon* both produce true

mycelia. The various cryptococcal species can be identified precisely by sugar and nitrate assimilation tests.

ANIMAL INOCULATION

Mice are susceptible to pathogenic strains. The routes of inoculation are intracerebral or intraperitoneal. Organisms are demonstrable in brain or lung lesions in one to three weeks.

SEROLOGY

A latex agglutination procedure is available as a test for antigen.

Tube agglutination, complement fixation, and indirect fluorescent antibody tests are used. False-positive and false-negative reactions are a problem.

TREATMENT

Amphotericin B is the drug of choice, although imidazole derivatives have shown some promise.

GEOTRICHOSIS

Geotrichosis caused by *Geotrichum candidum* is an uncommon disease rarely diagnosed clinically. This fungus is found widely in nature, and its isolation is not necessarily significant. Two cultural forms occur: (1) the glabrous or yeast-like form and (2) the fluffy form. The latter strains are sometimes given the name *Oospora.* The glabrous form of *G. candidum* is the one usually associated with disease.

PATHOGENICITY

Infections have been reported from cattle, dogs, fowl, and humans. They are usually identified on postmortem examination. The bronchi, lungs, udder (mastitis), and the mucous membranes of the alimentary tract are most frequently affected. The disease is usually mild and is characterized by the formation of granulomas that may suppurate. *G. candidum* is occasionally recovered from otitis externa in the dog.

DIRECT EXAMINATION

Purulent material or scrapings from lesions are examined in wet mounts. The organism appears as rectangular or spherical arthrospores. They are thick-walled, nonbudding, and in stained smears strongly gram-positive.

ISOLATION AND IDENTIFICATION

The organisms grow fairly rapidly at room temperature on Sabouraud agar. The colonies are membranous, with radial furrows, and soft, with a dry, granular surface. The mycelium is made up of septate hyphae that fragment, producing chains of characteristic rectangular to round arthrospores (see Fig. 35–1).

Differentiation from other fungi is based upon cultural and morphologic characteristics. *G. candidum* can be distinguished from *Coccidioides immitis* and *Blastomyces dermatitidis* by the fact that the latter two species produce cottony, filamentous colonies at room temperature. *G. candidum* produces a soft, yeast-like colony at room temperature.

TREATMENT

Specific treatment is rarely administered.

Malassezia (Pityrosporum)

Species of this genus of lipophilic yeasts are associated with the skin of humans and animals. *Malessezia furfur* causes blepharitis, seborrhea, dandruff, and tinea versicolor in human beings. The yeasts that have been called *Pityrosporum canis* and *P. felis* and similar organisms from other animals are now called *M. pachydermatis.* This species occurs as a commensal on the oily areas of the skin and ears of dogs. Strains may also be recovered from the ears of cats. In some cases of otitis externa, they appear to be present in larger numbers than usual and some veterinarians think they may have etiologic significance.

Malassezia are bottle-shaped, small budding cells that reproduce by a process known as bud fission in which the bud detaches from the parent cell by the production of a septum (see Fig. 35–1). They can be demonstrated in wet mounts (10% NaOH) of clinical material from dog's ears.

They can be readily recovered on Sabouraud agar after 2 weeks' incubation at room temperature. Growth is increased if sterile olive or coconut oil is applied to the surface of the medium.

SUGGESTED CLINICAL EXAMPLES

Genital candidiasis in the mare.

Intestinal candidiasis in the cat and dog.

An outbreak of crop mycosis in young chickens.

Cases of cryptococcosis in the cat, dog and horse.

SOURCES FOR FURTHER READING

(Note: See also References for Chapter 31.)

Bistner, S., de Lahunta, A., and Lorenz, M.: Generalized cryptococcosis in a dog. Cornell Vet., *61*:440, 1971.

Bowman, P.I., and Ahearn, D.G.: Evaluation of commercial systems for the identification of clinical yeast isolates. J. Clin. Microbiol., *4*:49, 1976.

Cross, R.F., Moorhead, P.D., and Jones, J.E.: *Candida albicans* infection of the forestomachs of a calf. J. Am. Vet. Med. Assoc., *157*:1325, 1970.

Gedek, B., et al.: The role of *Pityrosporum pachydermatis* in otitis externa of dogs: Evaluation of a treatment with miconazole. Vet. Rec., *104*:138, 1979.

Gross, T.L., and Mayhew, I.G.: Gastroesophageal ulceration and candidiasis in foals. J. Am. Vet. Med. Assoc., *182*:1370, 1983.

Kade, W.L., Kelley, D.C., and Coles, E.H.: Survey of yeast-like fungi and tissue changes in esophagogastric region of stomachs of swine. Am. J. Vet. Res., *30*:401, 1969.

Krogh, P., Basse, A., Hesselholt, M., and Bach, A.: Equine cryptococcosis: A case of rhinitis caused by *Cryptococcus neoformans*. Sabouraudia, *12*:272, 1974.

Lincoln, S.D., and Adcock, J.L.: Disseminated geotrichosis in a dog. Pathologia Vet., *5*:282, 1968.

Lodder, J. (ed.): The Yeasts, A Taxonomic Study. 2nd Ed. Amsterdam, North Holland Publishing Co., 1970.

Mayeda, B.: Candidiasis in turkeys and chickens in the Sacramento Valley of California. Avian Dis., *5*:232, 1961.

Mills, J.H., and Hirth, R.S.: Systemic candidiasis in calves on prolonged antibiotic therapy. J. Am. Vet. Med. Assoc., *150*:862, 1967.

Silva-Hutner, M., and Cooper, B.H.: Yeasts of medical importance. *In* Manual of Clinical Microbiology. Edited by E.H. Lennette, A. Balows, W.J. Hausler, Jr., and J.P. Truant. 3rd Ed. Washington, D.C., American Society of Microbiology, 1980.

Smith, J.M.B.: Candidiasis in animals in New Zealand. Sabouraudia, *5*:220, 1967.

34

Subcutaneous Mycoses

SPOROTRICHOSIS

Sporotrichosis is caused by *Sporothrix (Sporotrichum) schenckii*, a fungus that occurs in nature and is associated with soil, wood, and vegetation. Infections are exogenous and worldwide in distribution. The portal of entry is usually wounds.

PATHOGENICITY

Infections in humans and some animals are characterized by the formation of subcutaneous nodules or granulomas. The organisms usually enter through wounds in the skin, and spread is via the lymphatics. The nodules eventually ulcerate and discharge pus. Involvement of bones and visceral organs with fatal termination is rare but has been reported in the dog and horse. Infections have been described in humans and in the dog, horse, donkey, mule, camel, cattle, fowl, and rodents.

DIRECTION EXAMINATION

In pus and tissue the organism appears as a single-celled cigar-shaped body, usually within neutrophils. These structures are very difficult to demonstrate in stained smears and wet mounts of pus and tissue scrapings. Fluorescent antibody staining of clinical materials frequently yields positive results.

ISOLATION, CULTIVATION, AND IDENTIFICATION

Sporothrix schenckii is readily grown on brain heart infusion agar, blood agar (37°C), and Sa-bouraud C and C agar (25°C) in one to three weeks.

Tissue Phase. At 37°C, colonies are yeast-like, smooth, soft, and cream to tan color.

There is no mycelium. Colonies are composed of the same elements that occur in pus and tissue, i.e., cigar-shaped cells and spherical or oval budding cells. Some large pyriform cells may also be seen (Table 34–1).

Mycelial Phase. At 25°C colonies appear early, but the characteristic structures are not evident until the aerial mycelium is produced. Colonies are white and soft at first, and then become tan to brown to black. The texture is leathery, wrinkled, and coarsely tufted.

The mycelium consists of fine, branching septate hyphae that bear pyriform or ovoid microconidia, which are borne in clusters from the ends of conidiophores or as sessile forms directly on the sides of hyphae (see Fig. 34–1). Thick-walled, large, chlamydospores may be seen in old cultures.

ANIMAL INOCULATION

Mice are susceptible. Suspected material or cultures are inoculated intra-peritoneally. The mice are sacrificed in three weeks and if infected, cigar-shaped bodies can be seen in smears from the peritoneal exudate and granulomata.

SEROLOGY

A latex agglutination test and a tube agglutination test are used to detect antibodies in hu-

236

	Growth in tissues at 37°C	Growth on blood agar at 37°C	Growth on Sabouraud's at 25°C
Sporothrix schenckii	Cigar bodies	Yeast cells	Hyphae, microconidia in "flowerette" arrangement
Blastomyces dermatitidis	Yeast cells	Yeast cells	Hyphae, chlamydospores
Histoplasma capsulatum	Small, intracellular yeast cells with a dark central area	Yeast cells	Tuberculate chlamydospores
Coccidioides immitis	Intra- or extracellular spherules containing round endospores	Hyphae, arthrospores with collarettes	Hyphae, arthrospores with collarettes

mans. The immunodiffusion test is reliable and easy to perform.

TREATMENT

Potassium iodide is administered orally to the point of producing iodinism. It is continued for several weeks after apparent recovery in order to prevent recrudescence. Other drugs that have been useful are amphotericin B, 5-fluorocytosine, miconazole, and griseofulvin.

PHAEOHYPHOMYCOSIS (CHROMOMYCOSIS)

This name denotes infrequent opportunistic fungal dematiaceous infections of humans, dogs, and horses caused by a number of species of dematiaceous fungi. The infections, which begin in wounds or abrasions, result in nodular and frequently ulcerating lesions of the skin of the feet and legs, with regional granulomatous lymphadenitis. Ocular infections and systemic disease in turkeys have been reported. The following species of fungi have been incriminated: *Dactylaria gallopava, Exophiala pisciphila, E. salmonis, Scolecobasidium humicola,* and *S. tshawytschae.*

DIRECT EXAMINATION

Material from granulomatous or ulcerous lesions is examined in 10% sodium hydroxide. Organisms are single-celled or clustered, spherical, and thick-walled, with a black or dark brown pigment. They multiply by cross-wall formation or splitting rather than budding.

ISOLATION AND CULTIVATION

The organisms will grow on Sabouraud agar at room temperature. Growth is slow, up to a month being required.

IDENTIFICATION

Identification of the genus is usually not difficult. The aid of a specialist may be required to identify the species.

MYCOTIC SWAMP CANCER

This disease is considered a phaeohyphomycosis by Rippon.

More than 40 cases of this disease have been reported in Texas and Florida. It has also been seen in Australia, New Guinea, and India.

The fungus involved is a *Pythium* (formerly

called *Hyphomyces destruens*). It gains entrance via wounds involving the hoof, hock, fetlock, head, neck, and lips. There is a granulomatous reaction, with necrosis and the formation of fistulous tracts. Masses of branching, sparsely septated fungi are seen in the yellow necrotic lesions. The disease is progressive but not usually systemic, and there have been no remissions in the absence of treatment, which involves radical surgery. Several cases have been reported in dogs.

Identification after cultivation is rather involved and may require the assistance of a mycologist.

MADUROMYCOSIS (EUMYCOTIC MYCETOMA)

Maduromycotic mycetomas (subcutaneous mycotic abscesses) consist of granulomatous processes produced by several species of fungi. Microcolonies that frequently are pigmented can sometimes be seen grossly in lesions and exudate. There have been several reports of these infrequent infections in horses, cattle, dogs, and cats. The lesions occur most commonly on the extremities but may also be found involving the nasal mucosa (e.g., bovine nasal granuloma), the peritoneum, and the skin in various locations.

The following species of fungi have been recovered: *Pseudoallescheria boydii, Curvularia geniculata,* and *Cochliobolus spicifer.*

Incision of the lesions in the case of the dematiaceous fungi reveals discrete brown or black fungal microcolonies embedded in a large mass of granulation tissue.

The first species mentioned above is a "hyaline" nonpigmented fungus, while the other two are dematiaceous (black or brown pigment) fungi. The first grows rapidly, while the others require several weeks. Some additional species and genera have been recovered from human maduromycosis.

DIRECT EXAMINATION

Scrapings or biopsy tissue are examined grossly for the characteristic microcolonies, which are small (0.5 to 3.0 mm), irregularly shaped, and variously colored. These colonies or "grains" are placed in 10% sodium hydroxide and then pressed out by means of a coverslip and observed microscopically. The grains of maduromycosis reveal mycelia that are usually 2 to 4 μm in width in contrast to the narrower filaments found in the actinomycotic granule. Also of significance is the presence of chlamydospores in the grains.

ISOLATION, CULTIVATION, AND IDENTIFICATION

The species involved grow readily but slowly (two to three weeks) on Sabouraud agar at room temperature. Cultures are usually submitted to a mycology laboratory for confirmation of identification.

CHROMOBLASTOMYCOSIS

Chromoblastomycosis occurs in horses, dogs, cats, and humans, but only a small number of cases have been reported in animals. The fungi enter tissues at the site of some trauma or wound. A granulomatous mass develops that may spread peripherally and on occasion to the lymphatics and other tissues and organs. The disease is chronic and if not treated persists and frequently progresses.

Some of the dematiaceous fungi that have been implicated are *Fonsecaea pedrosoi, Exophiala spinifera, Cladosporium carrionii,* and *Phialophora* spp.

Standard mycology texts should be consulted for the laboratory diagnosis of this disease.

HYPHOMYCOSIS

This is an uncommon opportunistic fungous disease of animals and humans caused by species of the genera *Penicillium, Beauveria, Acremonium, Fusarium,* and *Paecilomyces.*

EPIZOOTIC LYMPHANGITIS

This disease is caused by *Histoplasma farciminosum (Cryptococcus farciminosum).* It occurs in horses, mules, and donkeys in parts of Europe, Africa, and Asia. Mycologists claim that this organism does not belong in the genus *Histoplasma.*

PATHOGENICITY

H. farciminosum causes a chronic disease involving the lymph nodes, superficial lymph vessels, and skin of mainly the limbs. It is characterized by the formation of nodular, ulcerating lesions along the lymphatics of the legs. A pulmonary form has also been described.

DEMONSTRATION AND CULTIVATION

The oval or pear-shaped cells can be seen in pus from fresh lesions. The organism is dimorphic, growing in the mycelial phase at room temperature and in the yeast phase at 37°C.

IDENTIFICATION

Details relating to cultural and morphologic characteristics and identification are provided in the references.

TREATMENT

Potassium iodide, amphotericin B, and hamycin are reported to be effective.

RHINOSPORIDIOSIS

The agent that is considered the cause of this disease is *Rhinosporidium seeberi,* a fungus presumed to occur in nature (water) which as yet has not been cultivated.

PATHOGENICITY

R. seeberi causes a chronic, generally benign disease of cattle, horses, mules, dogs, and humans characterized by the formation of polyps on the nasal and ocular mucous membranes. The disease occurs mostly in tropical areas. Several cases of the infection have been reported in dogs in the United States.

DIRECT EXAMINATION

Wet mounts from nasal discharge and sections from polyps disclose large sporangia (200 to 300 μm). These develop in tissue from small globose cells (6 to 8 μm). The large sporangia contain and release thousands of spores.

TREATMENT

Surgical excision.

SUGGESTED CLINICAL EXAMPLES

A case of sporotrichosis in a horse.
A case of sporotrichosis in a dog.
A case of chromomycosis in a dog.
A case of maduromycosis in a horse.

SOURCES FOR FURTHER READING

(Note: See also References for Chapter 31.)

Bridges, C.H.: Maduromycotic mycetomas in animals. *Curvularia geniculata* as an etiologic agent. Am. J. Pathol., *33*:411, 1957.

Bridges, C.H., and Beasley, J.N.: Maduromycotic mycetomas. J. Am. Vet. Med. Assoc., *137*:192, 1960.

Davis, H.H., and Worthington, W.E.: Equine sporotrichosis. J. Am. Vet. Med. Assoc., *151*:45, 1964.

Kurtz, H.J., Finco, D.R., and Perman, V.: Maduromycosis (*Allescheria boydii*) in a dog. J. Am. Vet. Med. Assoc., *157*:917, 1970.

Londerno, A.T., et al.: Two cases of sporotrichosis in dogs in Brazil. Sabouraudia, *3*:273, 1964.

Myers, D.D., Simon, J., and Case, M.T.: Rhinosporidiosis in a horse. J. Am. Vet. Med. Assoc., *145*:345, 1964.

Refai, M., and Loot, A.: The incidence of epizootic lymphangitis in Egypt. Mykosen, *13*:247, 1970.

Singh, T.: Studies on epizootic lymphangitis: Study of clinical cases and experimental transmission. Indian J. Vet. Sci., *36*:45, 1966.

Singh, T., and Varmani, B.M.L.: Some observations on experimental infection with *Histoplasma farciminosum* (Rivolta) and the morphology of the organism. Indian J. Vet. Sci., *37*:47, 1967.

Stuart, B.P.: Rhinosporidiosis in a dog. J. Am. Vet. Med. Assoc., *167*:941, 1975.

35

Systemic Mycoses

ZYGOMYCOSIS (MUCORMYCOSIS)

Mucormycosis, hyphomycosis, and zygomycosis are caused by species of *Mucor*, *Absidia*, *Rhizopus*, and *Mortierella*. Strains of these genera occur widely in nature.

PATHOGENICITY

The mode of infection is by inhalation or ingestion.

These fungi frequently infect lymph nodes of the respiratory and alimentary tracts. Lesions are granulomatous and occasionally ulcerative; they are usually localized but may be generalized. Lymph nodes enlarge and become caseocalcareous. Ulceration of stomach and intestines has been attributed to zygomycosis.

Pigs. Lesions are found in mediastinal and submandibular lymph nodes; embolic "tumors" are seen in the liver and lungs. Fungi of this group may be found in gastric ulcers.

Cattle. Lesions are found in the bronchial, mesenteric, and mediastinal lymph nodes; there may be nasal and abomasal ulcers. Abortions are attributed to these fungi.

Horses. There are several reports of zygomycosis in this species.

Infections have also been reported in dogs, cats, sheep, mink, guinea pigs, and mice.

DIRECT EXAMINATION

Fragments and pieces of coarse, nonseptate, branching hyphae are seen. The coarseness or thickness of the pieces is especially significant.

These infections are frequently detected in tissue sections.

ISOLATION AND CULTIVATION

Fungi of this group grow rapidly at room temperature on Sabouraud agar. Because they are common contaminants, isolation alone is not necessarily considered significant. Repeated isolation, characteristic lesions and the presence of fungal elements in sections are clinically significant.

IDENTIFICATION

All have round sporangia borne on sporangiophores; sporangia contain numerous sporangiospores.

Identification to species may require the aid of a mycologist.

Mucor **Species.** There do not appear to be authenticated cases of zygomycosis caused by species of this genus. They have thick, colorless mycelium without rhizoids. Sporangiophores are simple or branched, and globose sporangia contain small spores (see Figure 35–1).

Absidia **Species.** *A. corymbifer* causes mucormycosis. In this genus the sporangiophores do not arise from the stolons opposite the rhizoids as in *Rhizopus*. However, *Absidia* resemble *Rhizopus* species grossly (Fig. 35–1).

Rhizopus **Species.** *R. oryzae* is one of the more common species causing disease. Another pathogenic species is *R. rhizopodoformis* and possibly *R. microsporus*. They have dense, cottony, aerial mycelium that are first white and then turn grey.

240

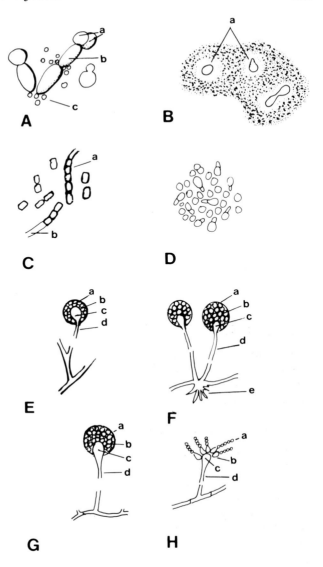

Figure 35–1. A, *Candida albicans:* a. chlamydospore, b. pseudohypha, c. blastospores. B, *Cryptococcus neoformans,* India ink preparation: a. large capsules. C, *Geotrichum candidum:* a. arthrospores, b. hypha. D, *Malassezia (Pityrosporum):* yeast cells showing budding (bottle-shaped). E, *Mucor:* a. sporangium, b. sporangiospores, c. columnella, d. sporangiophore. F, *Rhizopus:* a. sporangium, b. sporangiospores, c. columnella, d. sporangiophore, e. rhizoids, G, *Absidia:* same basic structure as *Mucor.* H, *Aspergillus:* a. conidia, b. sterigmata, c. vesicle, d. conidiophore.

Sporangiophores arise from the stolons where stolons contact the medium through rhizoids (see Fig. 35–1).

Mortierella **Species.** *Mortierella hygrophila* and *M. polycephala* have been recovered from zygomycosis in fowl and cattle, respectively. *M. wolfii* is an important cause of abortion (mycotic placentitis) in some regions. This condition is sometimes followed by an acute, frequently fatal pneumonia.

M. wolfii grows on blood agar and Sabouraud agar at 25 to 27°C and 37°C. The colonies on Sabouraud and blood agars are white, velvety, dense, and characteristically lobulated. The hyphae are hyaline, and sporangia are produced on special media. Definitive identification is based on the morphology of the sporangia and spores.

TREATMENT

Amphotericin B is the preferred drug. Surgical measures may be indicated.

ASPERGILLOSIS

The most prevalent pathogenic species of *Aspergillus* is *A. fumigatus.* Other potentially pathogenic species are *A. flavus, A. nidulans,* and possibly *A. niger.* Some workers think that the differences among these species are small and that they should all be called *A. fumigatus.* Species of *Aspergillus* are widely found in nature and are common contaminants in the laboratory.

PATHOGENICITY

Several manifestations of aspergillosis are seen in chickens, turkeys, and other avian species: (1) a diffuse infection of the air sacs; (2) a diffuse pneumonic form; and (3) a nodular form involving the lungs. The disease is called "brooder pneumonia" in chicks and poults; many birds may be affected. The spores are acquired by inhalation from the fungi growing on feed or litter. The principal gross lesion consists of yellow nodules found in the lungs and air sacs.

Cattle. Infections involve the uterus, fetal membranes, and fetal skin and on occasion result in abortion.

Horses. Infection causes abortion and guttural pouch mycosis.

Other Animals (Including Dogs, Cats, and Sheep). Infrequent infections occur, most often involving the lungs. Respiratory aspergillosis is common in penguins in captivity. Nasal aspergillosis is an important disease of dogs.

Humans. Primary and secondary infections occur in a wide variety of tissues and locations: lungs, skin, nasal sinuses, external ear, bronchi, bones, and meninges.

DIRECT EXAMINATION

Small pieces of tissue or deep scrapings are examined in 10% sodium hydroxide. Short pieces of thick, septate hyphae are characteristic. The typical conidial heads are seen only in the lungs and air sacs, where there is access to oxygen.

ISOLATION AND CULTIVATION

Aspergilli grow rapidly on blood and Sabouraud agars at room and incubator temperatures. Colonies are white at first but later turn green to dark green, flat, and velvety.

IDENTIFICATION

The genus is identified by the presence of the conidiophores with large terminal vesicles bearing sterigmata from which chains of spores or conidia are produced (see Fig. 35–1). Identification to species may require the assistance of a mycologist.

SEROLOGY

An agar gel immunodiffusion test has been of value in the diagnosis of nasal aspergillosis in dogs.

TREATMENT

Amphotericin B is the drug of choice.

BLASTOMYCOSIS (NORTH AMERICAN)

The causative agent, *Blastomyces dermatitidis*, occurs widely in the soil. Blastomycosis is widespread, and in the United States it is most common in the north-central and southeastern states.

PATHOGENICITY

The mode of infection is via the respiratory tract, and the initial lesions are found in the lung. The disease is characterized by the formation of granulomatous nodules and occurs principally in humans and dogs. It has also been described in the horse, cat, and sea lion, but it is uncommon in these animals. In dogs the lesions are usually found in the lungs and on the skin. Skin lesions and generalized blastomycosis result from hematogenous dissemination from the original pulmonary lesions. Unless treated, the disseminated disease terminates in death. The skin lesions, which are circumscribed and granulomatous, may ulcerate.

DIRECT EXAMINATION

The large, spherical, thick-walled cells (5 to 20 μm in diameter) are readily demonstrable in wet mounts. A single bud connected to the larger mother cell by a wide base is frequently seen. Some cells give a double contoured effect.

ISOLATION, CULTIVATION, AND IDENTIFICATION

The organism grows slowly at 25°C and 37°C on Sabouraud agar and blood agar, respectively.

On Sabouraud agar at 25°C, a moist, greyish, yeast-like colony is seen that develops a white cottony mycelium. As it ages, it becomes tan to dark brown to black. The septate hyphae bear small, oval, or pyriform conidia laterally, close to the point of septation. Older cultures form chlamydospores with thickened walls (see Table 34–1).

On blood agar at 37°C, creamy, waxy, wrinkled colonies, cream to tan in color, are observed. Thick-walled budding yeast cells similar to those in tissue sections and exudate are seen (see Table 34–1).

ANIMAL INOCULATION

Guinea pigs, mice, rats, and hamsters can be infected by intraperitoneal inoculation. They usually die within three weeks. Yeast-like cells are demonstrable in the peritoneal exudate and nodules.

The complement fixation test can be of value; rising titers are significant. A positive immunodiffusion test indicates recent or current infection.

TREATMENT

Amphotericin B is the treatment of choice. Dihydroxystilbamidine is less toxic and can be used in cases with limited lesions and in instances in which the more toxic amphotericin B is contraindicated. The imidazoles have been used in human beings, but the relapse rate has been high. They may have value if the disease is very limited.

HISTOPLASMOSIS

Histoplasmosis is caused by *Histoplasma capsulatum*, a dimorphic fungus that is found in soil and on decaying vegetation. A heavy concentration has been encountered in the feces of birds, e.g., starlings, and pigeons. Infection is exogenous, usually by inhalation and less frequently by ingestion. Apparently avian feces provide a favorable milieu for multiplication. It does not occur in the intestines of live birds. There are many subclinical, transient infections. The heaviest concentration of infections in the United States is in the northeast, central, and south-central states. The disease is worldwide in distribution.

PATHOGENICITY

Clinical histoplasmosis is a generalized disease involving the reticuloendothelial system. Infections have been reported from dogs, cattle, nonhuman primates, cats, horses, sheep, swine, humans, and various wild animals. Some of the lesions seen in dogs and cats are ulcerations of the intestinal canal; enlargement of the liver, spleen, and lymph nodes; and necrosis and tubercle-like lesions in the lungs, liver, kidneys, and spleen. Acute and chronic forms are seen. Although the clinical disease is generalized, it usually assumes either a predominantly pulmonary or an intestinal form in animals.

DIRECT EXAMINATION

Because *H. capsulatum* is small and rarely found extracellularly, it is extremely difficult to demonstrate in clinical materials. Smears are made from scrapings of uclers, from cut surfaces of lymph nodes, from biopsies, and from material from sternal puncture and buffy coat. They are stained by the Giemsa or Wright method and examined under oil immersion objective. The organisms occur intracellularly (mononuclear cells) as small, round or oval, yeast-like, single, or budding cells. A clear halo is seen around the darker staining central material. The characteristic small yeast cells can be seen in the cytoplasm of macrophages in stained sections of affected tissues.

ISOLATION, CULTIVATION, AND IDENTIFICATION

On Sabouraud agar at 25°C colonies are cottony white to cream at first, later becoming tan to brown. Two kinds of spores are borne on the septate hyphae: (1) small, smooth, round to pyriform microconidia, either on short lateral branches or attached directly by the base; and (2) small and large macroconidia or chlamydospores (7 to 18 μm in diameter) that are round, thick-walled, and may be covered with knob-like projections (tuberculate chlamydospores) (see Table 34–1).

On blood agar at 37°C colonies are small, white, and yeast-like and yield yeast-like cells (see Table 34–1).

ANIMAL INOCULATION

Mice can be infected by the intraperitoneal route. Mucin may be added to the inoculum to enhance pathogenicity and promote the conversion of the mycelial phase to the yeast phase. After four weeks, organisms can be recovered from the liver of successfully infected mice.

SEROLOGY

The complement fixation test is useful; rising titers are significant. The immunodiffusion test and counterimmunoelectrophoresis (if reaction is positive) indicate past or current infection.

TREATMENT

Amphotericin B is the preferred drug. The imidazoles (miconazole and ketoconazole) are still being evaluated. They can be given orally if the use of amphotericin B is contraindicated.

COCCIDIOIDOMYCOSIS

The causative agent of coccidiodomycosis is *Coccidioides immitis*. It occurs widely in the soil of certain arid areas of the southwestern United States and South America. Its occurrence is infrequent outside the Americas. There are many subclinical, transient infections in humans and animals. The mode of infection is by inhalation.

PATHOGENICITY

The disease is characterized by the formation of nodules or granulomas. It has been encountered in humans, cattle, sheep, dogs, primates, horses, swine, and various wild animals. The gross lesions in cattle resemble tuberculosis and are usually seen in the bronchial and mediastinal lymph nodes and less frequently in the lungs. Lesions have been found in the lungs, brain, liver, spleen, bones, and kidneys of dogs. Infrequent progressive disease in the dog runs a course of two to five months.

DIRECT EXAMINATION

In unstained wet mounts the organisms are seen as nonbudding, thick-walled sporangia having diameters varying from 5 to 50 μm. These large sporangia contain numerous endospores 2 to 5 μm in diameter. The large sporangia burst releasing the endospores and leaving "ghost" spherules.

ISOLATION AND CULTIVATION

Caution: C. immitis is highly infectious. It grows readily in one to two weeks at 25°C and 37°C on Sabouraud and blood agars, respectively. Colonies are flat, moist, and membranous at both temperatures, later developing a coarse, cottony, aerial mycelium, the color of which varies from white to brown. The tissue phase is not seen on artificial media but may be obtained by inoculating cultures into mice (see Table 34–1).

The thallus consists of branching septate mycelia that form chains of thick-walled, barrel-shaped arthrospores (2 to 3 μm long). When stained by lactophenol cotton blue, the chains of arthrospores are stained in a characteristic alternate fashion and may possess typical collarettes.

IDENTIFICATION

Definite identification is based upon cultural and morphologic characteristics. Some differential considerations are

1. *Geotrichum* species (glabrous or yeast-like form) remain yeast-like in appearance on Sabouraud agar (25°C). Arthrospores are characteristic; they do not have a collarette.
2. *Oospora* species (fluffy form of *Geotrichum*)

do not produce alternate stained arthrospores and are not pathogenic for animals.
3. *Coccidioides immitis* produces typical spherules filled with endospores. Characteristic arthrospores are seen at 25°C and 37°C.
See Table 34–1.

ANIMAL INOCULATION

In the guinea pig, when *C. immitis* is inoculated into the testicle, spherules are demonstrable in pus in five to six days. The mouse is inoculated intraperitoneally, and spherules are demonstrable in smears from the peritoneum and various organs.

SEROLOGY

The complement fixation test is useful; rising titers are significant. A positive immunodiffusion test and a positive reaction with counter-immunoelectrophoresis indicate a past or current infection.

TREATMENT

Amphotericin B is the preferred drug. The imidazole compounds are still being evaluated. Ketoconazole has shown some promise in treatment of nonsystemic coccidioidomycosis in human beings.

ADIASPIROMYCOSIS (HAPLOMYCOSIS)

Chrysosporium parvum and *C. crescens* cause respiratory infection in many species of rodents and other wild mammals, including insectivores, herbivores, and carnivores. The disease has been reported in humans and in a dog but is probably rare. The names *Chrysosporium parvum* and *C. crescens* have been given to the in vitro small forms of the fungus and to the form resulting in enormous growth of spores in vivo, respectively.

The causal fungi occur as thick-walled, spherical cells (up to 500 μm in diameter) in lung tissue. In histopathologic sections they have been confused with *Coccidioides immitis*. Light grey to yellowish granulomatous lesions have been found in the lungs of apparently healthy animals.

ISOLATION AND IDENTIFICATION

This dimorphic fungus grows on blood agar at 37°C and on Sabouraud agar at room temperature. Unlike *C. immitis*, it has a mycelial phase at 25°C. Additional characteristics for definitive identification are provided in the references.

SUGGESTED CLINICAL EXAMPLES

Mucormycotic abortion in a cow.

An outbreak of brooder pneumonia in chicks.

Abortion in a mare due to *Aspergillus fumigatus*.

A case of respiratory aspergillosis in the dog.

An outbreak of aspergillosis in 300 penguins.

A case of canine blastomycosis.

A case of canine histoplasmosis.

A case of histoplasmosis in a horse.

A case of progressive coccidioidomycosis in a dog.

A case of adiaspiromycosis in a dog.

SOURCES FOR FURTHER READING

(Note: See also References for Chapter 31.)

Balows, A., Ausherman, R.J., and Hopper, J.M.: Practical diagnosis and therapy of canine histoplasmosis and blastomycosis. J. Am. Vet. Med. Assoc., *148*:678, 1966.

Barsanti, J.A., Attleberger, M.H., and Henderson, R.A.: Phycomycosis in a dog. J. Am. Vet. Med. Assoc., *167*:293, 1975.

Bridges, C.H., and Emmons, C.W.: A phycomycosis of horses caused by *Hyphomyces destruens*. J. Am. Vet. Med. Assoc., *138*:579, 1961.

Brodey, R.S., et al.: Disseminated coccidioidomycosis in a dog. J. Am. Vet. Med. Assoc., *157*:926, 1970.

Cook, W.R., Campbell, R.S.F., and Dawson, C.: The pathology and etiology of gutteral pouch mycosis in the horse. Vet. Rec., *83*:422, 1968.

Cordes, D.O., Dodd, D.C., and O'Hara, P.J. Bovine mycotic abortion. N. Z. Vet. J., *12*:95, 1967.

DeMartini, J.C., and Riddle, W.E.: Disseminated coccidioidomycosis in two horses and a pony. J. Am. Vet. Med. Assoc., *155*:149, 1969.

Lane, J.G., and Warnock, D.W.: The diagnosis of *Aspergillus fumigatus* infection of the nasal chambers of the dog with particular reference to the value of the double diffusion test. J. Sm. Anim. Pract., *18*:169, 1977.

Legendre, A.M., Walker, M., Buyukmihci, N., and Stevens, R.: Canine blastomycosis: A review of 47 clinical cases. J. Am. Vet. Med. Assoc., *178*:1163, 1981.

Lingard, D.R., Gosser, H.S., and Monfort, T.M.: Acute epistaxis associated with gutteral pouch mycosis in two horses. J. Am. Vet. Med. Assoc., *164*:1038, 1974.

Maddy, K.T.: Coccidioidomycosis of cattle in the southwestern United States. J. Am. Vet. Med. Assoc., *124*:256, 1954.

Menges, R.W.: Canine histoplasmosis. J. Am. Vet. Med. Assoc., *119*:411, 1951.

Ohbayashi, M., and Ishimoto, Y.: Two cases of adiaspiromycosis in small animals. Jpn. J. Vet. Res., *19*:103, 1971.

Rose, M.N.: Aspergillosis in wild and domestic fowl. Avian Dis., *8*:1, 1964.

Stevens, D.A. (ed.): Coccidioidomycosis. New York, Plenum Publishing Corporation, 1980.

Stock, B.L.: Case report: Generalized granulomatous lesions in chickens and wild ducks caused by *Aspergillus* species. Avian Dis., *5*:89, 1961.

APPENDIX

A "Clinical Example" (Listeriosis) of the kind the author has found helpful in teaching

Clinical Example

Approximately 400 feeder lambs were brought to a farm in Michigan and placed on a ration of predominantly corn silage. Those lambs that became ill first appeared dull and stood quietly with drooping ears. Next they showed signs of impaired vision, and animals walked into objects; a number circled and appeared to be blind. Other signs were conjunctivitis, corneal opacity, and drooling from pendulous lips. In a little over a month, 45 lambs had died. Recoveries were few. An examination of the silage disclosed that pockets of it had spoiled, particularly around the poor sealing doors.

1. What diseases would you consider in your differential diagnosis?

2. What specimens would you submit to the laboratory?

3. How would you conduct the microbiologic examination?

4. a. What was the probable source of the organism?

   b. What circumstances probably contributed to this outbreak?

5. What forms of the disease are recognized, and what is the usual mode of infection in each?

6. What lesions are seen in the two forms of this disease?

7. In which animals is this disease usually seen?

8. How is this disease treated?

9. What is the nature of the immune response in this disease?

10. Why do you think autogenous bacterins are of little value?

11. What is the potential public health significance of this organism?

SUGGESTED SOURCES FOR REFERENCE AND SUPPLEMENTARY READING

1. Veterinary Bacteriology

Merchant, I.A., and Packer, R.A.: Veterinary Bacteriology and Virology. 7th Ed. Ames, Iowa, Iowa State University Press, 1967.

Soltys, M.A.: Bacteria and Fungi Pathogenic to Man and Animals. Baltimore, Williams & Wilkins Co., 1963.

Soltys, M.A.: Introduction to Veterinary Microbiology, Serdang, Selangor, Penerbit Universiti Pertanian Malaysia, 1979.

Gillespie, J.H., and Timoney, J.F.: Hagan and Bruner's Infectious Diseases of Domestic Animals. 7th Ed. Ithaca, New York, Comstock Publishing Associates, 1981.

Greene, C.E. (ed.): Clinical Microbiology and Infectious Diseases of the Dog and Cat. Philadelphia, W.B. Saunders Company, 1984.

Buxton, A., and Fraser, G.: Animal Microbiology. Vol. 1, Immunology, Bacteriology and Mycology. London, Blackwell Scientific Publications, 1977.

2. Veterinary Mycology

Dvorak, J., and Otcenasek, M.: Mycological Diagnosis of Animal Dermatophytoses. The Hague, Holland, Dr. W. Junk, N.V. Publishers, 1969.

Ainsworth, G.C., and Austwick, P.K.C.: Fungal Diseases of Animals. 2nd Ed. England, Commonwealth Agricultural Bureaux, 1973.

Jungerman, P.F., and Schwartzman, R.M.: Veterinary Medical Mycology. Philadelphia, Lea & Febiger, 1972.

Vanbreuseghem, R.: Guide Practique de Mycologie Médicale et Vétérinaire. Paris, Masson et Cie, 1966.

3. General and Human Microbiology

All except Topley and Wilson are usually superficial in their discussions of predominantly animal pathogens.

Davis, B.D., Dulbecco, R., Eisen, H.N., and Ginsburg, H.S.: Microbiology 3rd Ed. New York, Harper & Row, 1980.

Joklik, W.K., Willet, H.P., and Amos, D.B. (eds.): Zinsser Microbiology. 18th Ed. Norwalk, Conn., Appleton-Century-Crofts, 1984.

Wilson, G.S., and Miles, A.A.: Topley and Wilson's Principles of Bacteriology and Immunity. Vols. 1 and 2. 5th Ed. Baltimore, Williams & Wilkins Co., 1964.

4. General and Human Mycology

These books contain some material on animal mycoses and laboratory procedures.

Beneke, E.S., and Rogers, A.L.: Medical Mycology Manual. 4th Ed. Minneapolis, Burgess Publishing Company, 1980.

Conant, N.F., Smith, T.L., Baker, R.D., Callaway, J.L., and Martin, E.S.: Manual of Clinical Mycology. 3rd Ed. Philadelphia, W.B. Saunders Co., 1971.

Emmons, C.W., Binford, C.H., and Utz, J.P.: Medical Mycology. 3rd Ed. Philadelphia, Lea & Febiger, 1977.

Rebell, G., and Taplin, D. Dermatophytes: Their Recognition and Identification. Revised ed. Coral Gables, Florida, University of Miami Press, 1970.

Rippon, J.W.: Medical Mycology. 2nd Ed. Philadelphia, W.B. Saunders Co., 1982.

5. Laboratory Procedures in Bacteriology and Mycology (Veterinary and Medical)

Balows, A., and Hausler, W.J., Jr. (eds.): Diagnostic Procedures for Bacterial, Mycotic and Parasitic Infections. 6th Ed. New York, American Public Health Association, Inc., 1981.

Beneke, E.S., and Rogers, A.L.: Medical Mycology Manual. 4th Ed. Minneapolis, Burgess Publishing Co., 1980.

Carter, G.R. (ed.): Diagnostic Procedures in Veterinary Bacteriology and Mycology. 4th Ed. Springfield, Illinois., Charles C Thomas, 1984.

Cowan, C.T.: Cowan and Steel's Manual for the Identification of Medical Bacteria. 2nd Ed. Cambridge, Cambridge University Press, 1974.

Cruickshank, R. (ed.): Medical Microbiology. 11th ed. Baltimore, Williams & Wilkins Co., 1965.

Cruickshank, R., Duguid, J.P., Marmion, B.P., and Swain, R.H.A.: Medical Microbiology. Vol. 2: Practice of Medical Microbiology, New York, Churchill Livingstone, 1975.

Cottral, G.E.: Manual of Standardized Methods for Veterinary Microbiology. Ithaca, N.Y., Comstock Publishing Associates, 1978.

Gillies, R.R., and Dodd, T.C.: Bacteriology Illustrated. 3rd Ed. Baltimore, Williams & Wilkins Co., 1973.

Lennette, E.H., Balows, A., Hausler, W.J., and Truant, J.P. (eds.): Manual of Clinical Microbiology. 3rd Ed. Bethesda, Md., American Society for Microbiology, 1980.

6. Determinative Bacteriology

Buchanan, R.E., and Gibbons, N.E. (eds.): Bergey's Manual of Determinative Bacteriology. 8th Ed. Baltimore, Williams & Wilkins Co., 1974.

Krieg, N.R. (ed.): Bergey's Manual of Systematic Bacteriology. Vol. 1, Baltimore, Williams & Wilkins Co., 1984.

Sherman, V.B.D.: A Guide to the Identification of the Genera of Bacteria. 2nd Ed. Baltimore, Williams & Wilkins Co., 1967.

7. Veterinary Medicine

The Merck Veterinary Manual. 5th ed. Rahway, N.J., Merck & Co., Inc. 1979. This is probably the most useful book for veterinary students interested in practice. Its succinct but comprehensive presentations of the clinical manifestations, pathology, diagnosis, control, and treatment of infectious diseases provide excellent supplementary reading.

INDEX

Page numbers in **boldface** indicate illustrations; page numbers followed by "t" indicate tables.